The Exceptional Acacia Gum Arabic

RESEARCH EVOLUTION FROM ACACIA RESIN TO ACACIA FIBER TO ACACIA PREBIOTIC

Mohamad Alnoor

Printed in the United States of America.
ISBN (Paperback) : 979-8-9995916-3-0
First Edition: November 2025

For more information, or to book an event, contact:
www.AcaciaGumArabic.com

TABLE OF CONTENTS

PREFACE

I am not a doctor, scientist, or professional researcher. My background is far removed from medicine or nutritional science. Yet here I am, presenting you with a book analyzing over 140 scientific studies on a substance that has captivated me for years. The FDA calls it Acacia (Gum Arabic).

My journey to this book began not in a laboratory or medical library, but in a modest office in Khartoum, Sudan, during a meeting that would change my life forever. Ten years ago, I was a naïve but ambitious Sudanese American entrepreneur searching for business opportunities between the two countries I called home. At the time, Sudan was under comprehensive U.S. sanctions, with Gum Arabic as the only exception. It was exempted solely because major American beverage manufacturers depended on it. I thought I had found my opening. If Gum Arabic was the only legal export, surely Sudanese companies would welcome an American partner.

That's how I met Taric Khalil.

Taric was the general manager of Dar Savanna, an innovative company that had accomplished something remarkable. It transformed raw Acacia gum into refined powder products sold in pharmacies across Sudan, the Gulf States, and Iraq. I arrived expecting a straightforward business discussion. What I received instead was an education that would consume the next decade of my life.

Taric opened my eyes to a hidden universe. He told me about people with kidney disease avoiding dialysis by using Hashab (the local name for Acacia Senegal gum). He described investors from Kuwait and Iraq

1

competing to secure supplies of this "medicine". He spoke of research studies being conducted throughout Sudan and the Arab world with a vast body of scientific work virtually unknown in the West.

Through Taric, I met his boss, Dr. Isam. Dr. Isam was a man of unrelenting vision and, frankly, audacious stubbornness. In a decision that stunned the industry, he halted all raw gum exports; sacrificing millions of dollars in revenue. His reasoning was simple but radical. It was the only way to force his European buyers to acknowledge the true value of the product. He refused to sell raw material any longer. From that point forward, he would only sell refined prebiotic powder.

The financial consequences were devastating in the short term. However, Dr. Isam's gamble achieved something more important, it forced the conversation. He collaborated with researchers, partnered with universities, and courted foreign investors. He launched an international awareness campaign about Acacia's prebiotic properties. His persistence paid off. His brands became the regional standard, and the industry was forever changed.

Over the years, Dr. Isam, Taric, and their colleague Fawaz Abbaro continued my education. I couldn't stop researching. I followed every publication, tracked every study, and absorbed everything I could find. And the more I learned, the more perplexed I became.

In Sudan, this knowledge was common. Families knew about Hashab's benefits. Doctors recommended it. Pharmacies stocked it. Yet in the West, where most of the scientific research was actually being published, almost no one had heard of it. Researchers were validating what Sudanese grandmothers had known for generations, yet the information never reached the people who needed it most.

How could something so well researched remain so unknown?

This question haunted me and ultimately launched me on a years-long investigation. I began systematically compiling studies and what I discovered astonished me. Study after study demonstrating benefits across a breathtaking range of health conditions, from diabetes to cardiovascular disease, from kidney function to immune health, from inflammation to oral care. Yet despite this mountain of evidence, Acacia (Gum Arabic) remained largely invisible to Western consumers and underutilized by healthcare providers. The Pharaohs had known its value. Medieval physicians prescribed it. Modern scientists had validated it. However somehow, in our age of instant information, this knowledge remained hidden in plain sight.

The more I learned, the more convinced I became that Acacia (Gum arabic) represents a solution to one of the most pervasive health crises of our time which is dysbiosis. This term (referring to an imbalance in gut bacteria) may be unfamiliar to many, yet it underlies countless modern health problems. Our Western diet, antibiotic use, stress, and processed foods have created an epidemic of disrupted gut health, and with it, a cascade of inflammatory and metabolic diseases that plague developed nations.

Acacia (Gum arabic), I discovered, is not just another supplement or health fad. It is a prebiotic fiber with thousands of years of history and hundreds of modern studies supporting its ability to restore balance to the gut microbiome. What began as an industrial food additive has emerged through rigorous scientific investigation as one of nature's most powerful tools for supporting digestive health and, by extension, whole-body wellness.

After reaching this conclusion, I then discovered how difficult it was to explain these benefits. Explaining Acacia's benefits is challenging because

3

understanding requires foundational knowledge. You need the prerequisite understanding of how gut bacteria influences inflammation, how prebiotics differ from probiotics, how the microbiome affects distant organs, and how fiber fermentation produces healing compounds. Without grasping these interconnected systems, Acacia's remarkable effects can seem too confusing to be believable.

This book is the result of my deep dive into that research. I have read and analyzed 540 studies and decided to include 140+ of them in this book. Each chapter examines a different aspect of health; from inflammation and cardiovascular function to kidney disease, diabetes, immunity, and beyond.

I present the evidence as objectively as possible, including studies that showed limited or contradictory results, because honest inquiry demands we examine all the data, not just what confirms our beliefs. I want to be clear about what this book is and what it isn't. This is not medical advice. I am not qualified to tell you what to do about your health conditions, and I strongly encourage you to work with qualified healthcare professionals for any health concerns. What I offer instead is information; a comprehensive compilation of scientific research that you and your healthcare providers can use to make informed decisions.

My hope is that this book serves as a bridge connecting ancient wisdom with modern science. Whether you discovered Acacia through an online search about digestive issues, kidney health, or inflammation, or you're simply curious about this substance's potential, I believe you'll find the evidence compelling. The story of Acacia (Gum arabic) is one of rediscovery. It's about uncovering a treasure that was never truly lost, just overlooked.

Welcome to the story of the exceptional Acacia (Gum arabic).

CHAPTER 1

How bureaucrats, botanists, and regulatory agencies conspired (whether by design or negligence) to bury an ancient healer under layers of deliberate confusion.

P icture yourself at the computer, trying to make a simple purchase.

You've read about the gut-health benefits of "Gum arabic"; something about feeding beneficial bacteria, producing those short-chain fatty acids that researchers can't stop talking about. So, you type the words into a search bar and wait. What arrives is not clarity but chaos. You find "Gum arabic," yes, but also "Acacia gum," "Arabic gum," "Senegal gum," "Sudanese gum," and something called "Hashab." One listing specifies "Acacia senegal," another "Senegalia senegal," and a third simply says "Acacia." The prices vary wildly as some bottles cost twice as much as others for ostensibly the same thing. A label mentions "Talha." While another emphasizes that it's "from Kordofan". You have a graduate degree, you can read ingredient lists, and yet you find yourself paralyzed by a product that humans have consumed safely for thousands of years.

This is not an accident. This is bureaucratic negligence masquerading as complexity. This is what happens when trade cartels, colonial naming systems, territorial botanists, and lazy regulatory agencies refuse to fix problems they have the power to solve. They have buried a treasure that is one of the most studied, most functional, most quietly ubiquitous ingredients in modern food and medicine. It's the dried exudate from a particular tree that grows in the Savanna belt across the African Sahel and is known to Sudanese farmers for generations as Hashab. Sourced primarily from the Kordofan region, and responsible for the overwhelming majority of what the world incorrectly calls "Gum arabic".

The First Veil: An Ethnic Label Nobody Will Correct

Let's start with the name itself. "Gum arabic" sounds straightforward like a gum from Arabia. Except the trees don't grow in Arabia, at least not in meaningful commercial quantities. The name is a fossil from medieval trade routes, when European merchants encountered the material at Arabian ports like Jeddah and Alexandria which are transshipment points for goods moving from Nubia to the Mediterranean world. The gum itself came from Acacia trees growing in the belt of the semi-arid savanna that stretches from Mauritania to Somalia. Here's what makes this inexcusable; by the eighteenth century, when French and British traders established direct access to production regions, they knew perfectly well that the gum does not came from Arabia.

The term "Gum arabic" entered official standards, regulations, and eventually the scientific literature as if repetition could transform a lie into truth. The FAO and WHO Joint Expert Committee on Food Additives codified the misnomer in 1999, defining Gum arabic as the dried exudation obtained from the stems and branches of Acacia senegal or closely related species (Acacia seyal) [1]. That sounds precise, until you notice these are 2 different species of plants producing two different types of gum with different effects.

The International Numbering System codes Gum arabic as INS 414. It appears on ingredient labels worldwide. However, in actual commerce, the term has never mapped cleanly to a single botanical source or a single production geography. Sudan produced approximately 66 percent of the world's so-called Gum arabic in the years 2014-2016 [2]. Chad and Nigeria produced the vast majority of the remaining 34% with Senegal itself a minor player in global markets. Yet the name Acacia Senegal persists which I'm sure you will laugh when you realize neither Acacia nor Senegal have much to do with the esteemed ingredient anymore.

The Second Veil: A Country Name for a Species That Grows Elsewhere

Now that we discussed the arabic in Gum arabic, we arrive at Acacia senegal, the species name. Surely "senegal" points to Senegal the country? Not quite. The botanical epithet senegal was assigned in the eighteenth century when European naturalists cataloged specimens from the Senegambia region; a vague geographical descriptor that included parts of modern Senegal, Mauritania, and Mali. But the economically dominant form of Acacia senegal, the one that produces the premium-grade gum historically known as Hashab gum, grows in the Kordofan belt of Sudan, a region located more than two thousand miles east of Dakar.

This is not a small detail. Kordofan province alone has historically accounted for about seventy percent of Sudan's gum production, and Sudan accounts for up to 66% of the world trade. The tree is locally known in Sudan as the Hashab tree. The gum it produces has been the gold standard for food-grade applications since antiquity and used to stabilize soft drinks, bind pharmaceuticals, and emulsify everything from printing inks to confectionery coatings. When researchers write about Gum arabic in clinical or food-science papers, they are almost always referring to material sourced from Sudanese Acacia trees, not from the modern nation of Senegal.

So we have a species named for one place, economically centered in another, and marketed under an ethnic label from a third. If you were designing a system to obscure the origins and identity of a globally traded commodity, you could hardly do better, and yet no one fixes it. The name could be changed. Botanical names are changed all the time and this name was changed but unfortunately only to bury it further.

The Third Veil: The Great Acacia Heist

Then came the taxonomists, and here is where incompetence gives way to something that looks suspiciously like theft. In the early 2000s, phylogenetic studies confirmed what botanists had long suspected. The genus Acacia, as traditionally conceived, was not a single evolutionary lineage. It was a huge tally containing over thirteen hundred species scattered across Australia, Africa, Asia, and the Americas that share similar-looking flowers and seed pods but were only distantly related [3].

Standard practice in such cases is to split the genus and assign new names. The logical move, following the rules of botanical nomenclature, would have been to keep the name Acacia for the group containing the original type species; Acacia nilotica, an African tree first documented in Egypt. That would have meant renaming the roughly one thousand Australian species to something else, perhaps Racosperma, a name that had been proposed two centuries earlier in 1835 by von Martius and elevated to generic rank by Pedley in 1986 [4]. Most Australian botanists hated this because Australian "Acacia" species (known as wattles) were thought to be of national interest and they argued that renaming them would create widespread disruption in forestry, horticulture, and conservation.

So in 2003, Australian botanists Anthony Orchard and Bruce Maslin filed a formal proposal to conserve the name Acacia with a new type specimen. It sought to retypify the genus Acacia with a new type specimen (an Australian species) to replace the original African/Asian type [5]. This was not a scientific decision. This was a political maneuver, a request to override the normal rules of priority because Australia had more money and clout than Africa in international botanical circles. What ensued was a taxonomic theft of unprecedented proportion and this heist was documented in detail in "The Acacia Heist" book.

In summary, let's be clear about what happened here. A group of wealthy-country botanists, facing inconvenience, lobbied an international body to transfer a name away from its rightful owners (Egyptian trees that had been called Acacias for more than two thousand years) to Australian trees that already had a perfectly good common name. The theft result is that Acacia senegal and Acacia seyal, the two species that produce commercial gum arabic, were reclassified into new genera names called Senegalia and Vachellia. So the tree that produces the substance millions of people know as Acacia gum is no longer, technically, an Acacia. These trees are now called Senegalia Senegal and Vechallia Seyal. It's ok to laugh, or cry!

Try explaining that to a consumer searching for Acacia gum on a health-food website. There is some good news; the Acacia heist can be reversed. botanical nomenclature is not written in stone. The International Code of Nomenclature for algae, fungi, and plants is amended regularly. A proposal to restore the name Acacia to African species could be submitted, voted on, and ratified at the next International Botanical Congress. It would take political will, international coordination, and a willingness to prioritize a two thousand year heritage over the convenience of Australian botanists. That's apparently too much to ask.

To learn the full story and join this initiative, check out the book "The Acacia Heist" because "Acacia" deserves to be saved.

The Fourth Veil: Two Gums, One Shelf, One Deliberate Lie

Now we come to the functional distinctions that regulatory agencies actively refuse to acknowledge. Even within the legal definition of Gum arabic as the exudate of Acacia senegal or Acacia seyal, there are profound differences. These are not interchangeable materials, and everyone in the industry knows it.

Acacia senegal (Hashab Gum) produces a gum that is richer in protein content (2.7% vs. 1.0%), including the arabinogalactan-protein fraction responsible for its superior emulsifying properties and functional value. Acacia seyal (Talha Gum) has higher average molecular weight (8.2×10^5 vs. 6.8×10^5 g/mol) but more compact, less viscous molecules and poorer emulsifying properties that limit its commercial applications [6].

Chemically, both are arabinogalactan polysaccharides, both are composed of the same monosaccharide units (arabinose, galactose, rhamnose, glucuronic acid and 4-O-methyl-glucuronic acid) but in different proportions and different branching architectures. Acacia senegal gum has more extensive branching, shorter arabinosyl side chains, and a higher galactose-to-arabinose ratio. Acacia seyal has more 4-O-methyl-glucuronic acid and less rhamnose [6]. These are not trivial distinctions. They affect viscosity, emulsification capacity, and fermentability by gut bacteria.

In-vitro colon models have shown that both gums are fermented by human microbiota to produce short-chain fatty acids (acetate, propionate, butyrate) [7]. However, given the kinetics and different chemical composition, the microbial populations involved in fermentation most likely also differ. Clinical studies of Gum arabic's prebiotic effects have predominantly used Hashab (Acacia Senegal) material even when they only refer to it as "Gum Arabic" or "Acacia Gum". When we talk about Gum arabic promoting Bifidobacteria proliferation, or modulating bile acid metabolism, or improving stool consistency in people with IBS, we are usually talking about Hashab, not Talha. The evidence base is not identical and individual responses vary. Some consumers with inflammatory bowel conditions may not tolerate Talha Gum due to its higher tannin and polyphenol content. This vagueness has led to many disappointing trials with this ingredient. That is specifically why we decided to completely end this vagueness by exploring Hashab gum (Acacia Senegal) only in this book.

Yet the FDA, the European Food Safety Authority, and every other major regulatory body continue to classify both materials under the single code INS 414, as if they were functionally equivalent. This is not an oversight, this is policy. The agencies could create subcategories (INS 414a for Hashab gum, INS 414b for Talha gum) tomorrow if they chose to. They could require labels to specify botanical sources. They could demand that clinical claims be tied to specific gum types. They don't, because doing so would force suppliers to disclose what they're actually selling, and that transparency would destabilize a market that profits from this confusion.

On most retail shelves, you will find only the umbrella term Gum Arabic, Acacia fiber or Acacia Gum (which could now refer to poisonous wattle exudates). The consumer has no way to know which botanical source, which functional profile, which research lineage they are purchasing. This is not an accident.

The Fifth Veil: The Nationalist Rebranding That Solves Nothing

In recent years, Sudanese traders and producers have called for the term Gum Arabic to be replaced with Sudanese gum, in recognition of Sudan's overwhelming contribution to global supply. This is understandable. The country's gum sector supports millions of rural livelihoods and generates essential foreign exchange. Why should the product carry a name that credits Arabia when Sudan does the work?

However, this also presents another problem and not a solution, as it's a fifth veil. In Sudanese commerce, Sudanese gum can mean Hashab from Acacia senegal, or Talha from Acacia seyal, or sometimes lower-grade exudates from other local species like Acacia nilotica or kakamout gum from the Acacia Polyacantha. These materials do not have equivalent properties. Lumping them under a national umbrella obscures the very research-dominant material (Hashab) that Sudanese growers ought to be championing.

An umbrella term substitutes one confusion for another. It preserves the ambiguity that allows lower-grade material to ride the coattails of premium product. It makes it harder, not easier, for consumers and formulators to find what the scientific literature describes. This is what happens when well-meaning nationalists adopt the philosophy of their exploiters instead of demanding clarity.

Even if this logic succeeds, will Sudanese nationalists succeed in changing the names of the underlying chemicals derived from Gum Arabic? The sugar "Arabinose" was itself discovered and called that due to being first identified and extracted from "Gum Arabic". A feat we will discuss later in detail.

The Map Becomes Legible: Why "Hashab Gum" Is the Only Honest Name

So what is the solution? Precision and Transparency. A name that tracks the material to its botanical source, its functional profile, and its research lineage. A name that doesn't rely on the goodwill of international bureaucracies that have shown, for centuries, that they have none. When we talk about the top-quality, research-dominant gum tied to classical functionality and the preponderance of clinical literature then we are talking about Hashab Gum. This is Senegalia (Acacia) Senegal, historically sourced from the Kordofan belt of Sudan, corresponding to the

12

material with lower molecular weight, robust emulsification capacity, and demonstrated prebiotic activity. We will call it what everyone in the industry will be forced to call it when sourcing from the largest producer: Hashab gum.

This is not a neologism. It is the term Sudanese producers have used for hundreds of years. It is the word that appears in Sudanese gum auctions, in export classifications, in the technical monographs published by the Gum Arabic Company of Sudan. It is specific. It is traceable. It respects the people who grow and harvest the trees and it draws a clear line between the material most commonly studied in labs and clinics. It distinguishes (from the very source) the other lesser-quality exudates that may share the legal designation Gum arabic but do not share the same performance profile.

For purposes of clarity, this book will will only explore Hashab Gum even when the researchers and documenters label it as "Acacia gum", "Gum Arabic", "Gum Acacia", "Commercial grade gum" etc.. This means that as we explore the different studies, we will use the terms they used but always know and take for granted that the material being cited is the Hashab gum scientifically known today as Senegalia (Acacia) senegal. We will not cite any research about any other gum (only one exception at the end of the book) and this means all the following research in this book is Hashab specific. This is not pedantry. This is consumer protection. This is how you bypass a corrupt system.

The Treasure Unlocked

A naming reform this straightforward should not feel radical, but in a world where centuries of compounded confusion have been actively maintained by those who profit from it, clarity is an act of resistance. For too long, Hashab gum has been hidden. Not by accident, not by the innocent accumulation of historical quirks, but by the deliberate choices of

HOW TO HIDE A TREASURE

regulators who refuse to update outdated standards, botanists who prioritize their own convenience over scientific accuracy, and trade associations that benefit from keeping consumers confused. Each layer was avoidable. Each layer remains fixable. Stacked together, they form a nearly perfect system for making an ancient healer invisible to the very people who could benefit most from it.

The good news is that once you see the veils, you can rip them down. Once you know to ask for Hashab gum, the treasure hunt is over. You have found the map. In the essays to come, we will use that map to explore what Hashab gum actually does. How it feeds your microbiome, how those short-chain fatty acids it generates influence everything from gut barrier integrity to metabolic signaling. How a substance humans have consumed since the time of the pharaohs is quietly working inside millions of sodas, pills, and snack bars without most people ever knowing its name. We will examine the clinical evidence, the biochemical mechanisms, and the careful language scientists use when they explain what this polysaccharide can and cannot do for human health.

This book focuses primarily on the health benefits of Hashab gum. We will not delve deeply into the wider technological or formulation applications as that would go beyond the scope of a single volume. Instead, we will present these applications only where they naturally complement and reinforce our central priority; the health benefits of Hashab gum.

First, we needed to solve the naming problem, because you can't study a treasure you can't name. With "Hashab gum" we removed five centuries of deliberate confusion that rendered this health treasure invisible. Now you can see it. The veils are ripped away. The treasure is Hashab gum. Let's find out what it can do.

References

1. "Gum Arabic." Compendium of Food Additive Specifications: Addendum 7, Joint FAO/WHO Expert Committee on Food Additives, FAO Food and Nutrition Paper 52 Add. 7, Food and Agriculture Organization of the United Nations, 1999.
2. United Nations Conference on Trade and Development (UNCTAD). Commodities at a Glance: Special Issue on Gum Arabic. UNCTAD Secretariat, 2017.
3. Miller, J.T., and R.J. Bayer. "Molecular Phylogenetics of Acacia (Fabaceae: Mimosoideae) Based on the Chloroplast MATK Coding Sequence and Flanking TRNK Intron Spacer Regions." American Journal of Botany, vol. 88, no. 4, 2001, pp. 697-705.
4. Pedley, L. "Derivation and Dispersal of Acacia (Leguminosae), with Particular Reference to Australia, and the Recognition of Senegalia and Racosperma." Botanical Journal of the Linnean Society, vol. 92, no. 3, 1986, pp. 219–254.
5. Orchard, A.E., and Maslin, B.R. "Proposal to Conserve the Name Acacia (Leguminosae: Mimosoideae) with a Conserved Type." Taxon, vol. 52, no. 2, 2003, pp. 362–363.
6. Lopez-Torrez, L., Nigen, M., Williams, P., Doco, T., and Sanchez, C. "Acacia senegal vs. Acacia seyal gums – Part 1: Composition and structure of hyperbranched plant exudates." Food Hydrocolloids, vol. 51, 2015, pp. 41–53.
7. Rawi, M.H., Abdullah, A., Ismail, A., and Sarbini, S.R. "Manipulation of Gut Microbiota Using Acacia Gum Polysaccharide." ACS Omega, vol. 6, no. 26, 2021, pp. 17782–17797

CHAPTER 2

Acacia Gum is a 70,000-year-old proof of Human Intelligence and Ancient Egypt was the first to prescribe it as medicine 3,600 years ago

Deep Time: The Birth of Sticky Intelligence

Seventy thousand years ago, in what is now South Africa, someone mixed Acacia gum with red ochre and fire-dried the result into an adhesive strong enough to haft a stone blade to a wooden handle [1]. This act, documented in microfractures and residue traces on tools excavated from Sibudu Cave, represents more than clever craftsmanship. It represents abstract thought made manifest. To create a compound adhesive, you must hold multiple variables in mind simultaneously including the acidity of the gum (which fluctuates tree to tree), the mineralogy of the ochre (which changes outcrop to outcrop), the temperature of the fire, and the timing of application. You must understand that combining these elements will create something neither possesses alone. You must plan ahead, because the adhesive must be prepared before the hunt, not during it.

The people who made these adhesives were us. Homo sapiens in the Middle Stone Age, navigating the same cognitive architecture we carry today, but applying it to a world that demanded intimate knowledge of materials. Plant gums (sticky exudates from wounded trees) were everywhere in the southern African landscape, but recognizing which gums could be transformed to tools required observation across seasons and

16

experimentation across generations. When you add ochre to Acacia gum, you don't just color it red; you change its pH, you alter its mechanical workability, you strengthen its bond. Ancient artisans discovered this through trial and error, then passed the knowledge forward, embedding sticky intelligence into their culture.

This is where Acacia gum's 70,000-year arc begins. It serves as one of the oldest proofs of human intelligence articulated by the manipulation of materials to extend our capabilities. Glue-making required the same forward-thinking cognition that would later build cities, write laws, and develop pharmacopeias. It requires recognizing cause-and-effect across time, which is perhaps the most human thing we do. The fact that Acacia gums were part of this cognitive toolkit matters because it established a pattern; wherever humans were solving complex problems, Acacia was both witness and participant.

Egypt Revealed: The Workshops of Eternity

Fast-forward to Egypt around 2650 BC, the dawn of the Old Kingdom. At Saqqara, where the revolutionary Step Pyramid of Djoser rose in six tiers of white limestone, a new social order was taking shape; one that would define Egyptian civilization for the next five centuries. The construction of the first monumental stone structure in human history required not just engineering genius, but an unprecedented organization of specialized labor. Artists working in an array of mediums and techniques (stone, wood, precious metals, monumental statuary, reliefs, and wall paintings) created masterpieces during this first golden age of Egyptian culture, a period that determined the form and character of Egyptian art for millennia to come.

Their tools were elegantly simple including brushes made from chewed reeds, stone palettes with wells for red and black ink, copper chisels, wooden mallets, and pots of pigment ground from minerals hauled from distant quarries. Their binding medium was sophisticated. Plant gums (mostly Acacia gum harvested from the thorny trees that dotted the Nile valley), became the invisible matrix that held Egyptian visual culture together. Acacia gum bound mineral pigments to tomb walls, temple columns, and sacred objects, allowing colors to survive four thousand years in the dry Egyptian climate. This early technology enabled the Old Kingdom artists to illuminate human relationships and daily life with a sensitivity that still has the power to move us today [2].

The invisible chemistry that made Egyptian visual culture possible has long been overlooked. While scholars have catalogued the brilliant ochres, the luminous Egyptian blue, and the precious lapis lazuli that adorned temple walls and tomb paintings, they paid less attention to what held these pigments in place. The binder was Acacia gum harvested from the thorny trees scattered across the Nile valley and throughout Nubia to the south. Recent archaeological investigations at two pharaonic colonial settlements in Upper Nubia (the town of Sai) established around 1500 BCE have revealed something remarkable; paint palettes found in ordinary houses, not just elite tombs. For the first time, scientists have identified polysaccharide gums (most likely Acacia) as binding media in everyday vernacular architecture, demonstrating that this sophisticated adhesive technology pervaded all levels of colonial society [3].

This sounds technical, but an ancient Egyptian scribe would mix carbon soot with Acacia gum and water to create a black ink that would flow smoothly from a reed pen and remain legible for millennia. The Acacia gum would serve as a binder that held the carbon particles in suspension and fixed them to the papyrus surface after the water evaporated. For red ink, scribes used iron-based ocher pigments mixed with the same gum binder, though recent analysis has revealed they also added lead compounds not as pigments, but as driers to prevent the ink from spreading too much on the writing surface. This technique would be reused in

Renaissance Europe thousands of years later [4].

Then there were the bodies. Mummification required adhesives to secure
linen wrappings, to bind protective amulets into place, to seal and stabilize
the elaborate bandaging that transformed a corpse into an eternal vessel.
Acacia gum, biocompatible and stable, played a quiet but essential role in a
process designed to defeat time itself. It is no exaggeration to say that
Acacia gum was part of Egypt's strategy for immortality.

The Medical Turn: From Stomach Heat to Empirical Observation

Egypt did not use Acacia gum only on the outside of bodies. They used it
inside them, too. The Ebers Papyrus, compiled around 1550 BC and
preserved in a scriptorium attached to Thebes' House-of-Life (a
combination temple, medical school, and library) is one of the most
comprehensive medical texts to survive from antiquity. Among its 110
columns of remedies, spells, and anatomical observations, one entry stands
out for our purposes. It prescribes a treatment for "stomach heat," a
condition that seems to have encompassed what we might call gastritis,
heartburn, or general digestive inflammation. The remedy calls for *kʒmw*
(Acacia gum) among other ingredients [5]. The prescription does not
explain why Acacia gum soothes an inflamed stomach, only that it does.

We can now venture an explanation the Egyptians lacked the tools to
articulate. Acacia gum is a soluble fiber that, when dissolved in liquid and
consumed, forms a gentle mucilaginous coating. It does not irritate; it
soothes. It creates a temporary barrier that protects irritated tissue from
further insult. The ancient Egyptian observation was empirical and
outcome-based. Give this to people with stomach complaints and they feel
better. That observation, transmitted through the Ebers Papyrus, prefigures
by more than three millennia the modern understanding of Acacia gum as a

prebiotic fiber with mucosal-protective properties. The Egyptians didn't know about microbial fermentation or short-chain fatty acids, but they knew enough to keep using it.

This is worth pausing over. The same substance that made paint stick to walls also made stomachs calm. The same molecular architecture (a complex, branched polysaccharide) that created transparent, flexible films outside the body created soothing, protective films inside it. One material, two seemingly unrelated applications, united by the same physical properties: solubility, viscosity, film-forming capacity, and a profound compatibility with biological systems.

Greco-Roman Codification: How Knowledge Travels

Medical knowledge, like trade goods, followed routes. *De Materia Medica*, written between 50 and 70 AD, became the foundational pharmacological text for more than fifteen centuries. The work would circulate first in Syriac and then translated into Arabic in ninth-century Baghdad, with the translation supervised by the renowned physician-translator Hunayn ibn Ishaq. This ensured that Dioscorides' knowledge of approximately 600 plants and 1,000 medicines would shape both Islamic and European medical practice for millennia to come [6].

Dioscorides catalogued around six hundred plants and the medicines derived from them. Drawing on Egyptian, Greek, Persian, and Syrian sources. His entries on Acacia and related gum-producing trees codified what had been scattered regional knowledge into a portable, translatable reference work. *De Materia Medica* was translated into Arabic in ninth-century Baghdad, then into Latin in medieval Europe. Through it, Acacia gum's therapeutic uses (astringent, demulcent, wound-healing) entered the medical mainstream of three continents. This was not innovation; this was transmission. Dioscorides served as a bridge, carrying Egyptian empiricism into the Greek taxonomic tradition, which in turn fed into Islamic and later European medical practice [6].

Pliny the Elder, writing his *Naturalis Historia* in 77 AD, takes a slightly different angle. Pliny was an encyclopedist, a Roman nobleman with a fatal case of curiosity (he died investigating the eruption of Vesuvius), and his *Natural History* attempted to catalog everything knowable about the natural world. In Book XII, section 32, Pliny discusses "gummi" from Egypt and Arabia; the Acacia gums that arrived in Roman ports as trade goods. He notes their use in perfumes and varnishes, applications that leverage the same qualities Egyptian painters had exploited; clarity, adhesion, and the ability to blend disparate ingredients without altering their essential character [7].

Pliny's casual mention of gum in perfumes reveals something important. By the first century AD, Acacia gum had become a commodity as mundane as olive oil, yet its utility spanned cosmetics, medicine, art, and craft. It was a material so versatile that it appeared in nearly every corner of ancient technology, yet so reliable that it required little comment. The best technologies, after all, become invisible.

The Translator Metaphor: A Material That Mediates

Call Acacia gum a translator. Not metaphorically, but literally as it's a substance that mediates between incompatible worlds and makes them communicate. In art, it translates loose mineral pigment into durable color, allowing the visual imagination to survive the corrosive passage of time. In writing, it translates carbon soot and plant dyes into legible, permanent ink, allowing ideas to escape the fragility of memory. In medicine, it translates irritation into comfort by creating a soothing barrier between damaged tissue and the harsh chemistry of digestion. In trade, it translates fragile aromatic oils and resins into stable, transportable commodities by acting as a fixative and emulsifier.

This is not a metaphor we impose from outside. It is a description of what the molecule actually does. It creates interfaces, mediates boundaries, and allows incompatible phases to coexist. It is hydrophilic (water-loving) which allows it to dissolve and coat and spread but it dries into something stable and protective. It's a molecular handshake between the liquid and solid phases of matter.

Today, we extend this translator role into the interior landscape of the body. Modern microbiome science has revealed that Acacia gum, when consumed, becomes a substrate for beneficial bacteria in the colon. These bacteria ferment the gum's complex polysaccharides into short-chain fatty acids (acetate, propionate, and butyrate) metabolites that support intestinal barrier integrity, modulate inflammation, and signal satiety to the brain [8]. The ancient Egyptians who prescribed Acacia gum for "stomach heat" were observing downstream effects of this fermentation such as the soothing of inflamed tissue and the calming of digestive distress. They lacked the conceptual framework of microbiology, but they had the outcome data, and they trusted it enough to write it down.

What the Egyptians called *k3mw* and used empirically, we now call a prebiotic fiber and study mechanistically. The translator metaphor holds: Acacia gum mediates between what we eat and how our internal microbial community responds, just as it once mediated between pigment and stone, between soot and papyrus.

The Industrial Mirror: Ancient Virtues in Modern Systems

W alk into a modern food science laboratory and you will find Acacia gum everywhere. It is listed as E414 on ingredient labels, and it performs the same foundational work it did in Egyptian ateliers, just in different contexts. In beverages, it stabilizes emulsions and prevents the separation of oils and water which is the molecular equivalent of holding pigment in suspension. In confections, it prevents sugar crystallization and provides a smooth mouthfeel which is the same textural control that made ancient inks flow smoothly from reed pens. In pharmaceuticals, it encapsulates active ingredients and controls their release which is a direct descendant of its use in binding medicinal compounds into stable preparations.

Nubia: The Invisible Supplier

No discussion of Acacia gum in ancient Egypt is complete without acknowledging its geography. While Acacias grew along the Nile, the highest-quality gum (the clearest, most soluble grades) came from further south, from the lands the Egyptians called Kush or Nubia. Trade records and expedition accounts make clear that Nubia was a consistent supplier of Acacia products, along with gold, ebony, ivory, and incense. The Acacia trees of the sub-Saharan Sahel, particularly Hashab (Acacia Senegal), produced the gum that trade routes preferred, and Nubian merchants knew it.

This matters because it locates Acacia gum within the economic and political networks that sustained Egyptian civilization. Gum was not a luxury like lapis lazuli or a strategic material like copper. It was a utilitarian substance, essential to daily operations, procured through established trade routes that connected the Mediterranean world to the Sahel and the Savanna.

Why Acacia Gum Keeps Reappearing

Here is the central question: why does this one material keep showing up precisely where human capability expands? Part of the answer is biochemical. Acacia gum's molecular structure gives it properties that are difficult to replicate with simpler molecules. It dissolves easily but dries into a stable film. It increases viscosity at low concentrations without becoming thick or opaque. It is compatible with both water-based and lipid-based systems. It does not degrade quickly, does not become toxic, does not interfere with the things it binds or carries. These are rare virtues in a single substance.

However, part of the answer is also historical and cultural. Once a material proves useful, knowledge about it accumulates and travels. Egyptian scribes taught apprentices how to prepare ink, and those apprentices became master scribes and refined the technique. Medical practitioners observed outcomes and recorded them, and later practitioners read those records and tested them. Greek physicians catalogued the material properties they inherited from Egyptian and Near Eastern sources; Islamic scholars translated and expanded those catalogues; medieval and Renaissance Europeans built on both traditions. Each generation added a layer of understanding, and the material kept proving useful enough to preserve.

Acacia gum became what we might call "infrastructure of wisdom", a substance so reliable and so multipurpose that it was woven into the basic operating procedures of successive civilizations. You didn't question whether to use Acacia gum in ink or paint or medicine any more than you questioned whether to use copper in tools or wool in clothing. It was simply what worked.

The Signal in the Strata

Picture the conservator in her laboratory, lifting that fragment of Acacia gum from a mummy wrapping. She is holding a molecule that witnessed the cognitive revolution of the Middle Stone Age, that enabled the visual and written culture of pharaonic Egypt, that traveled through Greco-Roman pharmacies and medieval scriptoria, that today feeds the beneficial bacteria in millions of human colons. It is a time-traveler that appears in the archaeological and historical record wherever humans were building systems of communication, of preservation, of healing, and of trade. It appears because it made those systems work better.

Egypt did not invent Acacia gum; it systematized its use, institutionalized its knowledge, and left us the clearest early record of what a complex society could do with this plant exudate. The Egyptians showed us that this substance could be many things at once. A paint binder, a medicine, an ink stabilizer, a ritual adhesive, a trade good and a technological enabler. They showed us that materials with the right properties become indispensable not through marketing but through utility, not through novelty but through reliability.

In showing us this, the Ancient Egyptians taught us how to recognize a class of substances (gentle, versatile, biocompatible plant polysaccharides) that help civilizations cohere without dominating the narrative. Acacia gum does not shout. It binds, it soothes, it stabilizes, it ferments, it protects. It has done so for 70,000 years, and if we are wise, it will continue doing so for millennia to come.

References

1. Wadley, Lyn, et al. "Implications for Complex Cognition from the Hafting of Tools with Compound Adhesives in the Middle Stone Age, South Africa." Proceedings of the National Academy of Sciences, vol. 106, no. 24, 2009, pp. 9590–9594; Prinsloo, Linda C., et al. "Graphite and Multilayer Graphene Detected on ~70,000-Year-Old Stone Tools: Geological Origin or Constituent of Hafting Resin?" Journal of Raman Spectroscopy, vol. 54, no. 2, 2023, pp. 182–190

2. Arnold, Dorothea. When the Pyramids Were Built: Egyptian Art of the Old Kingdom. The Metropolitan Museum of Art/Rizzoli International Publications, 1999.

3. Fulcher, Kate, et al. "Polysaccharide Paint Binding Media at Two Pharaonic Settlements in Nubia." Heritage, vol. 5, no. 3, 2022, pp. 2028-2040

4. Christiansen, Thomas, et al. "Insights into the Composition of Ancient Egyptian Red and Black Inks on Papyri Achieved by Synchrotron-Based Microanalyses." Proceedings of the National Academy of Sciences, vol. 117, no. 43, 2020, pp. 27825–27835

5. Popko, Lutz, et al. Papyrus Ebers—English Translation Based on the German Edition by H. J. J. Jette and W. Wreszinski. Leipzig University, 2006.

6. Dio Greek Learning in the Arab World: The Materia medica of Dioscorides." Leiden University Libraries (Arabic translation by Stephanus/Istifān ibn Bāsīl, checked/supervised by Hunayn ibn Isḥāq, 9th-c. Baghdad).

7. Pliny the Elder. Natural History. Book 12, Chapter 32. Translated by H. Rackham, Loeb Classical Library, Harvard University Press, 1945.

8. Rawi, M. H., et al. "Manipulation of Gut Microbiota Using Acacia Gum Polysaccharide." ACS Omega, vol. 6, no. 28, 2021, pp. 17679–17691.

CHAPTER 3

ANCIENT KNOWLEDGE HIDDEN IN MIDIEVAL MEDICINE

Medieval monks and Islamic Scientists retain the Ancient Knowledge

The lamp burned low in the Monte Cassino scriptorium. Outside, the Italian night pressed against stone walls three feet thick. Inside, a Benedictine monk named Constantinus sat hunched over an Arabic manuscript, his right hand poised above a horn cup of ink. The ink itself was a small miracle. An iron gall suspension bound with three pea-sized lumps of Acacia gum dissolved in warm water until the liquid ran clear as mountain spring. He dipped his quill, tested the flow on a scrap, and began translating the Arabic word *samgh* into its Latin cousin, *gummi*. It was the year 1080, and Constantinus Africanus was about to change European medicine by doing something deceptively simple. He made a recipe legible [1].

It was at that moment where sap became a solution, Arabic translated to Latin, and ingredient turned to instructions is where our story picks up. You've already met Acacia gum in the caves of our ancestors 70,000 years ago and in the shadow of the pyramids where it soothed pharaonic bellies. Now watch it travel north, carried not by traders' caravans but by something stranger and more durable, the institutional memory of monks, physicians, and early printers. These are the professionals who turned this tree exudate into one of medieval Europe's most reliable instruments of care. This chapter argues that the medieval world did not simply copy the ancients; it stress-tested their observations. It built protocols and in doing so, it preserved Acacia gum not as a curio in a catalog but as a living technology. This technology was clear, safe, and miraculous for soothing inflamed tissues, stabilizing medicines, and literally holding knowledge together.

The story begins, as many medieval stories do, with a long journey across languages. Greek physicians (Dioscorides, writing his *De Materia Medica* in the first century, and Galen a century later) had cataloged Acacia gum (*kommi Aigyptiakon*) as a gentle astringent and vehicle for compounding. Their manuscripts, copied onto parchment in scriptoria from Alexandria to Byzantium, became the inheritance of Syriac-speaking Christian scholars in the Levant. By the seventh and eighth centuries, those Syriac texts fed into the great Arabic medical synthesis. Physicians working in Baghdad, Damascus, and Cordoba didn't just translate Greek sources. They tested them in hospitals (*bimaristans*), recorded outcomes, and wrote new books that cross-referenced centuries of observation.

Enter Avicenna (Ibn Sina to his contemporaries) whose *Canon of Medicine*, completed in 1017, became the single most influential medical text of the next six hundred years [2]. In Book II, under *samgh al-'Arabī* (gum arabic), from the "Aqaqiya" tree; Avicenna laid out something medieval Europe desperately needed. He documented a clear temperament profile (cooling, astringent), preferred dose forms (syrups, lozenges, electuaries), and a list of indications written in the spare language of humoral theory. Stomach heat, hoarseness, cough and fluxes. The Canon wasn't flowery; it was a field manual. When Latin translators in Toledo produced the "Latin Canon"; it quickly circulated to Salerno, and later Padua in the thirteenth century. They heavily incorporated Avicenna's clinical shorthand into their own pharmacopeias [3]. The gum that had soothed Egyptian priests now soothed Tuscan monks, not because of mystic lineage but because the instructions worked.

But how did those instructions survive the journey from Arabic hospitals to European infirmaries? The answer sits in two interlocking institutions: the monastery and the medical school. Let's start with the monks.

Benedictine and Cistercian houses were not just places of prayer. They were Europe's knowledge engines. The scriptoria is where scribes spent decades copying everything from Augustine to seed catalogs, and infirmaries where monk-physicians treated their own communities and, often, the sick poor who gathered at monastery gates. These two functions (preservation and practice) created a feedback loop. A scribe copying Dioscorides would note in the margin that the infirmary used Acacia gum to soothe Brother Anselm's throat ulcers last winter. That margin note might make it into the next copy, and the next. Over centuries, recipes became protocols, and protocols became institutional knowledge.

Take the *Schedula Diversarum Artium*, a twelfth-century Latin manual attributed to "Theophilus Presbyter," likely a Benedictine metalworker and scribe. Theophilus wasn't writing about medicine; he was writing about ink but his instructions are a clinic in quality control [4]. Dissolve Acacia gum in warm water, he writes, too little gum and the iron-gall pigment bleeds on parchment. Too much and the ink clots The Goldilocks zone (just enough to bind pigment particles into a stable suspension) required the same careful observation a physician would use compounding a syrup. Interestingly, if you can trust gum to keep your prescription legible (remember, recipes were written instructions, often in that same iron-gall ink), you can trust it to keep the dose itself consistent. Cistercian scriptoria across France and Germany used Acacia-based inks precisely because the material was reliable [5]. That trust transferred. When monks walked from the scriptorium to the infirmary, they carried not just a substance but a reputation.

In *Circa instans*, Matthaeus Platearius describes Acacia as a dried juice, imported and strongly astringent, "cold and dry in the third degree". He lists its uses in rapid, practical strokes stating that it is good against erysipelas (searing red skin infections), for excoriations of lips and gums, for dysentery and other "fluxes" [6].

If *Circa instans* gives you the "what" the *Antidotarium Nicolai* shows you the "how". Produced in the same Salernitan milieu, it alphabetically lists approximately 150 compound medicines and soon becomes "the essential pharmacopeia of the Middle Ages," copied, translated, and used as an official standard from Naples to Paris. Gum arabic (gummi arabici) appears throughout its recipes in syrups for stomach weakness and vomiting; in electuaries for lung complaints, in complex powders where its role is to bind fragrant resins, spices, and mineral drugs into a stable mass [7].

While Salernitan compilers were organizing the textbook tradition, monastic authors were weaving plants into theological and visionary frameworks. Hildegard of Bingen's *Physica* (12th c.) offers not only lists of simples but concrete, kitchen-table recipes rooted in daily care. Her flaxseed-and-gum plaster for side pain and burns is one of the clearest uses of Gum arabic in a monastic context. She instructs the healer to cook flaxseed with a smaller quantity of Gum arabic until it becomes like glue, then to add pear-mistletoe juice and more deer marrow than gum. The finished ointment is strained and stored in a wax-lined vessel, then applied warm and repeatedly while the patient sits by the fire [8].

By the high and late Middle Ages, Gum arabic has become a quiet constant. It appears in monastic herbals, learned commentaries, and vernacular remedy books. What is striking (modern historian Paula De Vos argues) is how little its medical role changes across more than fifteen centuries [9]. In other words, Gum arabic is not a marginal curiosity. It is an archetypal astringent, used whenever the body is too wet, too hot, or too lax. Its benefits are systemic as it helps keep fluids where they should be, calm surfaces that are inflamed, and support tissues that threaten to sag, prolapse, or ulcerate.

Cennino Cennini, writing his Libro dell'Arte around 1400 for Florentine painters, made the same point from a different angle. He notes that gum is used as a binder for water-based colors on parchment or paper in miniature/illumination work, helping the color mix properly and adhere to the surface. The emphasis is on workability and binding, not on theoretical claims about brilliance or transparency. [10]. Artists valued it for the same reason physicians did as it formed a thin, even film and then got out of the way. If you're mixing vermillion for a fresco, you need the binder to disappear. If you're mixing a pectoral syrup for a wheezing patient, you need the vehicle to soothe without masking the taste of the active ingredient. Same logic, different substrate. Parchment, plaster, mucosa; Acacia gum treated them all as surfaces in need of a gentle, invisible infrastructure.

One of the most beautiful artifacts of this era is the *Tractatus de Herbis*, an illustrated Latin herbal compiled in Italy around 1440 and often attributed to the Salernitan compiler Platearius [11]. Imagine a medical student in Padua flipping through its vellum pages. Each entry pairs a plant or gum with a small, vibrant painting (Acacia rendered as a thorny tree with pendulous golden pods) and a few terse lines of text. The illustrations weren't decorative; they were safety features. Misidentifying a plant could kill a patient. A clear image, standardized across copies, reduced that risk. The Tractatus is where medieval medicine began to look like a field guide that is portable, visual, and built for practitioners who might never see a live Acacia tree but needed to recognize the gum in an apothecary's jar.

In the 1542 Fuchs's "Basel folio", he presents hundreds of plants with large, precise woodcuts (roots, leaves, flowers, and seeds) paired with concise notes and names in Latin, Greek, and German, supported by indices and a glossary. His Acacia section fits this method: a careful image plus brief, practical remarks grounded in classical sources (especially Dioscorides) rather than speculative synonym chains. Later Renaissance usage sometimes labels African acacias as "Acacia Aegyptiaca vera" [12].

William Turner, an English botanist and Protestant reformer, published *A New Herball* between 1551 and 1568, first in Cologne (he was exiled under Mary I), then in London. Turner's tone is empirical and corrective: he criticizes superstition and error and favors what he has seen or confirmed. In the Acacia material he distinguishes the plant and its products, notes principal properties and uses, and describes preparations in straightforward terms (useful for physicians and apothecaries) without the polemics [13].

Let's pause and translate. What medieval physicians called "cooling" and "astringent" in humoral language, we would today describe as film-forming mucilage with mild adsorptive properties and gentle prebiotic fermentability that supports mucosal barrier function. The gum's highly branched polysaccharides dissolve in water to form a viscous but low-surface-tension solution that spreads easily over inflamed tissue, creates a temporary protective layer, and may buffer irritants through mild adsorption. Its near-neutral taste and lack of pharmacological activity made it an ideal vehicle for delivering other, less palatable medicines like bitter purgatives, astringent tannins, and aromatic oils in a form patients can endure. Medieval physicians didn't know the polymer chemistry, but they knew the effect. They had a thousand years of written observations and their own clinical experience. That's empiricism.

References:

1. Constantinus Africanus. Liber Pantegni. Circa 1080. Manuscript. Adapted from ʿAlī ibn al-ʿAbbās al-Majūsī. For a scholarly summary: Constantine the African. "Liber pantegni." Translated and adapted c. 1080. See also:
    Britannica, The Editors of Encyclopaedia. "Constantine the African." Encyclopaedia Britannica, 2024

2. Avicenna [Ibn Sīnā]. The Canon of Medicine (al-Qānūn fī al-Ṭibb). Book II, entry "samgh al-ʿArabī" [gum arabic]. Circa 1025. Manuscript. For English:
    Avicenna. The Canon of Medicine. Translated editions and facsimiles available, e.g., Laleh Bakhtiar, Kazi Publications, 1999

3. National Library of Medicine. "Islamic Medical Manuscripts: The Canon of Medicine." U.S. National Library of Medicine. (Notes Gerard of Cremona's 12th-century Latin translation and later revisions.).

4. Theophilus Presbyter. De Diversis Artibus (The Schedula Diversarum Artium). Circa 1120. Edited and translated by C. R. Dodwell, Clarendon Press, 1961.

5. Theophilus Presbyter. De diversis artibus (Schedula diversarum artium). Edited and translated by C. R. Dodwell, Clarendon Press, 1961; Lluveras-Tenorio, Anna, et al. "Iron-gall inks: a review of their degradation mechanisms and stabilization treatments." Heritage Science, vol. 10, 2022; Cistercian scriptoria of Burgundy, the Rhineland, and England.

6. Platearius, Matthaeus. Circa Instans (Liber de simplici medicina). c. 12th century. Facsimile in Practica Ioannis Serapionis…, Octavianus Scotus, 1497

7. Nicolaus of Salerno. Antidotarium Nicolai. Edited by Franco Brunello, Cavallino, 1975

8. Hildegard of Bingen. Hildegard's Healing Plants: From Her Medieval Classic Physica. Translated by Bruce W. Hozeski, Beacon Press, 2001.

9. De Vos, Paula. "European Materia Medica in Historical Texts: Longevity of a Tradition and Implications for Future Use." Journal of Ethnopharmacology, vol. 132, no. 1, 2010, pp. 28–47.

10. Cennini, Cennino d'Andrea. Il Libro dell'Arte. Translated by Daniel V. Thompson, Jr., as The Craftsman's Handbook, Dover Publications, 1954.

11. Tractatus de Herb is. Italy, c. 1440. Illuminated manuscript often attributed to the Salernitan compiler Platearius.

12. Fuchs, Leonhart. De Historia Stirpium Commentarii Insignes. Tübingen, 1542.

13. Turner, William. A New Herball. Cologne and London, 1551-68.

CHAPTER 4

Following trade routes - 15th Century to Industrial Revolution

As November fog hangs over the London docks, 1785. The East India Company factor walks the length of Warehouse Seven, his lantern swinging yellow arcs across bales stacked to the rafters. He stops at a cask marked with Arabic script and splits the seal with a pry bar. Inside, nested in straw, lie small chunks of Acacia gum which is brittle and translucent. He pinches a fragment between his teeth and its neutral. No bitterness, no sweet bite. He drops another piece into a tin cup of warm water and stirs with the handle of his penknife. Within minutes, the solid has vanished, leaving a clear solution, clear enough to read newsprint through. He nods, marks the manifest, and moves on. Forty sacks of Acacia gum, passed for sale.

That simple clarity; solid to solution, opaque to transparent, distant shore to London dispensary is about to reorganize two worlds at once. The first world is of medicine, where physicians and apothecaries are building standardized dose forms that soothe, bind, and carry relief across inflamed tissue. The other world is of industry; where textile printers, lithographers, and eventually photographers demand materials that perform the same way. The bridge between them is not philosophy, it is supply. Predictable, testable, repeatable supply hauled across oceans by chartered companies whose logbooks care nothing for humoral theory but everything for consistency.

By the time Acacia gum reaches the pharmacopoeia committees of Edinburgh, London, and Philadelphia in the early nineteenth century, it will have passed through the hands of Savanna producers, Arab traders, Portuguese factors, Dutch merchants, British dyers, French chemists, and American apothecaries. With each demanding that it behave exactly as advertised. That chain of custody, paradoxically, is what makes it safe to prescribe. When a substance survives the scrutiny of profit, it earns the trust of care.

Let's back up two centuries and follow the routes. Portuguese explorers, nosing down the West African coast in the fifteenth century, were hunting gold, slaves, and shortcuts to the spice islands. What they found was also "*goma*" harvested from Acacia groves of Senegal, Mauritania, and Mali. The "Senegal gum" traded through coastal entrepôts by Berber and Arab intermediaries who had been moving the stuff north for a thousand years. The early cargos were speculative (a bale here, a cask there) but by the sixteenth century, regular convoys were carrying these gums to Lisbon, Seville, and Antwerp. The Dutch and British followed. By 1700, Acacia gum was a line item in the ledgers of the Dutch East India Company and the English Levant trade, arriving in Amsterdam and London with the reliability of a tide.

Reliability is the hinge. Medieval monasteries had depended on gum, but their supply was episodic. With users waiting for a merchant caravan one year, nothing the next. Global trade didn't make gum available; it made it dependable and dependability is the first condition of clinical confidence. When a physician in Edinburgh knows she can walk into an apothecary's shop in January and find clear, soluble Acacia gum that behaves like the batch she used in July, she begins to write it into her standard repertoire. When that same physician publishes a case series or teaches an apprentice, the recipe travels. However, the recipe only works if the material is there, year after year, sack after sack, tested at the dock and cleared for sale. Now watch what happens when industry gets involved, because this is where the story takes a counterintuitive turn. You might think medicine and manufacturing live in separate worlds but in the eighteenth century, they shared a problem: *how do you make a process reproducible when you're working with natural materials that vary batch to batch?* The answer, for both, was measurement, documentation, and trusted ingredients. And one of those ingredients was Acacia gum.

Switzerland (Basel), 1766. A Swiss manufacturer's shop manual in 1766 records calico-printing recipes that thicken printed mordants with gum (gum arabic/"gomme du Sénégal" among the period options), including color processes such as blue and madder. Contemporary technical accounts explain that a gum thickener keeps the mordant's line sharp under the block and washes out after steaming, leaving only the metallic salt on the fibre [1].

Cut to Edinburgh, 1803. In a committee room of the Royal College of Physicians of Edinburgh, fellows finalize the new official pharmacopoeia; the standard Scottish apothecaries are expected to follow. This is regulation, not theory. When a physician in Glasgow prescribes Mucilago Acaciae (mucilage of gum arabic), the pharmacopoeia ensures the Glasgow apothecary compounds it to the Edinburgh formula. [2]. That consistency (across cities, across pharmacies, across years) is what allows clinical knowledge to accumulate. If every syrup is different, every patient is an experiment. If every syrup is the same, patterns emerge.

When Edinburgh physicians standardized the dispensary book, Mucilago Gummi Arabici is specified as equal parts by weight of powdered Gum arabic and boiling water, digested and strained; a single official preparation used as a soothing vehicle in other formulas (e.g., Potio Cretacea includes mucilaginis gummi Arabici) [2]. An apprentice in a frontier pharmacy, miles from a teaching hospital, can open the dispensatory and compound a demulcent syrup that matches the standard. Acacia gum, because it behaves predictably, becomes infrastructure.

Now shift scenes again, because something else is happening in the early nineteenth century that will make gum even more trustworthy as chemistry is learning to name it. Working as director of the botanical garden, Henri Braconnot extracts from mushrooms a tough, acid-resistant, nitrogenous substance he names fungine; the first description of what would soon be called chitin. Braconnot publishes a landmark memoir showing that vegetable fibre can be hydrolyzed with sulfuric acid to produce sugars, opening a sustained research path into the chemical breakdown of plant matter. His results connect workshop practice with emerging chemical explanations of polysaccharide conversion [3]. Braconnot's work is foundational, though he doesn't know it yet. He's glimpsing the molecular grammar of plants. The long-chain polymers built from repeating sugar units, branched and cross-linked in ways that give each gum its particular texture, solubility, and film-forming behavior. For physicians, this is more than curiosity. It's reassurance. The more we understand why a plant exudate behaves gently and predictably, the safer we feel prescribing it.

Braconnot's acids are a lens into structure, and structure explains function. In his 1820's *Lehrbuch der Chemie*, J. J. Berzelius gives organic substances a clear structure inside plant chemistry. He groups the "nearer constituents" of plants into practical classes (starch, gums-mucilage, sugars, and resins) and contrasts their behavior. Starch swells in water but does not truly dissolve; true gums (e.g., acacia) form clear aqueous solutions; resins are water-insoluble yet dissolve in alcohol. These are not mere bookish labels; they give buyers and dispensers a testable profile. If a shipment sold as "Gum arabic" fails to dissolve cleanly in cold water or leaves a resinous film, it signals mislabeling. Berzelius's taxonomy thus doubles as quality control, which, in medicine, is simply patient safety by another name [4].

Let's bring this forward into mid-century clinical practice in Paris, 1845.

This is clinical care in the age of professionalization. Hospitals are growing. Medical societies are meeting and journals are circulating. Across that network, Acacia gum appears again and again, not as a headline but as a reliable supporting player. Guérin's publications (representative of the French hospital tradition) confirm what the pharmacopoeias codified. Acacia gum is safe, versatile, and reproducible enough to trust with your patients' comfort.

This is the moment when industry offers medicine a mirror. In Paris, 1855; Alphonse Louis Poitevin, a chemist and lithographer, patents a photographic process using gum bichromate which is a mixture of Acacia gum and light-sensitive chromium salts [5]. The process works something like this: coat paper with gum-bichromate emulsion, place a negative on top, expose to sunlight. Where light strikes, the chromium cross-links the gum, making it insoluble. Wash away the unexposed areas, and you're left with an image. A photograph fixed not in silver but in stabilized gum. The technique becomes popular with art photographers because it allows hand-tinting and fine control of tone.

Why does this matter for medicine? Because it's another materials test passed. Photographic processes are exacting. A gum that doesn't coat evenly, or that degrades in light, or that leaves residue, ruins the plate. The fact that Acacia gum can hold a photographic image by forming a film fine enough to preserve delicate gradations of tone and stable enough to survive washing and drying; tells users something they already suspected but now see confirmed in a different domain: this material is reliable under stress.

This is the power of a material that crosses domains. The more contexts in which Acacia gum proves itself (dye house, scriptorium, studio) the more trust compounds and this compounded trust, by the mid-nineteenth century, has made Acacia gum a known ingredient in various applications.

We're back at the dock now, but it's 1850, not 1785. The crate is still stamped with Arabic script, but alongside it is a second mark: the seal of the Edinburgh Pharmacopoeia, confirming that this batch meets the published standard. The factor still tests a fragment in water, still watches it bloom clear, but now he's not guessing. He's verifying. The gum has crossed not just an ocean but a conceptual threshold. It's no longer a curiosity from a distant land. It's a standard that is listed in pharmacopoeias, named by chemists, quantified by dyers, trusted by physicians, and prescribed to patients from Manchester to Manhattan.

That's the gift of the age of exploration to the age of the dispensary. Empire built the routes. Industry demanded the quality. Chemistry gave it a name and medicine, taking all that accumulated trust, turned a tree's exudate into an instrument of care that worked the same way from London to Philadelphia.

References:

1. Ryhiner, Jean. Traité sur la fabrication et le commerce des toiles peintes. Manuscript begun 1766. Musée de l'Impression sur Étoffes (Mulhouse), Fonds SIM, cote 96 B 1517. (Modern scholarly transcription: Aziza Gril-Mariotte, ed., Les indiennes… Suivi de l'édition du manuscrit écrit par Jean Ryhiner, à partir de 1766, Silvana Editoriale, 2022.
2. Royal College of Physicians of Edinburgh. Pharmacopoeia Collegii Regii Medicorum Edinburgensis. Edinburgi: Bell & Bradfute, 1803.
3. Braconnot, Henri. "Sur la nature des champignons." Annales de Chimie (series 1), vol. 79, 1811, pp. 265–304.
4. Berzelius, Jöns Jacob. Lehrbuch der Chemie. N.p., 1825.
5. Poitevin, Alphonse-Louis. Brevet d'invention no. 24 592, "Procédé de gravure et d'impression photographiques sur pierre et sur métal (photolithographie et procédés aux colloïdes bichromatés)." Paris, 27 Aug. 1855

CHAPTER 5

CHEMICAL DETECTIVES

What is it? Unlocking the Complex Medical Code of Acacia Gum

The chemist sits on a slate bench in a Berlin laboratory. Let's call him by his proper name, Carl Scheibler. This is 1873, and Scheibler is trying to answer an old simple question by sugar refiners and pharmacists alike: *What exactly is this substance that the traders call "gum arabic" and that apothecaries dissolve into syrups that soothe inflamed throats as reliably as quinine breaks fevers?* The question is an ancient one, and the answer will require a relay team of the most inventive chemists in Europe and America (several of them bound for Stockholm and the Nobel ceremony) working with tools that range from primitive crystallization to light-scattering spectroscopy.

By the time they finish, in 1969, they will have cracked a molecular code so elegant that it humbles most synthetic polymers. The code lies in a protein-studded, uronic-acid-decorated, hyperbranched arabinogalactan architecture that forms films, stabilizes emulsions, feeds beneficial microbes gently, and does it all while tasting like nothing at all. The story of how they got there is a detective story set in laboratories from Berlin to Birmingham to Cape Town. Interestingly, every revelation maps back to a historical puzzle; Why does this ancient healer work so well?

The case opens with sugar. Not the common table sugar, sucrose, that Scheibler knew intimately from his work in beet-sugar refineries, but something stranger. It's a sugar no one had isolated or named before. When Scheibler hydrolyzed Acacia gum with dilute acid, he isolates a previously unnamed sugar, He called it *Arabinose*, "gum sugar," because it came from Gum arabic which is the traders' shorthand for Acacia exudates from Arabian ports [1]. The name stuck, and with it, Acacia gum moved from the category of "mysterious oriental resin" to "definable carbohydrate source" as Scheibler had given the ghost an address.

What kind of sugar was Arabinose? That question landed on the desk of Heinrich Kiliani in 1887. Kiliani, a specialist of carbohydrate degradation and chain-extension reactions, put arabinose through a gauntlet of tests (oxidation, reduction, derivatization) and concluded that it was a *pentose*, a five-carbon sugar [2]. This was a revelation. Most natural sugars known at the time were hexoses (glucose, fructose, galactose) six-carbon backbones that dominated starch, cellulose, and glycogen. Pentoses were rare, temperamental, and biologically mysterious. By fixing Arabinose in the five-carbon family, Kiliani gave structural chemists a map. Pentoses behaved differently from hexoses in their reactivity, their glycemic impact, and their digestibility. That difference would later explain why Acacia-based syrups sat so gently in the stomach compared to glucose-heavy medicaments. A clinical observation that now had a chemical rationale.

The next detective to enter the case was Emil Fischer, working in Germany in the 1890s. Emil was such a formidable chemist he would win the Nobel Prize in Chemistry in 1902 for his work on sugar and purine synthesis. Fischer isolated another pentose, L-ribose from Arabinose, via deduction from Gum arabic in 1891, confirming that Acacia wasn't just a sugar source but a rare sugar source [3]. Ribose, it would turn out decades later, is a building block of RNA and ATP which is the energy currency and genetic messenger of every living cell. Fischer couldn't have known that in 1890, but he recognized that Gum arabic sat at a biochemical crossroads. It was a trade commodity that yielded laboratory-pure samples of sugars essential to life's machinery. The caravan route had delivered a chemical Rosetta stone.

Fischer wasn't done. In 1891, working with his colleague Oscar Piloty at the University of Würzburg, he demonstrated that nature's Arabinose could be transformed into biology's ribose on a chemist's bench, proving that the boundaries between "natural product" and "laboratory synthesis" were permeable [4]. For pharmacists and physicians, this synthesis meant something practical. If Gum arabic was a renewable source of rare sugars with known reactivity and mild physiological impact, it became easier to justify its use as a therapeutic vehicle where its predictable chemistry breeds clinical confidence.

The pentose thread had been pulled and now the question shifted. If Arabinose is just one building block, how are those blocks assembled in the intact gum? What architecture turns a collection of five-carbon sugars into a substance that dissolves completely, coats smoothly, and stabilizes emulsions? That question required new tools and a new language. That new language was called colloid science.

F ast forward to New York, 1928. Alfred W. Thomas and Harry A. Murray Jr., working at Columbia University, approached Acacia gum not as a sugar problem but as a colloidal problem which is a question of how large molecules behave in water. They examined Gum arabic as a physico-chemical (colloidal) system, not a mixture of small sugars. Using acid–base titration (base-combining capacity) plus osmotic-pressure and viscosity measurements on alcohol-purified solutions, they showed it behaves as an

44

acidic macromolecular colloid (what we'd later call a polyelectrolyte) shifting attention from "sugar content" to solution behavior [5]. The viscosity was surprisingly low for such large molecules, meaning they coiled tightly in water rather than sprawling like linear chains. That compact coil explained a historical riddle. The riddle was why a small dose of gum (just a few percent by weight) can make a stable, pourable syrup that didn't turn gummy or stringy? The answer it turns out was in the shape. Branched polymers pack efficiently, hydrate evenly, flow smoothly, and don't tangle. Thomas and Murray's work opened the door to modern pharmaceutical and food formulation.

Rheology is how a gum solution flows, thins under shear, and recovers when stress is removed. Understanding rheology allows you to design syrups that pour easily from a spoon but coat the throat on contact. It shows how lozenges that dissolve at a controlled rate, and emulsions that stay stable in the bottle can release flavor cleanly on the tongue. The Columbia study gave formulators a dashboard of concentration, temperature, ionic strength, and pH. Adjust the knobs and predict the outcome. This was medicine as engineering, and Gum arabic had just earned its blueprint.

While Thomas and Murray were quantifying flow in New York, a group of carbohydrate chemists in Birmingham, England, was dismantling the molecule itself. Sydney W. Challinor, working under the legendary Walter Norman Haworth and Edmund Langley Hirst at the University of Birmingham, published the first systematic study of "arabic acid" (the acidic polysaccharide backbone of Acacia gum) in 1931 [6]. Their approach was forensic: 1-break the polymer into smaller pieces with controlled acid hydrolysis, 2-identify the fragments, 3-deduce the linkages. They identified the aldobiuronic acid as 6-O-β-D-glucuronosyl-D-galactose; the fuller arabinogalactan-type picture was established by later work. We now know that it wasn't a simple linear chain; it was a tree, with

45

a trunk of galactose and branches of arabinose, and the whole thing was studded with acidic groups that made it water-soluble and pH-sensitive. Haworth would go on to win the Nobel Prize in Chemistry in 1937 for his work on carbohydrate structures and the synthesis of vitamin C. His genius brought an architect's precision to the Acacia gum problem. He and Hirst didn't just identify sugars; they mapped connections. They uncovered which carbon on one sugar was bonded to which carbon on the next. Those connections (the glycosidic linkages) determine how the polymer folds, how enzymes recognize it, how it interacts with water, protein and bile salts. By 1931, the Birmingham group had moved the case from "gum is a mixture of sugars" to "gum is an arabinogalactan with uronic acid decorations." That's not a name; it's a structure class, and structure predicts function.

The breakthrough moment came in 1929, in the laboratory of Michael Heidelberger at Columbia University's College of Physicians and Surgeons. Heidelberger and his colleague Forrest E. Kendall crystallized an aldobionic acid obtained by hydrolyzing Gum arabic. This furnished direct evidence that uronic-acid residues are integral to the polysaccharide's makeup, rather than accidental impurities introduced during isolation. Subsequent studies confirmed and elaborated the linkage details [7]. We now know that those uronic acids (glucuronic acid, in this case) carried negative charges at physiological pH. Negative charges do things such as bind minerals (calcium, magnesium), interact with bile salts, modulate fermentation by gut bacteria, and they create a slippery, hydrated surface that resists protein adsorption. In clinical terms, those charged sugars explained why Acacia syrups calmed "stomach heat" (the historical term for acid reflux or gastritis) and why thick mucilage painted onto oral ulcers formed protective films that resisted bacterial adhesion. The chemistry was specifying the care.

However, the most elegant clue came a decade later, in 1939, from Fred Smith, a young chemist who had trained at the University of Leeds and completed his Ph.D. at the University of Cape Town. Smith isolated the disaccharide 3-D-galactosido-L-arabinose from Gum arabic, providing direct evidence for a galactose→arabinose (1→3) linkage in the polysaccharide [8].

Acacia gum is a type-II arabinogalactan-protein with a β-(1→3)-galactan backbone and β-(1→6) side chains ending largely in α-L-arabinofuranose. It also bears glucuronic/4-O-methyl-glucuronic acid residues that make it polyanionic. This highly branched, compact architecture explains its unusually low viscosity at high solids compared with other gums. In water it forms hydrated macromolecular dispersions that act as demulcents; traditionally described by the ancients as soothing (cooling and moistening) by lightly coating irritated mucosa. Additionally, its carboxylate groups contribute negative charge and electrostatic interactions (with proteins/mucins), which may aid its gentle mouth/throat feel.

By mid-century, the chemical structure was becoming clear, but a new question arose: *How do you turn lab knowledge into procurement logic?* A substance as complex as Acacia gum doesn't come off the tree in pharmaceutical-grade purity. It varies by species, season, geography, tapping method, and post-harvest processing. Someone needed to bridge the field and the bench, and that someone was Alexander Jacob Charlson, a South African chemist who completed his Ph.D. at the University of Cape Town in 1954.

Charlson's thesis, Chemistry of Acacia Gums, is a masterclass in applied natural-product chemistry. He collected samples from different Acacia species, from different regions and provided an early, rigorous comparison of Acacia species rather than a catch-all "gum arabic". Working chiefly on Acacia cyanophylla and A. karroo (with a commercial A. senegal sample for reference), he used electrophoresis, specific rotation, and classical carbohydrate degradations (methylation, hydrolysis, chromatography) to show that so-called "gum arabic" encompasses distinct macromolecular families. His take-home: if you want consistent performance (from pharmacy syrups to beverage stabilization) you must specify the Acacia source, not just buy "Gum arabic" [9].

Charlson's work transformed the market. Before his thesis, purchasing Gum arabic was a gamble as you relied on the trader's word, and a visual inspection. After Charlson, you could write a specification asking for Acacia senegal, hand-picked, dry-season harvest, maximum 4% ash, minimum 90% solubility at 25°C. Suddenly, formulators could reproduce batches year over year, and regulatory agencies could set standards. This was the hinge between colonial commodity and modern ingredient specification. Charlson gave the industry a quality language, and quality language enables trust at scale.

The final act of the detective story unfolded between 1966 and 1969, in a series of papers that read like the closing chapters of a drama series. Every loose thread tied, every suspect cleared, every mystery resolved. The first breakthrough came from Brian Warburton at the University of London, who published a paper in 1966 for the Society of Chemical Industry on the rheology and physical chemistry of Acacia systems [10]. Warburton built on the Thomas and Murray foundation but added precision by mapping how concentration, temperature, and added salts (ionic strength) influence solution viscosity and documented interfacial film/rheology at the air-water (and related) interfaces. This helped shift Acacia gum discussions from sugar content toward macromolecular colloid behavior.

His work gave beverage scientists and tablet formulators a control panel. Need a syrup that stays pourable at refrigerator temperature? Adjust the calcium level. Need an emulsion that resists creaming under heat? Use a specific fraction of the gum with higher protein content. Warburton's rheograms became the formulator's Rosetta stone. Simply translate the product requirement into a processing parameter, and the gum will deliver. Then came the Anderson series; a decade-long investigation led by Douglas M. W. Anderson. Anderson and his collaborator J. F. Stoddart used molecular-sieve chromatography (a technique that separates molecules by size as they flow through a porous gel) to fractionate Acacia gum into distinct populations [11]. What they found was revelatory and it was the foundation for what we know now. The gum wasn't a homogeneous polymer but a mixture of three main fractions. The largest fraction (about 90% by weight) was a neutral-to-slightly-acidic arabinogalactan with modest molecular weight. A smaller fraction (around 10%) was a *protein–polysaccharide conjugate*; a hybrid molecule where a polysaccharide chain was covalently attached to a small protein. A minor fraction has very high molecular weight and highly branched.

The protein–polysaccharide conjugate was the key to emulsification as the protein provided hydrophobic patches that anchored to oil droplets, while the polysaccharide provided a hydrophilic shell that stabilized the droplet in water. This was nature's surfactant, and it explained why Acacia gum could stabilize citrus oils in soft drinks, essential oils in pharmaceutical emulsions, and fat droplets in flavor encapsulation. All were applications that synthetic gums struggled to match.

Anderson and Haworth's successor, Sir Edmund Hirst, followed up in 1967 with light-scattering studies that measured the molecular weight and conformation of these fractions in solutions. Light scattering is a physical

49

technique that tells you how large a molecule is and how it's shaped. The data confirmed the compact, branched architecture that Thomas and Murray had inferred in 1928 [12]. Future discoveries concluded that Acacia gum molecules were hyperbranched spheroids, not extended chains, which explained the paradox of low viscosity at high molecular weight. A branched sphere tumbles through solution without tangling; a linear chain snags and drags. That difference is why you can dissolve 50% Gum arabic in water and still pour it, but 5% linear gum (like xanthan) turns into a gel. Formulation scientists read those light-scattering curves and saw possibility; high solids loading, clean mouthfeel, no slime.

The culmination came in two papers from 1968 and 1969. Anderson, working with I. C. M. Dea, K. A. Karamalla, and J. F. Smith, published an exhaustive analytical study comparing different forms of gum from Acacia harvested under varying geographic conditions and demonstrated that while the core structure was conserved, the fine details (protein content, uronic acid ratio) varied within characteristic ranges [13]. This was applied chemotaxonomy demonstrating that if you know which tree you're tapping and when, you can predict the gum's performance. This was gold for procurement managers and quality-control labs as it was testable, reproducible, and tied to supply-chain reality.

Finally, in 1969, Anderson and Dea published a chemotaxonomic review of Acacia gum exudates that compared analytical data across thirty species. Using sugar-composition profiles, specific optical rotation, nitrogen (protein) content and uronic acids. They showed these measures reliably differentiate species, including A. senegal (commercial gum arabic/hashab) from A. seyal (talha) [14]. This wasn't just academic botany; it was authenticity testing. Regulators, formulators, and buyers now had a chemical passport. If your shipment's sugar profile doesn't match the A. senegal standard, you're not getting what you paid for. Anderson and Dea's work closed the loop from laboratory to ledger, from molecular structure to trade honesty. The detectives had not only cracked the code but also taught the world how to read it in the real world of variable harvests, competitive markets, and regulatory scrutiny.

We're in a modern formulation facility now. A food scientist in Zurich, a pharmacist in São Paulo, a biotech researcher in San Francisco. Each warms a beaker; each watches a brittle amber resin dissolve into clarity. However now, unlike Scheibler a century and a half ago, they know what they're looking at. They see a hyperbranched arabinogalactan core, molecular weight around 300,000 Da, decorated with arabinose side chains and glucuronic acid caps, studded with protein patches that anchor hydrophobic guests. They see a compact coil that hydrates without tangling, a neutral-tasting film-former that soothes without smothering, a selectively fermentable prebiotic that feeds the right microbes gently. They see the code.

The code explains everything. It explains why Acacia gum soothed Pharaohs, Monks and Victorian consumptives. It did so not through mysticism or luck, but through a molecular architecture that forms protective films on inflamed tissue, buffers chemical irritants, and stabilizes fragile actives so they reach their target intact. It explains why textile printers and photographers trusted it. It explains why modern beverage chemists and pharmaceutical formulators still reach for it when they need emulsification that tastes clean, stabilization that lasts, and safety that's been verified by centuries of human use and decades of analytical chemistry.

The century-long investigation didn't just decode Acacia gum. It gave us a template for how to approach any complex natural polymer. Break it into pieces, name the pieces, map the linkages, measure the behavior, tie the structure to function, authenticate the source, and build the quality standards that make trust scalable. That template now guides how we evaluate seaweed polysaccharides for drug delivery, how we engineer pectin for targeted-release capsules, how we design next-generation prebiotics that feed specific microbial guilds without collateral gas and bloating. The detectives who chased arabinose crystals and aldobionic acids across a century of labs weren't just solving an academic puzzle. They were building the foundation of modern biopolymer science, one clear solution at a time.

From then on, when the modern formulator tilts her beaker and watches that invisible film creep up the glass, she's reading a code that took a hundred years and some of the century's brightest chemists to crack. The code says: I am branched, hydrated, charged, and gentle. I form films without residue. I carry oils without tasting oily. I feed good microbes without distress. I have been tested by empires, standardized by pharmacopoeias, mapped by Nobel laureates, and authenticated by chemotaxonomists.

Tomorrow's therapeutics such as targeted nano-delivery, mucosal vaccines, precision prebiotics, and bio-responsive emulsions will build on that code. First, the detectives had to solve the case and in solving it, they proved something deeper. They proved that sometimes, the world's gentlest, oldest, most transparent solution is also the most brilliantly complex.

References:

1. Scheibler, Carl. "Ueber das Vorkommen der Arabinsäure (Gummi) in den Zuckerrüben und über den Arabinzucker (Gummizucker)." Berichte der Deutschen Chemischen Gesellschaft, vol. 6, 1873, pp. 612–622. (Paper states he had reported related findings five years earlier in Berichte vol. 1.)

2. Kiliani, Heinrich. "Ueber die Zusammensetzung und Constitution der Arabinosecarbonsäure bezw. der Arabinose." Berichte der deutschen chemischen Gesellschaft, vol. 20, no. 1, 1887, pp. 339–346.

3. Fischer, Emil, and Oskar Piloty. "Reduction der Zuckersäure." Berichte der Deutschen Chemischen Gesellschaft, vol. 24, 1891, pp. 521–28. doi:10.1002/cber.18910240199. (Work from Fischer's lab in 1891 that includes the L-ribose synthesis program from arabinose.)

4. Fischer, Emil, and Oskar Piloty. "Ueber eine neue Pentonsäure und die zweite inactive Trioxyglutarsäure." Berichte der deutschen chemischen Gesellschaft, vol. 24, 1891, pp. 4214–4225. (Describes the arabinose → ribose route via pentonic acids/epimerization.)

5. Thomas, Alfred W., and Harry A. Murray, Jr. "A Physico-Chemical Study of Gum Arabic." The Journal of Physical Chemistry, vol. 32, no. 6, 1928, pp. 676–697.

6. Challinor, Sydney W., Walter N. Haworth, and Edmund L. Hirst. "XXXIV.—The compound uronic acids. Structure of the aldobionic acid from gum arabic." Journal of the Chemical Society (Resumed), 1931, pp. 258–265.

7. Heidelberger, Michael, and Forrest E. Kendall. "A Crystalline Aldobionic Acid Derived from Gum Arabic." Journal of Biological Chemistry, vol. 84, no. 2, 1929, pp. 639–653.

8. Smith, F. (Fred). "The Constitution of Arabic Acid. Part I. The Isolation of 3-d-galactosido-1-arabinose." Journal of the Chemical Society, 1939, pp. 744–753.

9. Charlson, Alexander Jacob. Chemistry of Acacia Gums. 1954. University of Cape Town, PhD dissertation, 1954.

10. Warburton, Brian. "The Rheology and Physical Chemistry of Some Acacia Systems." The Chemistry and Rheology of Water Soluble Gums and Colloids: Comprising Papers (with Discussions). Society of Chemical Industry, 1966. S.C.I. Monograph no. 24, pp. 118–130

11. Anderson, D. M. W., and J. F. Stoddart. "Studies on Uronic Acid Materials. Part XV. The Use of Molecular-Sieve Chromatography

in Studies on Acacia senegal Gum (Gum Arabic)." Carbohydrate Research, vol. 2, 1966, pp. 104–14

12. Anderson, D. M. W., E. L. Hirst, S. Rahman, and G. Stainsby. "Studies on Uronic Acid Materials. Part XVIII. Light-Scattering Studies on Some Molecular-Weight Fractions from Acacia senegal Gum." Carbohydrate Research, vol. 3, 1967, pp. 308–317

13. Anderson, D. M. W., I. C. M. Dea, K. A. Karamalla, and J. F. Smith. "Studies on Uronic Acid Materials. Part XXIV. An Analytical Study of Different Forms of the Gum from Acacia senegal Willd." Carbohydrate Research, vol. 6, no. 1, 1968, pp. 97–103

14. Anderson, D. M. W., and I. C. M. Dea. "Chemotaxonomic Aspects of the Chemistry of Acacia Gum Exudates." Phytochemistry, vol. 8, no. 1, 1969, pp. 167–176.

CHAPTER 6

THE PARADIGM SHIFT

The Research that transformed Acacia from harmless exudate
to Fiber

By the early 1960s, chemists had decoded Acacia's architecture. The next question that dominated scientists was simpler and more urgent. *What can this gentle, branched biopolymer do for human health?* The answer arrived not in a single eureka moment but a timeline of careful studies. These studies transformed Hashab gum; known in factories as a safe emulsifier, listed on labels as E 414, and traded globally as Gum arabic into something more substantial. Hashab gum was transformed into a well-tolerated dietary fiber with measurable physiological benefits and the regulatory credentials to scale. This chapter tells that transformation as a story, each anchored to a study that asked a harder question than the one before.

Albany, California, 1963. The USDA Western Regional Research Laboratory is where federal scientists spend their days safeguarding the American food supply. In the early 1960s, that supply is rapidly changing. Synthetic polymers and additives are flooding into food formulations as stabilizers, thickeners, and emulsifiers. Someone needs to figure out whether they're safe to eat at the doses consumers will actually encounter.

A. Norman Booth, A. P. Hendrickson, and Floyd Deeds drew the assignment for three polysaccharides. They designed a straightforward rat study where they feed the gums at practical dietary concentrations. They then monitor the body weights, feed intake, serum chemistry, organ weights and Histology. This is civil-service science trying to catch a problem before it becomes a public-health disaster.

Before we follow their results, let's pause for context, because the term "dietary fiber" (coined by Hipsley, 1953) meant something different in 1963 than it does today. Back then, fiber was mostly synonymous with roughage. The indigestible plant material (cellulose, lignin) that added bulk to stool and prevented constipation. The idea that some fibers might be *fermentable* and that gut bacteria could break them down into metabolically active compounds was known in physiology but was just beginning to take shape in nutrition science. In other words, the distinction between "dietary fiber" (the fiber naturally present in whole foods) and "functional fiber" (isolated, purified fibers added to foods for specific health benefits) didn't yet exist in regulatory language. Acacia gum was known in factories as a stabilizer, an emulsifier, and a binder. It was an industrial ingredient with a long history of use but no reputation as a fiber.

Booth and his colleagues were testing it not because anyone thought it was a superfood, but because they needed to confirm it wasn't poisonous. Booth's findings showed no overt toxicity and that was reassuring and, in retrospect, revealing. Rats were fed these polysaccharides at levels much higher than human diet equivalence. The vast majority grew normally, ate normally, and showed no signs of distress. However, at the highest doses, some groups showed looser, bulkier stools and slower weight gain, but no organ damage or classic signs of toxicity. The data also hinted at something more interesting. They noticed shifts in fecal output, subtle physiological signals that didn't look like inert passage through the gut. These were exactly the footprints you would expect from a fermentable, non-laxative fiber rather than an indigestible filler [1]. The results didn't make headlines, but they did something more important. They signaled to industry and regulators that more research was warranted.

Two decades pass. The baton moves across the Atlantic to Britain, where the Rowett Research Institute in Aberdeen and the University of Birmingham have become hubs of modern nutrition toxicology. By 1982, the scientific bar has risen. Companies want ingredients that are not only safe but defensible. Meaning they are backed by the kind of rigorous, multiweek exposure studies that regulatory agencies trust. Douglas M. W. Anderson (the same chemist who spent the 1960s decoding Acacia's structure) teams up with clinical biochemist Peter Ashby, pathologist Andrew Busuttil, and colleagues to run a subchronic rat study on Gum arabic.

Let's define subchronic exposure, because the term carries weight with regulators. Acute toxicity studies last hours to days and catch poisons that act fast. Subchronic studies run for weeks to months and catch problems that emerge with repeated dosing. They monitor organ damage, metabolic disruption, and subtle carcinogenic signals. The gold standard outcome from a subchronic study is a *NOAEL* (a No Observed Adverse Effect Level) at the highest dose at which nothing bad happens. Regulators use the NOAEL to set safety margins. The NOAEL anchors confidence.

Anderson's team fed rats purified Acacia gum at doses spanning practical food-use levels up to levels far exceeding what any human would consume. They run blood panels. They weigh organs. They examine tissues under the microscope, looking for inflammation, necrosis, dysplasia and anything that would raise a red flag. The result, published in 1982, is as clean as the gum solution itself. No carcinogenic signal, no organ-specific toxicity, just physiological shifts consistent with a fermentable fiber [2]. Stool weight increases modestly. Cecal weight increases, a sign that microbial fermentation is happening in the hindgut. Serum lipids show minor, favorable changes. No histological evidence of tissue damage and only adaptive, fiber-like changes at the highest doses. The NOAEL is high enough that even the most fiber-enthusiastic formulator would struggle to reach it.

The incentives here are worth naming explicitly, because they explain why this work got funded and published. Confectionery companies (makers of gum drops, lozenges, soft candies) wanted a clean-label stabilizer that could also improve the nutrition profile of their products without causing embarrassing gastrointestinal side effects. Beverage formulators wanted an emulsifier that could hold citrus oils and clouding agents in stable suspension while adding soluble fiber to the label. Public-health researchers wanted evidence that isolated fibers could be deployed at scale without unintended consequences and regulators wanted data they could cite when approving new uses or updating specifications. The 1982 study gave all of them what they needed, a green light backed by necropsy.

Edinburgh, 1983. The scene shifts from rat cages to a metabolic kitchen at the University of Edinburgh Medical School. Alison H. Ross, working with the distinguished gastroenterologist Michael A. Eastwood, is about to execute the clinical pivot. It's the moment when Acacia gum stops being an animal-tested ingredient and starts being a human-validated fiber. The study design is elegant. A small, tightly controlled before–after study, meaning each participant serves as their own control, cycling through periods of high-fiber diet and low-fiber baseline

Before we narrate the findings, let's clarify what the team was measuring and why it mattered. Controlled feeding studies are the clinical-research equivalent of a chemistry experiment. You control all inputs (diet composition, timing, portion size), collect all outputs (stool, urine, blood), and measure what changes. Ross and Eastwood were tracking stool weight, fecal bile acids, neutral sterols, breath hydrogen, serum lipids, and glucose tolerance. They were also tracking something less quantifiable but clinically crucial which is tolerance. Did participants experience gas, bloating, cramping, and diarrhea; the side effects that make even beneficial fibers unusable for real people?

The results, published in 1983 in the American Journal of Clinical Nutrition, were quietly transformative. Participants tolerated Gum arabic at doses of 25 grams per day (a robust intake by fiber standards) with minimal gastrointestinal distress. Glucose tolerance and stool weight were minimally affected. No Gum arabic was recovered in stool, consistent with microbial fermentation and the excretion of bacterial biomass which is evidence that gut microbes were indeed metabolizing the gum. Serum lipids improved showing total cholesterol dropped significantly and low-density lipoprotein (LDL) cholesterol trended downward [3].

Although not reported or understood at the time of this study; these observed changes fit a coherent mechanistic picture, one that loops back to the chemistry we learned in the previous chapter. Hashab's uronic acids (those negatively charged sugar groups decorating the polysaccharide branches) can bind bile acids in the gut lumen. Bile acids are cholesterol-derived detergents that help digest fats. When you trap those bile acids in fiber and excrete them in stool, the liver has to pull cholesterol from the bloodstream to make more bile. That's one pathway to lowering serum cholesterol. Meanwhile, the slow, selective fermentation by colonic bacteria generates short-chain fatty acids (SCFAs) and specifically acetate, propionate, and butyrate. These molecules are not waste products; they're signaling molecules. Acetate and propionate enter the bloodstream and modulate hepatic lipid and glucose metabolism. Butyrate feeds colonocytes (the cells lining the colon) and supports barrier integrity. Together, SCFAs help explain the glycemic and lipid improvements Ross and Eastwood documented.

What made the 1983 paper a watershed moment? It was the tolerance data. For decades, fiber recommendations ran into the same practical wall as people wouldn't eat enough fiber because it made them feel bloated, gassy, and uncomfortable. Some fibers, especially rapidly fermentable oligosaccharides trigger symptoms in sensitive individuals and produce benefits in theory but misery in practice. Gum arabic, by contrast, fermented slowly and selectively. Its compact, branched structure and specific β-linkages meant that gut microbes processed it like a slow-release fuel, generating SCFAs over hours rather than minutes, minimizing the sudden gas production that causes cramping. The Edinburgh data made that visible. For clinicians and dietitians, Hashab gum could now be framed not just as a food-industry workhorse or an E-number on a label, but as a dietary fiber that patients would actually tolerate. What you might call "benefit without bloat".

Let's pause here to unpack the fermentation piece, because it bridges chemistry, microbiology, and human comfort in ways that matter for every fiber story to come. Think of gut microbes as a quiet night shift working in your colon. When fermentable fiber arrives, certain bacterial guilds get to work, cleaving sugar linkages and metabolizing the fragments. The end products of that fermentation are SCFAs, carbon dioxide, hydrogen, and bacterial biomass (which becomes part of your stool). If fermentation happens too fast or involves the wrong substrates, you get a sudden surge of gas and cramping. If fermentation is slow, selective, and steady, you get the metabolic benefits of SCFAs. These benefits include energy for your colonocytes, favorable shifts in lipid and glucose metabolism, and support for a healthy gut barrier without any distress. Acacia's branched arabinogalactan structure with β-linkages and protein conjugates makes it a "slow-release" fiber in exactly this way. The microbes that ferment it do so at a measured pace, producing a gentle rise in SCFAs rather than a spike. That's why the Edinburgh participants could consume 25 grams per day and still go about their lives.

York and London, 1986. D. M. W. Anderson (by this point the scientific architect of Acacia gum's identity) compiled a brief review in Food Additives and Contaminants that collates chemical, toxicological, and human data. It concludes that Gum arabic (Hashab gum from Acacia Senegal) requires no numerical ADI when it conforms to established identity and purity criteria, thereby providing a regulator-oriented synthesis. It situates safety within formal specifications that define the additive (E 414) and require conformance to identity and purity limits set by JECFA and later EU monographs, with A. Senegal (Hashab) as the benchmark source (A. Seyal came later under different JECFA specifications) and with defined purity tests (e.g., ash, acid-insoluble matter, heavy metals, microbiological criteria). The review's safety conclusions are supported by subchronic animal studies and early human data showing cholesterol lowering, minimal effects on glucose tolerance, and good short-term tolerability at studied doses [4].

In plain terms, this review connects the question "What is it?" to the question "What happens when people eat it?" and insists that the material be what it says on the label. This is where chemotaxonomy stops being an academic exercise and becomes a public-health safeguard. If you're going to declare that Gum arabic (E 414) is safe and functional, you need to define which Acacia species you're talking about (Acacia senegal being the gold standard, with A. seyal sometimes permitted but characterized separately), what purity criteria it must meet (nitrogen content below a threshold to limit excess protein, ash content controlled to minimize mineral contaminants), and what molecular profile it should have

61

(molecular-weight distribution, uronic acid content, protein-polysaccharide ratio). Without that specificity, a trader could substitute an inferior or adulterated gum and still call it "Gum arabic," undermining both safety and function.

Anderson's 1986 review does exactly this. It lays out the identity and purity monograph, summarizes the subchronic animal data showing no adverse effects up to high doses, and integrates the early human studies showing favorable lipid and glycemic shifts with high tolerability. The dose ranges tested in animals and humans are aligned with the concentrations used in real-world food applications such as confectionery coatings, beverage clouding, and dietary supplements. This is so formulators know they're working within a tested and characterized window. The review makes explicit what had been implicit. Acacia gum is not just presumed safe based on long historical use (the "generally recognized as safe" or GRAS rationale); it's demonstrated safe through modern toxicology and characterized through modern analytical chemistry.

The incentives driving this synthesis are easy to see. Rowntree-Mackintosh, the British confectionery giant that partly funded Anderson's work, wanted to deploy Acacia gum widely in lozenges, gums, and sugar-free candies. All are products where soluble fiber could add bulk, improve mouthfeel, and support a health claim without compromising taste or texture. Public-health reviewers wanted assurance that widespread adoption wouldn't introduce hidden risks such as organ toxicity, carcinogenicity, and nutrient malabsorption. The 1986 BNF review gave both sides a common language and shared confidence. It also paved the next, inevitable step which is submission to the international gatekeepers.

Geneva 1982 and Rome 1989. The Joint FAO/WHO Expert Committee on Food Additives (JECFA) meets at its 26th and then its 35th sessions to consider Gum arabic. JECFA is the global arbiter of food-additive safety, a panel of toxicologists, chemists, and clinicians drawn from member countries who review dossiers and issue verdicts that shape international trade and national regulations. For an ingredient like Acacia gum, which crosses borders in every soft drink, candy, and supplement, JECFA's opinion is the difference between niche use and global scale.

The committee of toxicologists, chemists and clinicians reviews the full package. The chemistry and chemotaxonomy establishing identity and purity; the rat studies from 1963 and 1982 establishing a high NOAEL; the human studies from Edinburgh showing tolerability and physiological benefit; and the British Nutrition Foundation synthesis showing that all the pieces fit together. They debate dose limits, purity thresholds, labeling requirements, and the need (or lack thereof) for a numerical cap on intake.

At its 26th meeting in 1982, JECFA allocated an ADI 'not specified' for Gum arabic. In the 35th meeting in 1989, it confirmed this conclusion, as summarized in the 1990 WHO Food Additives Series 26 monograph. ADI stands for Acceptable Daily Intake, the amount of a substance that a person can consume every day for a lifetime without appreciable health risk. For many additives, JECFA sets a specific ADI like 10 milligrams per kilogram of body weight per day based on the NOAEL from animal studies divided by a safety factor. However, for a small number of substances, those with exceptionally low toxicity, long histories of safe use, and consumption patterns that make overexposure implausible, JECFA issues an "ADI not specified," meaning the committee saw no necessity to set a numerical cap at the intended ranges of use, given the totality of evidence. It's the safety equivalent of a gold star. It says: this material is so well tolerated that setting a limit is unnecessary [5].

JECFA pairs the ADI ruling with detailed identity and purity specifications including nitrogen content limits (to control residual protein and microbial load), ash limits (to control mineral contaminants), species authentication criteria (*Acacia senegal* as the reference standard), and molecular-weight expectations. These specs become the passport for global trade. A confectionery plant in São Paulo, a beverage bottler in Manila, and a supplement manufacturer in Toronto can each source Acacia gum, verify it against the JECFA monograph, and use it with regulatory confidence. Labeling as E 414 (the European number) or simply as "Acacia gum" or "Gum arabic" is harmonized across jurisdictions. The identity-and-purity framework built over decades of chemotaxonomy now pays off as quality assurance at planetary scale.

Who benefits? Everyone in the supply chain. Acacia gum growers gain access to premium markets with clear quality benchmarks. Ingredient traders gain a harmonized spec they can contract against. Food and pharmaceutical companies gain de-risked R&D. Once JECFA green-lights a material, national agencies from the FDA to EFSA typically follow, smoothing the path to commercial launch. Importantly, consumers gain transparency and the "Acacia gum" or "Gum arabic" or "E 414" on the label is a defined substance, not a mystery powder. Most importantly for our story, the global safety runway means that higher-dose nutritional uses in the emerging fiber-supplement market become commercially rational to study and launch. When regulators say "no limit needed," innovators hear "explore the ceiling".

By 1990, Acacia gum occupied a rare position. It was a food additive with Millenia of safe use, reconfirmed through modern toxicology. It was a characterized biopolymer with a known structure, authenticated by chemotaxonomy, and reproducible batch to batch. It was a fiber; a material that, when isolated and consumed, produced measurable physiological benefits in humans without the tolerance problems that plagued other fibers. Most remarkably, it was all three at once.

What remained were the deeper questions, the ones that only become answerable once you have safe, tolerable doses deployed in real humans over weeks and months. Questions like: Which microbial species does Acacia gum favor, and why? What are the dose-response curves for SCFA production, and do those SCFAs translate into durable metabolic improvements like lower cholesterol, better glycemic control, and reduced inflammation? Can Acacia gum support gut barrier function in stressed populations such as athletes, elders, and people with metabolic syndrome? Does it modulate appetite or satiety through gut-brain signaling? These are the questions of the prebiotic era, the era we're about to enter. However, they only became answerable because the paradigm had already shifted. Acacia was no longer "just an emulsifier." It was gentle, clear, safe, effective and truly exceptional fiber. The next chapters will explain why.

References:

1. Booth, Albert N., A. P. Hendrickson, and Floyd Deeds. "Physiologic Effects of Three Microbial Polysaccharides on Rats." Toxicology and Applied Pharmacology, vol. 5, no. 4, July 1963, pp. 478–484.
2. Anderson, D. M. W., et al. "Subchronic Effects of Gum Arabic (Acacia) in the Rat." Toxicology Letters, vol. 14, no. 3-4, 1982, pp. 221-27.
3. Ross, Alison H. M., Michael A. Eastwood, William G. Brydon, J. R. Anderson, and D. M. W. Anderson. "A Study of the Effects of Dietary Gum Arabic in Humans." The American Journal of Clinical Nutrition, vol. 37, no. 3, Mar. 1983, pp. 368–375.
4. Anderson, D. M. W. "Evidence for the Safety of Gum Arabic (Acacia senegal (L.) Willd.) as a Food Additive—A Brief Review." Food Additives and Contaminants, vol. 3, no. 3, 1986, pp. 225-30.
5. Joint FAO/WHO Expert Committee on Food Additives. "Gum Arabic." Toxicological Evaluation of Certain Food Additives and Contaminants. WHO Food Additives Series, no. 26, World Health Organization, 1990

CHAPTER 7

THE RESEARCH AVALANCHE BEGINS

Hashab Prebiotic Power Revealed

A kitchen counter in the morning light. Someone adds tea to a mug with clear powder. The powder dissolves instantly, leaving no cloud, no thickness, no taste. Just a faint shimmer as the spoon circles. In another house, a parent folds the same powder into yogurt for a toddler; it vanishes on contact, invisible even to a suspicious three-year-old. In a hospital metabolic ward, a research volunteer drinks a measured dose mixed into orange juice, logs the time in a notebook, and goes about the day feeling nothing in particular. No bloating, no urgency, and no drama. That invisibility, that gentle disappearance into daily life, is a big advantage. The point is while the powder leaves no trace in the glass, it sets a careful tempo deep in the colon, where trillions of beneficial bacteria are about to get the boost they need to keep everything working properly.

This is Hashab gum, The most premium Acacia gum also known vaguely as Gum arabic, or E 414. It's an amazing natural product that is as tasteless and colorless as it gets in the therapeutic world. So far, we have followed it through millennia of medicine and a century of chemistry. We've learned its arabinogalactan-protein conjugated architecture. We've seen it earn the regulatory green light as a safe, well-tolerated fiber. Now we're going deeper, into the most elegant question: *What happens when you feed this gentle, clear, branched biopolymer to the ecosystem inside a human gut?* The answer, built across nearly four decades of research from Norwich to

Nebraska, transformed Hashab gum from "dietary fiber" into "potent prebiotic"; a material that reshapes the entire body in ways that support health. This chapter tells the story of how clarity in the glass became calm in the gut, and how calm in the gut became measurable change in multiple organs and systems.

Norwich, England, 1986. The AFRC Food Research Institute is a public-interest lab where scientists work at the intersection of agriculture, food safety, and human nutrition. G. M. Wyatt, C. E. Bayliss, and J. D. Holcroft are running a modest feeding study, the kind that rarely makes headlines but sometimes changes fields. They recruit a healthy volunteer, feed him diets supplemented with Gum arabic, and then do something that in 1986 is still relatively novel. They culture and count the bacteria in fecal samples, trying to see if dietary fiber can shift the composition of what they call the "*faecal flora*" [1].

Let's pause on that term, because language shapes how we think. In 1986, scientists spoke of "faecal flora" which is the cultivable bacteria recovered from stool samples and identified by colony morphology, staining, and biochemical tests. It was a narrow window into a vast world, because most gut microbes can't be cultured on standard agar plates; they're strict anaerobes that die on contact with oxygen, or they require growth factors we didn't yet know how to provide. So, when Wyatt and colleagues reported changes in faecal flora in response to Gum arabic, they were peering through a keyhole, seeing only the microbes that happened to grow on their plates. However, what they saw was enough. Adding Gum arabic to the diet reshaped the recoverable bacterial populations, sharply increasing the fraction of bacteria able to break down the gum (mainly species of *Bacteroides* and *Bifidobacterium*) and this shift reversed after supplementation stopped [1].

The idea that a *soluble* fiber could selectively feed beneficial microbes without causing gastrointestinal chaos was just beginning to crystallize. Wyatt's paper gave Acacia gum a new identity. It wasn't just an emulsifier that happened to be fermentable; it was a material that could gently, intentionally, reshape the gut ecosystem. That realization invited clinicians, formulators, and researchers to look beyond stabilization and start asking: "*What else can this do?*"

To understand what happened next, we need a shared definition that would let scientists around the world know they were studying the same phenomenon. That rulebook arrived in 1999, when Glenn R. Gibson, Robert A. Rastall, and Marcel B. Roberfroid published a landmark chapter titled "*Prebiotics*" in a volume on colonic microbiota, nutrition, and health. In that chapter, they restated their earlier definition from 1995: a prebiotic is "a non-digestible food ingredient that beneficially affects the host by selectively stimulating the growth and/or activity of one or a limited number of bacteria in the colon". In later papers, the same group refined this into the now-familiar wording that prebiotics are 'selectively fermented ingredients' that cause specific, beneficial changes in the gastrointestinal microbiota [7].

Let's unpack that definition, because every word carries weight. *Selectively fermented* means the ingredient isn't a free-for-all buffet; it favors certain microbial groups over others, ideally beneficial ones like bifidobacteria and lactobacilli over potentially harmful ones like sulfate-reducing bacteria or gas-producing clostridia. *Specific* changes in composition means you can measure shifts in which bacteria are present and how abundant they are. What we now call the microbiota profile. *Activity* means metabolic outputs like the short-chain fatty acids (SCFAs), vitamins, and other metabolites the microbes produce. So, in other words, prebiotics are what

69

your beneficial gut bacteria (including many of the species often known as probiotics) consume to produce helpful metabolic outputs (sometimes called postbiotics or metabiotics). "Benefits upon host well-being and health" [7] means the changes aren't just academic; they translate into measurable improvements such as better stool consistency, lower cholesterol, improved glycemic control, reduced inflammation, or simply the comfort and dignity of a gut that works without drama.

This definition, formalized in 1999, retroactively explained why the 1986 Norwich finding mattered. Wyatt's team had shown that Gum arabic met the first criterion of being selectively fermented by beneficial groups. The second criterion was that participants tolerated it well with benefits to host well-being. These are the experimental metrics that Acacia gum would have to be measured against over the next two decades.

Nantes, France, 2003. A clinical research unit at the French National Institute for Agricultural Research has become a hub for prebiotic science. Christine Cherbut and her colleagues design a controlled human trial to test whether Gum arabic can deliver on the promise suggested by the 1986 work, using the tools and standards of the new millennium. They recruit healthy volunteers, dose them with Acacia Gum at escalating levels (ten grams per day, then fifteen grams per day) and a separate dose-escalation from 10 to 70 g/day for tolerance to track two things rigorously: *bifidogenicity* and *tolerance* [2].

Let's define both, because they're the twin pillars of prebiotic validation. *Bifidogenicity* is the capacity to increase the population of *Bifidobacterium* species in the gut. Bifidobacteria are Gram-positive, anaerobic bacteria that dominate the infant gut during breastfeeding and remain important throughout life. They produce acetate and lactate (which other microbes can convert to butyrate), they outcompete pathogens for nutrients and adhesion sites, they modulate immune signaling, and they're associated with favorable metabolic and inflammatory profiles. A prebiotic that consistently raises bifidobacteria across diverse individuals is doing something important. *Tolerance*, meanwhile, is assessed through symptom diaries such as participants log flatulence, bloating, abdominal pain, stool frequency, and stool consistency on standardized scales. High tolerance means people can take meaningful doses without the side effects that make them stop.

The Nantes team reports their punchline in clear language. Acacia gum produces significant, dose-dependent increases in fecal bifidobacteria at doses of ten and fifteen grams per day, with remarkably few gastrointestinal complaints [2]. At commonly used doses (up to about 30 g per day), participants reported very few and mostly mild digestive symptoms, comparable to sucrose. Reports of bloating or cramps were infrequent and, when present, stayed in the mild range, with no signal of serious intolerance. Stool weight and water content increased modestly, suggesting slightly softer but still normal stools, without a clear laxative effect at the doses tested. The bifidogenic effect is measurable, reproducible, and, crucially, gentle. This is Gum arabic's signature comfort profile, what we might today describe as "low-FODMAP-like" despite being highly fermentable, a paradox we'll explain mechanistically later.

Why does public-sector leadership matter here? Because INRA was not a company trying to sell a product; it was a research institute trying to understand how fibers affect public health. When Cherbut's team declares Acacia gum arabic a bifidogenic prebiotic with high digestive tolerance, that declaration carries institutional credibility. It gives beverage formulators, pediatric nutritionists, and medical-food developers permission to explore higher doses and broader applications, knowing the safety and efficacy has been validated by scientists whose incentives align with consumer welfare. The 2003 paper reframed Gum arabic as it was no longer a niche ingredient looking for a health story; it was a validated prebiotic looking for the right applications.

Almere, **Netherlands, 2008.** The Kerry Group (a global ingredients company) funds a dose-response study that asks the most practical question a formulator or clinician can ask: *How much is enough*? Wim Calame and colleagues recruit healthy adults and dose them with Gum arabic at five, ten, twenty and fourty grams per day for four weeks, then measure bifidogenicity, and tolerance using validated questionnaires [3].

Before we report the findings, let's talk about why dose-response curves matter. A prebiotic that only works at thirty grams per day is hard to use as it requires multiple servings, adds bulk and cost to formulations, and may push tolerance limits. A prebiotic that works at five grams per day is programmable and you can titrate it into a single beverage serving, a meal replacement bar, or a probiotic capsule blend without overwhelming the host ingredient. Dose-response data also help clinicians personalize because some patients may thrive at five grams, others may need ten, and a few sensitive individuals may need to start at two and work up. Knowing the curve is knowing how to deploy the tool.

The Almere study delivers exactly that curve. After 4 weeks, Gum arabic at 10 g/day produces a clear prebiotic signal. Bifidobacteria, lactobacilli, and bacteroides all rise significantly compared with water, and at this same 10g dose Gum arabic actually outperforms 10g inulin for these three groups. Higher doses (20 and 40 g/day) do not boost bifidobacteria further; their numbers more or less plateau from 10g upward, which is why the authors conclude that the optimal effective range for prebiotic action lies around 5–10 g/day. For lactobacilli and bacteroides, the best responses are also seen at the lower doses, with some decline at 20 and 40 g. On the tolerance side, all Gum arabic doses, even 40 g/day, are described as very well tolerated. Reported symptoms like bloating, cramps, and diarrhea remain minimal and alleviate over time. In practice, that means 10 g/day sits at a sweet spot with strong, measurable increases in beneficial bacteria and very little digestive downside. This is an unusually friendly dose–response profile for a fermentable fiber [3].

This is the "actionable" moment, the point where Gum arabic moves from promising to programmable. The study uses contemporary molecular readouts (quantitative PCR for specific bacterial groups, HPLC for SCFA profiling) giving formulators and clinicians a modern evidence base. It also clarifies the practical sweet spot. Ten grams per day is where benefit, tolerance, and feasibility converge. That dose becomes the benchmark for the next wave of applications.

Muscat, Oman, 2009. Badreldin H. Ali, working at Sultan Qaboos University with colleagues Amal Ziada and Gerald Blunden, publishes a narrative review in Food and Chemical Toxicology that steps back from the microbiota-centric view and asks: *What are the broader biological effects of Gum arabic, and how might they connect to health beyond the gut?* The review synthesizes animal and early human data, touching on renal function, hepatic markers, serum lipids, glycemic control, and hints of antioxidant and anti-inflammatory activity [4].

We'll use this review sparingly here, deferring the deep dive on inflammation and metabolic endpoints to the next chapters, but it serves a narrative purpose and it legitimizes the higher, fiber-level dosing that the Nantes and Almere studies validated. Once you demonstrate that ten grams per day of a prebiotic is safe and shifts the microbiota favorably, the next question is: *Do those microbial shifts translate into systemic effects?* Ali's review suggests plausible pathways. SCFAs (especially propionate and butyrate) enter the bloodstream and modulate hepatic glucose and lipid metabolism. Bile-acid binding by Gum arabic's uronic acids could shift cholesterol recycling and excretion, lowering serum LDL.

The review doesn't make disease claims (it's careful to frame findings as mechanistic hints and associative data from controlled studies) but it connects dots. It tells clinicians and formulators that Gum arabic isn't just about comfort and regularity; it's about metabolic calm, about a gut ecosystem that supports the whole organism. That's the kind of ingredient story that opens doors to medical nutrition, functional beverages, and clinical trials in populations under metabolic or inflammatory stress.

Khartoum, Sudan, 2013. The story pivots from healthy adults to children who need help. M. W. Ali and colleagues at Sudanese universities recruit constipated children and then identify those with functional constipation. Functional constipation being a common miserable condition with no structural cause, where stool is infrequent and painful. Caregivers are desperate for something that works without tears, without the laxative urgency that makes someone afraid to eat or leave the house. The researchers treat one group with a laxative (lactulose) only and the other group with daily lactulose plus Gum arabic (about 20–40 g) for several months and compares overall clinical improvement and tolerability between the two treatment groups [5].

Pediatric endpoints require translation, because children can't fill out adult questionnaires. Stool frequency is counted by caregivers answering how many bowel movements per week? Consistency is assessed visually using the Bristol Stool Scale adapted for children, aiming for types three and four (formed but soft, easy to pass). Tolerance is gauged by whether the child

74

will continue taking the supplement and whether parents report adverse effects like crying during defecation, visible bloating, or refusal to eat.

The Khartoum team reports clear benefits and high tolerance over the intervention period. The proportion of children whose constipation improved is higher in the Gum arabic plus lactulose group than in the lactulose-only group, especially by three months [5]. No serious adverse effects related to Gum arabic were reported in the study. This is real-world validation in a population where fiber interventions often fail because compliance is poor. Gum arabic works not just because of its bifidogenic and SCFA-generating properties, but because it's invisible and kind. These two attributes matter profoundly when you're asking a four-year-old to drink something every morning.

Ghent, Belgium, 2015. We shift from clinical outcomes to mechanistic clarity, from what happens to why it happens. D. Daguet and colleagues at ProDigest (a Belgian contract research organization specializing in gut models) use validated in-vitro systems to test how fermentation products (generated by gut microbiota) from Acacia gum influence the gut barrier. They culture intestinal epithelial cell lines in co-culture with immune cells and expose them to fermentation supernatants produced when gut microbes break down Acacia gum (and, for comparison, fructo-oligosaccharides). They combine the SHIME® model (a dynamic simulator of the human intestinal microbiota) with a co-culture of human intestinal epithelial cells (Caco-2) and immune-like cells (THP-1) grown on Transwell inserts. Fermentation supernatants from SHIME, generated when gut microbes break down Acacia gum or fructo-oligosaccharides, are then applied to this cell model while the team measures two key readouts: transepithelial electrical resistance (TEER) and inflammatory cytokines [8]. Let's translate TEER in one friendly image. Imagine the lining of your intestine as a cobblestone street, each cell a stone, and the gaps between cells sealed with molecular zippers called tight junctions with proteins like claudin, occludin, and ZO-1 that lock neighboring cells together. When those zippers are closed, the barrier is strong whereby nutrients and water can pass through cells in controlled ways, but bacteria, toxins, and undigested food particles can't slip between cells into the bloodstream. When the zippers weaken (through inflammation, stress, dysbiosis, or poor diet) the barrier becomes "leaky," and unwanted molecules cross, triggering immune activation and low-grade inflammation. TEER measures how electrically resistant the cell layer is. High resistance means tight zippers and strong barrier while low resistance means loose zippers and leaky barrier.

Daguet's team finds that Gum arabic improves TEER and the effect is reproducible, suggesting that Gum arabic or more precisely the SCFAs and other metabolites its fermentation generates helps maintain or restore barrier integrity [8]. The mechanism likely involves butyrate, which is a preferred energy source for colonocytes and a signaling molecule that promotes tight-junction assembly. However, the effect may also involve the physical presence of Gum arabic mucilage coating the epithelium (providing a protective film) or modulation of mucus production by goblet cells. The study doesn't resolve every pathway, but it provides mechanistic support for a key claim. The gentle fermentation of Gum arabic leads not just to more bifidobacteria and more SCFAs, but to a calmer, stronger gut barrier.

Omdurman, **Sudan, 2016.** Another pediatric story, this time with even higher stakes. Duria A. M. A. Omer and Faiza M. A. Hilali, working at Omdurman Islamic University, study malnourished children aged six to fifty-nine months. These are toddlers and preschoolers whose growth has faltered due to inadequate nutrition, infection, or both [6]. In this population, every calorie must count, every intervention must be gentle, and caregiver acceptance is non-negotiable because compliance determines whether a child thrives or deteriorates.

Malnutrition is not just about insufficient calories; it's about a disrupted gut that can't absorb nutrients efficiently, a weakened immune system that can't fight infections, and a microbiota that's often dysbiotic. *Dysbiotic* means that your gut is overgrown with bad harmful bacteria, pathobionts and depleted of beneficial commensals and probiotics. Interventions that add fermentable fiber have theoretical appeal. SCFAs provide energy for colonocytes, support barrier function, and may improve nutrient absorption and immune tone. However, in practice, fibers can backfire if they cause bloating or diarrhea, which parents interpret as "making the child worse". The fiber must be tolerable and acceptable above all else.

Omer gave malnourished children Gum arabic as a daily supplement, in addition to the standard WHO malnutrition protocol, and measured weight-for-height, diarrhea, edema, and activity/mood over 2 weeks. The findings were very encouraging, showing diarrhea largely resolved in the Gum arabic group [6]. Growth outcomes show modest improvements over the intervention period, though longer studies with larger samples are needed to assess sustained catch-up growth. What the study demonstrates most clearly is feasibility. In a resource-limited setting where options are few and adherence is everything; Gum arabic proves to be a practical, well-tolerated adjunct in this setting. The study showed no serious problems reported which is a rare and valuable attribute in medical nutrition.

Reading, England, 2018. We're back in the lab, this time with tools that would have seemed magical to the Norwich team in 1986. Sehad Alarifi,

Alan Bell, and Gemma Walton at the University of Reading use batch in vitro fermentation to ask a deceptively simple question: *Which Bacteria and other microbes eat Acacia gum, and what do they produce*? [9].

Let's define *batch fermentation* briefly, because it's a workhorse method in prebiotic research. You take fecal samples from healthy volunteers (pooled to average out individual variation), dilute them in an anaerobic medium that mimics the colon environment (nutrients, salts, pH buffers, no oxygen), add your test ingredient (in this case, Acacia gum) and incubate for twenty-four to forty-eight hours in sealed vessels that simulate the oxygen-free world of the hindgut. Periodically, you sample the broth and measure bacterial populations (by culture or molecular methods), SCFA concentrations (by gas chromatography), pH, and sometimes gas production. The system is a simplified snapshot (it can't replicate the three-dimensional architecture, mucus layer, immune signaling, or peristaltic flow of a living colon) but it's reproducible, cost-effective, and lets you test hypotheses before investing in human trials.

Alarifi's team finds that Acacia gum drives a robust bifidogenic response in vitro, just as predicted, but also reveals something richer. The major discovery is that Gum Arabic supports a consortium of fermenters, not just one species [9]. The study concluded that Acacia gum is selectively fermented by a range of beneficial gut bacteria, especially Bifidobacterium spp., the Lactobacillus/Enterococcus group, Atopobium, and Bacteroides.

Although this was beyond the scope of this study; we can deduce why this might be the case. This wide array of beneficial microbe fermentation of Acacia gum can be due to *cross feeding* where certain microbe strains latch onto Acacia gum early to cleave off arabinose and galactose sugars from the polysaccharide backbone. Other microbes (butyrate-producing clostridia, for instance) don't use Acacia gum directly but feed on the lactate and acetate released by the early fermenters, a process called cross-feeding. The result would be a cascade where primary degraders break down complex polysaccharides into simpler molecules, secondary fermenters convert those intermediates into end products like butyrate, and the overall community shifts toward a metabolically cooperative, SCFA and Metabiotic rich profile.

Malaysia, 2019. Hammad Ahallil and colleagues take the next logical step as they move from batch fermentation to a more advanced version of the classic batch-fermentation approach. Instead of a simple bottle assay, they run anaerobic, pH-controlled faecal batch cultures designed to mimic the distal colon of obese adults. Human stool from four obese male donors is pooled, diluted into an oxygen-free medium, and incubated at 37 °C in glass vessels, each kept at a constant pH of 6.8. Into this they add either Hashab gum (Acacia senegal from Sudan) at 1 % w/w or inulin as a positive prebiotic control and follow the system over 36 hours. Using fluorescence in situ hybridization (FISH), they track four key bacterial groups: *Bifidobacterium*, Bacteroidaceae/Prevotellaceae, *Lactobacillus/Enterococcus*, and the *Clostridium histolyticum* group, along with microbial metabolites.

These in-vitro colon models are useful because they let you watch, hour by hour, how a microbial community responds to a new fiber, under tightly controlled conditions that mimic part of the gut. If a substrate is fermented very quickly, you may see rapid overgrowth of certain species and sharp changes in acidity that, in a real colon, could translate into discomfort. If it is fermented more gradually, you see a slower, steadier shift in the community, which usually predicts better tolerance in humans. Time-course data like this also tell you whether a prebiotic mainly feeds early colon residents or continues to provide fuel deeper into the distal colon, where cells are often most starved of energy.

In this distal-colon model, Hashab gum shows a clear prebiotic signature. At the start, Bacteroides-type bacteria dominate, while *Bifidobacterium* counts are relatively low. Under Hashab gum fermentation, *Bifidobacterium* numbers begin to rise significantly after around 12 hours and stay high through 36 hours. Bacteroidaceae also increase, but later, with noticeable growth only after 24 hours. *Lactobacillus/Enterococcus* barely move, while the *Clostridium histolyticum* group shows a slight bump at 6 hours followed by a significant drop at 12, 24, and 36 hours. The pattern is exactly what you hope to see from a selective prebiotic. A clear sustained support for beneficial groups like *Bifidobacterium* and Bacteroidetes, alongside a reduction or no-effect in potentially less desirable clostridial species (some strains within the clostridial species are good and produce butyrate while others are harmful and produce toxins). Although this conference paper focuses on microbial counts rather than detailed SCFA profiles, the authors conclude that Hashab gum meaningfully reshapes obese microbiota in vitro and may be a useful nutritional tool for managing obesity when combined with human data showing good tolerance at realistic daily doses [10].

Kagoshima, Japan, 2022. We reach the mechanistic smoking gun. Yuki Sasaki and colleagues at Kagoshima University ask the molecular question that underpins everything: *How, exactly, do bifidobacteria break down Gum arabic's (Hashab gum from Acacia Senegal) complex arabinogalactan-protein structures, and why are they so good at it?* [11]. The team isolates Bifidobacterium longum (one of the most common and beneficial bifidobacteria in the human gut) and uses a combination of gene-cluster analysis, recombinant expression, and carbohydrate enzymology to map the tools the bacterium uses. They showed that the bacterium keeps three tiny "scissors" on its surface (special sugar-cutting enzymes) that snip off small sugars from the side branches so the fiber can be used as food without pulling the whole large molecule into the cell. One enzyme removes Gal-Ara caps, another trims arabinose side chains (including $\alpha 1,3$ and $\alpha 1,4$ links), and a third nibbles down the $\beta 1,3$-galactan backbone, leaving a distinct tetrasaccharide that other gut bacteria can use, which helps cooperation in the gut community [11].

Why does this matter for human health and comfort? Firstly, it's a step towards proving the "crossfeeding mechanism" we touched upon earlier in the chapter. Secondly, the cooperative surface enzyme system helps explain three signature traits of Gum arabic fermentation: *selectivity* (only bacteria with the right enzyme toolkit can efficiently degrade arabinogalactan-proteins, so beneficial species are favored), *slow fermentation* (the multi-step enzymatic cascade takes time, preventing sudden substrate depletion and gas spikes), and *low side effects* (gradual, controlled breakdown means steady, moderate SCFA production without overwhelming the system). The Kagoshima study gives us the biochemical "how" behind the clinical "what"; proving that Gum arabic's gentle prebiotic profile reflects its molecular complexity and the specialized enzymes of its degraders.

Los Angeles and Athens, 2022. The narrative takes a translational turn.

Marlène Maeusli, working with colleagues at the University of Southern California and collaborators in Greece, publishes a striking finding in a mouse model. Their study finds that Acacia fiber (Brand is Renewlife – Hashab from Acacia Senegal) protects the gut from colonization by extended-spectrum beta-lactamase-producing *Escherichia coli* (antibiotic-resistant opportunistic pathogens) in animals whose microbiota has been disrupted by antibiotics [12].

81

Let's unpack this carefully, because it introduces two concepts. *Colonization resistance* is the phenomenon by which a healthy, diverse microbiota prevents pathogenic or opportunistic microbes from establishing a foothold. The mechanisms are multiple: 1-competition for nutrients and attachment sites, production of antimicrobial compounds (like bacteriocins - small peptides that kill or inhibit competitors), 2-maintenance of favorable pH and redox conditions, and 3-stimulation of immune defenses. When antibiotics wipe out large swaths of the commensal community, colonization resistance collapses, and opportunists like Clostridium difficile, vancomycin-resistant enterococci, or ESBL-E. coli can bloom. The translational question is: *Can a prebiotic restore colonization resistance by rebuilding a protective community?*

Maeusli's team finds that in antibiotic-disrupted mice, adding Hashab gum to the diet reduces ESBL-*E. coli* colonization significantly compared to controls. Mechanistic analysis suggests the effect involves *colicin M* (a bacteriocin produced by certain native *E. coli* strains that kills competing *E. coli*) and partly through shifts in the broader community that make the environment less hospitable to ESBL colonizers [12].

The study doesn't claim Hashab gum is a replacement for antibiotics or that it treats infection. However, it provides proof-of-concept that a well-chosen prebiotic can support ecosystem resilience under stress. Hashab gum helps the gut resist opportunistic colonization during and after antibiotic disruption. This is the kind of finding that opens doors to clinical trials in high-risk populations like patients on prolonged antibiotics, travelers at risk of diarrhea, and individuals undergoing chemotherapy where maintaining colonization resistance could prevent serious secondary infections.

Malaysia, 2023. Muhamad H. Rawi returns with a follow-up study using anaerobic enrichment culture, a technique that's essentially microbial fishing. The team takes pooled human fecal samples, inoculates them into anaerobic media containing Acacia gum (Hashab gum from Acacia Senegal) as the main added carbohydrate source, and serially transfers the cultures to enrich for bacteria that can use Hashab gum efficiently. After several rounds of enrichment, they isolate and identify the survivors [13].

The Malaysian team showed that fermentation shifted from acetate toward butyrate across serial transfers. They isolated five butyrate-producing strains identified as Escherichia fergusonii, confirming that specific gut bacteria can directly ferment Hashab gum to butyrate in vitro [13]. The study confirmed that Acetate was the most prevalent metabiotic during stage 1 and 2 while butyrate was the most abundant in stage 3. Propionate was also available only in stage 1 and 2 and in lesser quantities than Acetate.

Knowing the roster helps researchers design targeted probiotic pairings (*synbiotics*) and predict individual variation. This helps explain why different people may respond differently to Hashab gum, depending on which microbial populations they harbor within them versus which ones will take longer to build those populations from scratch.

Global, 2023. The Global Prebiotic Association (an industry organization that brings together brands, ingredient suppliers, researchers, and other stakeholders in the prebiotic sector) publishes a "Prebiotic Type Spotlight" on Acacia fiber, summarizing the state of the science and how practitioners are using it [14]. This is not a peer-reviewed study but a practice snapshot, reflecting how the previous two decades of research have translated into real-world applications. The spotlight notes that Acacia fiber shows prebiotic efficacy at 10 g/day, and that most published studies use daily doses between 5 and 30 grams for up to three months with no safety or tolerability concerns. It's favored in products targeting digestive comfort, regularity, metabolic wellness, and sports hydration because it dissolves clear, tastes neutral, and rarely causes bloating. The document emphasizes tolerance as a key strength, highlighting that Acacia fiber is effective at typical prebiotic doses and that clinical studies report good safety and digestive tolerance over a 5–30 gram per day range.

Why does a practice snapshot matter in a scientific narrative? Because it shows adoption and points to the moment when research escapes the lab and becomes a tool that people actually use. The GPA spotlight, together with the broader clinical and product literature, suggests that formulators trust Acacia fiber enough to build products around it, and that it is being used in real-world practice.

This is your philosophical landing. Acacia gum didn't just tick yesterday's boxes; it reshaped the boxes. It showed the field that a prebiotic could be gentle and powerful, invisible and effective, simple and cooperative. It proved that you don't need to punish the gut to help it, and that the best interventions feel like nothing while quietly rebuilding the neighborhood.

Let's pull the thread and ask: Why does Hashab gum overperform other fibers as a prebiotic? The answer, distilled from hundreds of studies across 4 decades, is a convergence of traits with chemistry, biology, and ecology working in concert.

- First, *slow, cooperative fermentation.* The arabinogalactan-protein architecture requires a multi-enzyme toolkit to dismantle, and only certain bacteria possess the full set needed break it down That selectivity drives bifidogenicity. This complexity also means

THE RESEARCH AVALANCHE BEGINS

fermentation happens gradually, over hours, through cross-feeding.
- Second, *high bifidogenicity* with dose-response at practical intakes. Five to ten grams per day reliably doubles fecal bifidobacteria in most people, with effects plateauing around ten to fifteen grams.
- Third, *barrier support*. Hashab gum fermentation products improve transepithelial electrical resistance and upregulate tight-junction proteins, A stronger, better-fed barrier means less translocation of bacterial fragments (endotoxins) into the bloodstream, less systemic inflammation, and a calmer immune tone.
- Fourth, *pediatric feasibility*. People refuse bad-tasting supplements, they complain loudly about belly aches, and their caregivers stop interventions at the first sign of trouble. Hashab gum passes the pediatric test because it's invisible, tasteless, and gentle.
- Fifth, *resilience under stress*. Hashab gum can support colonization resistance against antibiotic-resistant pathogens. This isn't a cure, but it's a shield. It's a way to help the ecosystem defend itself when external stressors (antibiotics, travel, illness) punch holes in its defenses.
- Finally, *generalizable evidence*. Study trials from Europe, Asia, Africa, and the Middle East, across ages from children to elders, in healthy volunteers and clinical populations, using doses from five to forty grams per day. The consistency of findings across that diversity of contexts tells you something profound: Hashab gum works broadly and it's a reliable tool for most people, most of the time.

So, here's the line you underline: Hashab *gum is the prebiotic that behaves like a good houseguest; it arrives quietly, tidies as it goes, and leaves the place stronger than before.*

We close with a promise and an invitation. You've just watched Hashab gum transform from "harmless additive" to "fiber" to "potent prebiotic" through a cascade of evidence that built trust, mechanism, and practice one study at a time.

The following chapter will take you deeper into the inflammation cascade explaining how Hashab gum helps people with irritable bowel syndrome find relief as it calms an overactive immune response, and how the gut-brain axis carries those signals upstream to affect cognition, mood, and metabolic regulation.

References

1. Wyatt, G. M., C. E. Bayliss, and J. D. Holcroft. "A Change in Human Faecal Flora in Response to Inclusion of Gum Arabic in the Diet." British Journal of Nutrition, vol. 55, no. 2, 1986, pp. 261–66

2. Cherbut, Christine, et al. "Acacia Gum Is a Bifidogenic Dietary Fibre with High Digestive Tolerance in Healthy Humans." Microbial Ecology in Health and Disease, vol. 15, no. 1, 2003, pp. 43-50.

3. Calame, Wim, et al. "Gum Arabic Establishes Prebiotic Functionality in Healthy Human Volunteers in a Dose-Dependent Manner." British Journal of Nutrition, vol. 100, no. 6, 2008, pp. 1269-75.

4. Ali, Badreldin H., Amal Ziada, and Gerald Blunden. "Biological Effects of Gum Arabic: A Review of Some Recent Research." Food and Chemical Toxicology, vol. 47, no. 1, 2009, pp. 1–8

5. Ali, M. W., et al. "Gum Arabic in Treatment of Functional Constipation in Children in Sudan." Sudan Journal of Medical Sciences, vol. 8, no. 2, 2013, pp. 73–76

6. Omer, Duria Abdelraheim M. A., and Faiza M. Ahmed Hilali. "Effect of Gum Arabic in Management of Malnourished Children Aged 6–59 Months." Journal of Biology, Agriculture and Healthcare, vol. 6, no. 24, 2016, pp. 7–14

7. Gibson, Glenn R., Robert A. Rastall, and Marcel B. Roberfroid. "Prebiotics." Colonic Microbiota, Nutrition and Health, edited by Glenn R. Gibson and Marcel B. Roberfroid, Kluwer Academic Publishers, 1999, pp. 101–124

8. Daguet, David, et al. "Acacia Gum Improves the Gut Barrier Functionality In Vitro." Agro Food Industry Hi-Tech, vol. 26, no. 4, 2015, pp. 29–33; Daguet, David, et al. "Arabinogalactan and Fructooligosaccharides Improve the Gut Barrier Function in Distinct Areas of the Colon in the Simulator of the Human Intestinal Microbial Ecosystem." Journal of Functional Foods, vol. 20, 2016, pp. 369–79

9. Alarifi, Sehad, Alan Bell, and Gemma Walton. "In Vitro Fermentation of Gum Acacia—Impact on the Faecal Microbiota." International Journal of Food Sciences and Nutrition, vol. 69, no. 6, 2018, pp. 696–704

10. Ahallil, Hammad, et al. "Fermentation of Gum Arabic by Gut Microbiota Using In Vitro Colon Model." AIP Conference Proceedings, vol. 2111, 2019, 050004

11. Sasaki, Yuki, et al. "Mechanism of Cooperative Degradation of Gum Arabic Arabinogalactan-Protein by Bifidobacterium longum Surface Enzymes." Applied and Environmental Microbiology, vol. 88, no. 6, 2022, e02187-21

12. Maeusli, Marlène, et al. "Acacia Fiber Protects the Gut from Extended-Spectrum Beta-Lactamase (ESBL)-Producing Escherichia coli Colonization Enabled by Antibiotics." mSphere, vol. 7, no. 3, 2022, e00071-22

13. Rawi, Muhamad Hanif, Hui Yan Tan, and Shahrul Razid Sarbini. "Identification of Acacia Gum Fermenting Bacteria from Pooled Human Feces Using Anaerobic Enrichment Culture." Frontiers in Microbiology, vol. 14, 2023, article 1245042.

14. Global Prebiotic Association. "Prebiotic Type Spotlight: Acacia Fiber." Global Prebiotic Association, June 2023, prebioticassociation.org/prebiotic-type-spotlight-acacia-fiber/

CHAPTER 8

INFLAMMATION SPILLOVER

Why Hashab Gum became the best natural long-term solution to Inflammation

---

We already learned from the previous chapter that Hashab gum is a slow, selectively fermented prebiotic that produces amazing short-chain fatty acids and strengthens the gut barrier without causing the bloating and cramping that define other fibers. We know it feeds probiotics preferentially, supports cross-feeding networks, and does all of this with a comfort profile that works in children, elderly, healthy volunteers and sensitive patients. Now we're asking the next, harder question. If the gut is the switchboard of inflammation and the place where barrier breaches, microbial signals, and immune activation first intersect; *what happens when you quietly stabilize that wiring, day after day, week after week*? What shows up downstream, in tissues and blood tests far from the colon?

This chapter answers that question through multiple waypoints. These will include drug-induced intestinal ulcers in rats, autoimmune inflammation in human joints, obesity-linked cytokines and double-blind trials in irritable bowel syndrome with constipation. Each study is a lens into the same phenomenon of prebiotic spillover. The process by which a gentle, local microbial intervention in the gut cascades into systemic anti-inflammatory effects that reshape how the body handles stress, injury, and chronic immune activation.

Along the way, we'll explain new concepts at exactly the moments they unlock understanding. You'll learn what NSAID enteropathy is and why it's a common modern trigger of "leaky gut." You'll see why brush-border enzymes and histology slides are hard evidence of tissue healing, and not just symptom relief. You'll understand formulation leverage explaining how Hashab can tame the fast, chaotic fermentation of other fibers to produce smoother, more anti-inflammatory metabolite profile. You'll grasp disease-activity scores and cytokine tone; the languages clinicians and immunologists use to track whether inflammation is winning or losing.

Importantly, you'll see how all of this stacks into a translational ladder that builds confidence for long-term use. The following in vitro models predict animal outcomes, animal outcomes predict human trials, and human trials (especially double-blind, placebo-controlled ones in sensitive populations) give us permission to believe the effect is real and durable. By the end, you'll understand why Hashab gum became not just a natural inflammation modulator, but one of the best ones. That's because it's gentle enough for daily use, broad enough to reach tissues beyond the gut, and backed by a stack of evidence that runs from microscopic slides to randomized controlled trials.

Let's start where inflammation often begins in modern life and that's with the unintended consequences of the medicines we take to alleviate pain. Assiut, Egypt, 2011. Ahmed M. A. Abd El-Mawla, working with colleague Husam E. H. Osman, slides a thin section of rat small intestine under the microscope and adjusts the focus. The tissue has been stained with hematoxylin and eosin (standard histological dyes that make cell nuclei purple and cytoplasm pink) and what he sees is not pretty. The *villi*, the finger-like projections that line the small intestine and maximize nutrient absorption, are blunted and ragged. The *lamina propria* (the connective tissue beneath the epithelium) is swollen with inflammatory cells. There

90

are patches where the epithelial layer has eroded completely, exposing raw submucosa. This is the intestine of a rat that's been dosed with meloxicam, a common nonsteroidal anti-inflammatory drug, or NSAID, used worldwide to treat arthritis, muscle pain, and fever.

Let's pause to explain NSAID enteropathy, because it's a silent epidemic hiding in plain sight. NSAIDs (aspirin, ibuprofen, naproxen, meloxicam, diclofenac) are among the most widely used medications on earth. They work by inhibiting cyclooxygenase enzymes that produce prostaglandins. These are inflammatory signaling molecules that cause pain and fever. The problem is that prostaglandins also protect the gastrointestinal lining by stimulating mucus production, maintaining blood flow to the mucosa, and supporting epithelial barrier integrity. When you block prostaglandins systemically, you inadvertently weaken the gut's defenses. The stomach gets most of the damage while the small intestine and colon suffer quietly.

The epithelial barrier becomes more permeable, and tight junctions loosen. This leads to bacteria and bacterial fragments (endotoxins) that should stay safely in the lumen, instead, begin to slip between cells into the bloodstream. This "leaky gut" triggers low-grade systemic inflammation, worsens the very pain the NSAID was meant to treat, and can accelerate chronic diseases like cardiovascular disease and metabolic syndrome. Millions of people take NSAIDs daily for chronic conditions, meaning millions of people are living with subclinical intestinal injury.

Abd El-Mawla and Osman designed their experiment to test whether Acacia gum could protect the intestinal lining from meloxicam-induced damage. They divided rats into four groups: meloxicam alone, gum acacia alone, meloxicam plus gum acacia, and an untreated control group. After several weeks, they harvested the intestines and pancreas, measured tissue enzymes, and prepared histological sections. The results were striking. Rats given meloxicam alone showed all the hallmarks of enteropathy including ulceration and inflammatory infiltrate [1].

Let's explain *brush-border enzymes* briefly, because they're a window into mucosal health. The brush border is the fringe of microvilli on the surface of intestinal epithelial cells, and it's studded with enzyme disaccharidases like lactase, sucrase, peptidases, and phosphatases that complete the final steps of nutrient digestion. When the mucosa is damaged, brush-border enzyme activity drops, a signal that the tissue is struggling. When the mucosa heals, enzyme activity normalizes.

Acacia's protective story in this model is tissue-level, not just symptomatic. When rats received meloxicam, the small intestine showed villus atrophy, epithelial desquamation, inflammatory cell infiltration, and ultrastructural damage, whereas meloxicam plus Acacia gum displayed "great improvement," with many enterocytes retaining intact long microvilli and overall better-preserved architecture. Acacia alone and meloxicam plus Acacia significantly increased these pancreatic enzymes above control levels, indicating recovery of exocrine function relative to NSAID damage. The authors conclude that Acacia gum provides protection and defense against meloxicam's harmful effects, consistent with an anti-injury effect [1]. The anti-inflammatory mechanisms are inferred from reduced mucosal injury.

A similar story emerged later the same year from Menoufia University, where Walaa A. Nasif, Mohamed Lotfy, and Mahmoud R. Mahmoud ran a parallel study with aspirin, the oldest and most ubiquitous NSAID [2]. Aspirin's gastrointestinal toxicity is legendary and it's why low-dose aspirin for cardiovascular protection often comes with *proton-pump inhibitors* (reduces stomach acid) to protect the stomach. However, the small intestine bears a hidden burden.

In a 21-day rat model, co-administering Acacia gum (1 g/day) with aspirin attenuated aspirin-induced intestinal injury and pancreatic suppression. The result is pancreatic amylase and lipase rebounded, intestinal enzymes shifted, and histology showed protection compared with aspirin alone, indicating Acacia gum mitigates NSAID-related gastrointestinal and pancreatic alterations [2]. The fact that two independent Egyptian research groups, using two different NSAIDs with slightly different protocols, arrived at the same conclusion strengthens the idea that Acacia gum helps via broad protective effects against NSAID-induced intestinal injury.

The specific mechanisms aren't fully resolved, but the prebiotic logic we've already learned points to several plausible drivers. Acetate and propionate (the SCFAs that acacia's slow fermentation generates) are directly anti-inflammatory. They bind to receptors on immune cells and epithelial cells, dialing down pro-inflammatory signaling. Butyrate, produced directly or by cross-feeding bacteria downstream of bifidobacteria, is the preferred energy source for colonocytes and promotes tight-junction assembly, literally zipping the barrier tighter. Acacia's mucilage coating may provide a physical buffer on the mucosal surface, reducing direct contact between luminal irritants and the epithelium. Importantly, as you feed the good bacteria in your microbiome they increase significantly while the bad harmful bacteria get crowded out overtime. This reduces the pool of bacteria producing harmful metabolites like hydrogen sulfide and secondary bile acids that can damage the mucosa. Together, these effects create a gentler luminal environment and a stronger, better-fed barrier which is exactly what you need to weather the prostaglandin-blocking storm of an NSAID.

The NSAID studies give us the first arc change which is barrier and tolerance groundwork. They show that Acacia gum doesn't just change lab values; it reduces NSAID-induced tissue damage in the intestine and pancreas, which is consistent with better barrier protection. Importantly, they do it as a model of everyday, real-world stress. The kind of stress

93

millions of people experience when they reach for a pain reliever. If a prebiotic can protect the gut from drug-induced injury, it has earned the right to be called a barrier guardian. Now let's see what happens when you pair that guardian with other fibers.

Ghent, **Belgium, 2015**. A laboratory at Ghent University houses a remarkable piece of equipment: the SHIME®, or Simulator of the Human Intestinal Microbial Ecosystem. Massimo Marzorati and his colleagues are running an experiment that tests a hypothesis with profound practical implications: *Can you blend fibers to get the best of both worlds; the rapid bifidogenic punch of fructo-oligosaccharides and inulin combined with the smooth, sustained fermentation of Acacia gum?* [3]

Let's introduce the concept of *formulation leverage*, because it's central to understanding why this study matters. Some fibers (especially short-chain fructo-oligosaccharides (FOS) and inulin) are metabolic sprinters. Gut bacteria ferment them quickly, releasing large bursts of SCFAs and gases within the first few hours after ingestion. That speed has benefits like getting a strong bifidogenic signal fast, but it also has costs like pH drops and gas spikes that lead to bloating, cramping, and discomfort. This is especially problematic in people with sensitive guts or dysbiosis.

Other fibers, like Hashab gum, are metabolic marathoners. They ferment slowly and steadily over twelve to forty-eight hours, producing a smoother SCFA curve with less gas. The trade-off is that you need higher doses to see quick robust effects. Formulation leverage is the idea that you can pair a sprinter and a marathoner in the same product, letting the marathoner discipline the sprinter by blunting the chaotic peaks while preserving the overall metabolic output. It's microbial traffic control, and if it works, it opens the door to products that deliver bifidogenic and anti-inflammatory benefits without the side effects that make people stop taking them.

The SHIME® team compared a rapid-fermenting FOS/inulin blend with the same blend partially substituted with Acacia gum. In the SHIME®, adding Acacia slowed and spread fermentation from an early, boosted peak into a more gradual, distal-colon profile, while maintaining total SCFA production (including propionate and butyrate) and showing bifidogenic effects. Summaries of the work also note less early gas with the Acacia-enriched blend. These kinetics suggest that combining fast and slow fermenters can deliver SCFAs throughout the colon and may reduce reliance on proteolysis later in the run [3].

Let's talk briefly about propionogenic versus butyrogenic balance, because the choice of which SCFAs dominate has downstream consequences. Propionate is produced mainly by bacteria in the *Bacteroides* and *Veillonella* groups, often through cross-feeding on lactate released by bifidobacteria. Propionate enters the bloodstream and travels to the liver, where it modulates glucose and lipid metabolism by dampening gluconeogenesis (the liver's production of new glucose) and cholesterol synthesis. It also signals immune cells and fat cells through receptors, tilting them toward anti-inflammatory, insulin-sensitive states. Butyrate, by contrast, is produced by certain *clostridia* and stays mostly local, feeding colonocytes and supporting barrier function. Both are good, but propionate's systemic reach makes it especially valuable for metabolic and inflammatory conditions that extend beyond the gut. The SHIME® data showed that adding Acacia gum to a FOS/inulin blend favored more gradual kinetics with maintained propionate and butyrate, a profile associated with anti-inflammatory benefits and lower local irritation.

Underline this sentence: Acacia doesn't just act; it conducts, turning a noisy chorus of fibers into a steadier, soothing harmony. For formulators

95

designing products for IBS, IBD, or metabolic syndrome; populations where tolerance is fragile and dropout rates are high, this kind of kinetic smoothing is the difference between a supplement that sits in the cupboard and one that people actually use.

We've covered tissue protection and fermentation kinetics. Now we're ready to ask whether these gut-level effects spill over into systemic inflammation, into tissues and conditions that seem far removed from the colon. Khartoum, Sudan, 2018. A rheumatology clinic at the Military Hospital in Khartoum, with investigators Ebtihal Kamal and Lamis Abdelgadir Kaddam from the University of Khartoum and Alneelain University. Patients shuffle in, many of them middle-aged women with swollen, painful joints which are the hallmarks of *rheumatoid arthritis*, or RA. RA is an autoimmune disease in which the immune system attacks the synovial lining of joints, causing chronic inflammation, pain, stiffness, and eventually joint destruction. The standard treatment is disease-modifying antirheumatic drugs (methotrexate, hydroxychloroquine, biologics like TNF-alpha inhibitors) but these drugs are expensive, have significant side effects, and don't work for everyone. The question Ebtihal Kamal and her colleagues set out to answer was: *Can a food-grade prebiotic fiber, taken daily, reduce the inflammatory burden in an autoimmune condition* [4]? Before we report the findings, let's teach the clinical language.

Rheumatologists use disease-activity scores to track how patients are doing week to week. The most common is the DAS28, which combines tender-joint count, swollen-joint count, patient-reported pain, and an inflammatory marker (usually C-reactive protein (CRP) or erythrocyte sedimentation rate (ESR)) into a single number. Lower is better. CRP is an acute-phase protein made by the liver in response to inflammatory signals like interleukin-6; it rises within hours of an inflammatory insult and falls when inflammation is resolved. ESR measures how fast red blood cells settle in a test tube; inflammation makes blood proteins sticky, causing cells to clump and settle faster. Both are crude but useful. If CRP and ESR are high, something inflammatory is happening. If they drop, the inflammation is calming.

In a 12-week, single-arm phase II trial in Khartoum, 49 adults with rheumatoid arthritis were enrolled; 40 completed Gum arabic (Hashab gum from Acacia Senegal) supplementation at 30 g/day (three of them for 10 weeks). Compared with baseline, patients showed significant reductions in TNF-α, ESR, tender/swollen joints, and DAS-28, consistent with an anti-inflammatory signal in the context of stable background therapy [4].

Feed the microbes, and the immune system often follows. One plausible spillover pathway runs through SCFAs and the gut barrier. Hashab gum fermentation yields acetate, propionate and butyrate, SCFAs that can support epithelial function and signal through GPR43/GPR41 on immune cells to favor regulatory responses (e.g., increased IL-10) over pro-inflammatory signaling. In vitro SHIME® work suggests Hashab gum can improve epithelial barrier metrics, which would be expected to limit translocation of bacterial products such as LPS, a driver of low-grade systemic inflammation. This Phase II trial in Khartoum RA patients reported lower inflammatory markers and improved disease scores with GA as adjunct therapy, consistent with systemic immunomodulation.

Let's pause here and introduce a meta-concept, because it helps explain why this particular sequence of studies is persuasive. Scientists talk about the *translational ladder* which is the sequence of evidence types that build confidence for moving an intervention from lab bench to bedside. At the bottom of the ladder are in-vitro studies: cells in dishes, and bioreactor models like the SHIME®. These are controlled, reproducible, and cheap, but they lack the complexity of a living organism. One rung up are animal models like rats, mice, and pigs. These add biological complexity (immune systems, gut-brain-liver axes, metabolism) but they're not human; findings don't always translate. The next rung is small human trials such as pilot studies with dose-finding Phase-II trials like the Khartoum RA study. These give you signals in real patients but often lack the statistical power or rigor to convince skeptics. At the top of the ladder are large, randomized, double-blind, placebo-controlled trials in well-characterized populations. This is the gold standard for proving causality and magnitude of effect. Each rung reinforces the one below and makes the one above feel inevitable. By the time we reach the top, the evidence is no longer suggestive; it's compelling.

Bonn, Germany, 2021. The University of Bonn's Institute of Pharmaceutical Technology. Henusha D. Jhundoo and colleagues are working on a problem that sits at the intersection of pharmacology and nutrition: *Can you pair a drug with a fiber to create something better than either alone?* [5] The drug is 5-aminosalicylic acid (5-ASA, also called mesalamine) the cornerstone treatment for mild-to-moderate inflammatory bowel disease (IBD), conditions like ulcerative colitis and Crohn's disease where the gut lining is chronically inflamed. 5-ASA works locally, in the bowel, by inhibiting inflammatory signaling pathways and scavenging free radicals. However, it has limitations as it requires high doses because much of it is absorbed in the upper gut before reaching the colon. Additionally, it doesn't address the underlying dysbiosis (the microbial imbalance) that perpetuates IBD.

Jhundoo's team formulated 5-ASA with Acacia gum (and, separately, guar gum) and tested the combinations in an experimental colitis model where mice with chemically induced intestinal inflammation mimic aspects of human IBD. The Bonn study found that colitis-afflicted rats treated with the 5-ASA-plus-Acacia formulation showed less macroscopic and microscopic tissue damage than those treated with 5-ASA alone [5]. This enhanced effect is attributed to Acacia gum acting as a colonic drug delivery agent, ensuring more 5-ASA reaches the target area, and its intrinsic anti-inflammatory properties, including suppressing pro-inflammatory cytokines and supporting gut barrier function as a prebiotic.

One more thread to tie before we close. The inflammation story we've told in this chapter rests on a foundation of barrier integrity, SCFA signaling, and cytokine modulation which are all gut-centric mechanisms. Amazingly, those mechanisms connect directly to the next frontier of cardiovascular and cardiometabolic health. SCFAs, especially propionate and acetate, don't stop at the gut wall. They enter the portal vein, travel to the liver, and modulate lipid and glucose metabolism at the source. They result in dampening cholesterol synthesis, improving insulin sensitivity, and reducing hepatic fat accumulation.

The next chapter will unpack those connections in detail, walking you through clinical trials that measure lipid panels, blood pressure, and vascular markers in people taking Hashab gum. You'll see how bile-acid binding (a property of Hashab's uronic acids) shifts cholesterol trafficking and excretion, lowering LDL without the side effects of statins. You'll see how steady propionate production improves postprandial glycemia and fasting insulin, reducing the spikes and crashes that damage blood vessels over time. Importantly, you'll see how the anti-inflammatory spillover we've traced in this chapter (from gut to joints) extends to the arterial wall, where it slows plaque formation and stabilizes vulnerable lesions. That's where we're headed next; the place where prebiotic spillover becomes cardiovascular protection, and where Acacia gum's story intersects with the biggest killers in modern medicine. Sometimes, the best intervention is the one that starts in the colon, with a clear powder added to the morning tea.

References:

1. Abd El-Mawla, Ahmed M. A., and Husam Eldien H. Osman. "Effects of Gum Acacia Aqueous Extract on the Histology of the Intestine and Enzymes of Both the Intestine and the Pancreas of Albino Rats Treated with Meloxicam." Pharmacognosy Research, vol. 3, no. 2, 2011, pp. 114–121. doi:10.4103/0974-8490.81959.

2. Nasif, Walaa A., Mohamed Lotfy, and Mahmoud R. Mahmoud. "Protective Effect of Gum Acacia Against the Aspirin-Induced Intestinal and Pancreatic Alterations in Male Albino Rats." European Review for Medical and Pharmacological Sciences, vol. 15, no. 3, 2011, pp. 285–292.

3. Marzorati, Massimo, et al. "Addition of Acacia Gum to a FOS/Inulin Blend Improves Its Fermentation Profile in the Simulator of the Human Intestinal Microbial Ecosystem (SHIME®)." Journal of Functional Foods, vol. 16, 2015, pp. 211-22.

4. Kamal, Ebtihal, et al. "Gum Arabic Fibers Decreased Inflammatory Markers and Disease Severity Score among Rheumatoid Arthritis Patients, Phase II Trial." International Journal of Rheumatology, vol. 2018, Article ID 4197537, 2018, 6 pp.

5. Jhundoo, Henusha D., et al. "Anti-inflammatory Effects of Acacia and Guar Gum in 5-amino Salicylic Acid Formulations in Experimental Colitis." International Journal of Pharmaceutics: X, vol. 3, 2021, article 100080.

CHAPTER 9

THE CARDIOVASCULAR CONNECTION

How Hashab Gum became the natural long-term
Cardiovascular ally

We left the previous chapter with the promise that Hashab gum's prebiotic spillover (the way it steadies the microbiome, tightens the gut barrier, and quiets inflammatory cytokines) doesn't stop at the intestinal wall. Those effects radiate outward, and one of the places they land most powerfully is the cardiovascular system. The same short-chain fatty acids that feed colonocytes and dial down TNF-alpha also travel through the portal vein to the liver, where they modulate the machinery that makes cholesterol. The same bile acids that Hashab's uronic groups bind in the gut lumen are the bile acids the liver must replace by pulling cholesterol from the bloodstream. The same calmer inflammatory tone (lower C-reactive protein, fewer endotoxin leaks) means less irritation of the arterial lining which prevents the kind of chronic vascular inflammation that seeds plaques and drives blood pressure upward. If you calm the gut's signals every day, what happens to the vessel walls mood (cholesterol, triglycerides, blood pressure)? This chapter answers that question through nearly four decades of research, from a surprising 1985 discovery in Delhi to a 2023 study that watched the liver's cholesterol-making machinery wind down.

Before we begin the journey, let's teach two concepts that will recur throughout, because they're the twin engines of Hashab gum's cardiovascular effect. First, *hepatic cholesterol synthesis*. Your liver is a cholesterol factory, and the rate-limiting enzyme (the faucet handle that controls how much cholesterol flows out of the production line) is called HMG-CoA reductase. *Statins* work by jamming that handle in the "off" position, forcing the liver to pull cholesterol from your bloodstream to meet the body's needs, which lowers LDL. However, there are other ways to turn the handle down, and one of them is metabolic signaling from the gut. Short-chain fatty acids like propionate, produced when beneficial microbes ferment soluble fiber, can cross into the liver and dial down HMG-CoA reductase activity. Meaning less synthesis, lower blood cholesterol, quieter cardiovascular risk and no prescription required.

Second, *bile-acid sequestration and the hepatic "pull"*. Bile acids are cholesterol-derived detergents made by the liver and stored in the gallbladder; they're released into the small intestine after meals to help digest fats. Normally, about ninety-five percent of bile acids are reabsorbed in the terminal ileum and recycled back to the liver, a thrifty loop called *enterohepatic circulation*. However, if a fiber in the gut lumen binds bile acids and escorts them out in the stool, the liver's bile-acid pool shrinks. The liver responds by pulling cholesterol from the bloodstream to synthesize new bile acids, and that pull nudges LDL-cholesterol downward. It's the same principle behind bile-acid sequestrant drugs like cholestyramine, but gentler, slower, and without the gastrointestinal side effects that make those drugs hard to tolerate long-term.

Hashab gum through its branched arabinogalactan structure decorated with uronic acids and its slow, cooperative fermentation by bifidobacteria and propionate-producing partners, does both. It binds bile acids in addition to generating propionate. Amazingly, it does both continuously, day after day, as long as you keep stirring that spoonful into your morning tea. That dual action, combined with tolerability so high that people actually stick with it, is why Hashab gum became not just a natural cardiovascular intervention, but the best one in my opinion. It's the fiber that moves the needle on cholesterol, blood pressure, and vascular inflammation without asking patients to endure discomfort or complexity. Let's see how the evidence for that claim stacked up, study by study, decade by decade.

India, 1985. Rakesh D. Sharma is running a small trial that will (in hindsight) open a door most cardiologists didn't know existed. They recruit men with elevated cholesterol and give them fifteen grams of Acacia gum twice per day, dissolved in water, for 30 days. No diet changes, no drugs, just the gum. At the end of four weeks, they draw blood and run lipid panels. The results are surprising: total serum cholesterol has dropped significantly [1]. In 1985, before statins dominated the market and when dietary interventions were still seen as marginal, this was a quiet bombshell. A "food additive," the industrial stabilizer that kept soft drinks cloudy and candies from sticking, was lowering cholesterol in real people.

Sharma didn't have the tools to prove any mechanisms. The Delhi finding was preliminary (small sample, short duration, no placebo control) but it landed in a moment when the cardiology world was hungry for alternatives to drugs and desperate low-fat diets that patients hated. If a well-tolerated, tasteless fiber could move cholesterol down in such a short period, what would happen over months? Over years? And was Acacia gum unique, or did it belong to a broader class of cholesterol-lowering fibers? Those questions were later explored in Stanford.

Before we continue further, let's clarify what the lipid numbers mean, because precision here matters. *Total cholesterol* is the sum of all cholesterol in your blood including HDL (the "good" cholesterol that ferries excess cholesterol back to the liver), LDL (the "bad" cholesterol that deposits in artery walls), and VLDL (very-low-density lipoprotein, which carries triglycerides). *LDL-cholesterol* is the workhorse for cardiovascular risk; it's the particle that oxidizes, gets trapped in vessel walls, and seeds plaques. *Non-HDL cholesterol* is total cholesterol minus HDL, capturing all the atherogenic (plaque-forming) particles in one number. When we say a fiber "lowers cholesterol," what matters most is whether it lowers LDL and non-HDL.

The 1990s were also the era when researchers began asking: *Can you blend fibers to get additive benefits*? If Gum arabic works and apple pulp works, does a mix work better? David Gee and Mee, working in the United States, tested exactly this in a 1997 trial with men who had mild hypercholesterolemia (cholesterol elevated enough to worry about but not high enough to justify drugs). They gave participants a daily supplement combining apple pulp and Gum arabic, at doses low enough to fit into a cereal serving or a beverage and tracked lipids over several weeks.

The Mee and Gee trial showed that the Apple-Acacia blend produced additional reductions in total and LDL cholesterol compared to baseline, with excellent tolerability [2]. The doses were practical (amounts you could deliver in a breakfast bar or a sports drink) and the lipid benefits were meaningful. Abstracts of this study claimed the effect is believed to have resulted from the supplemental dietary fiber only. This was translatable science and not a feeding study where every meal is controlled, but a real-world supplement added to regular diets.

Khartoum, Sudan, 2015. In the Omdurman hospital of Sudan, where resources are constrained. R. E. Mohamed, M. O. E. Gadour, and colleagues enroll newly diagnosed hyperlipidemic patients. The patients are randomized to 4 weeks of atorvastatin 20 mg/day with or without nightly Gum arabic reported as 30 grams, with 110 completing the study and comparable baseline characteristics between arms. Lipid panels were measured at baseline after 4 weeks, and the combination group experienced markedly greater reductions in total cholesterol (−25.9% vs −7.8%), triglycerides (−38.2% vs −2.9%), and LDL-cholesterol (−30.8% vs −8.1%) compared with statin alone (all P < 0.001), while HDL(good cholesterol) did not change significantly in either group. The design included weekly compliance checks, bedtime dosing, and instructions for controls to avoid Gum arabic, with diet and exercise kept under control in both groups [3].

The authors conclude that Gum arabic exerts a lipid-lowering effect (except for HDL) in patients with hyperlipidemia, aligning with prior reports that soluble fibers can reduce atherogenic lipids. Although the study evaluates Gum arabic as an adjunct rather than a stand-alone therapy and spans only 4 weeks; the magnitude and consistency of the changes across total cholesterol, triglycerides, and LDL provide clinically meaningful proof-of-concept from this source alone [3].

This study introduces the concept of *special-population stress tests*, and it's worth pausing to explain why results in dyslipidemic patients carry extra weight. When you test a cholesterol-lowering intervention in healthy people with borderline-high cholesterol, you're working in a relatively forgiving metabolic environment. The liver is functioning well, inflammation is low, the gut barrier is intact. However, when you test people with established dyslipidemia (often accompanied by insulin resistance, low-grade systemic inflammation, and oxidative stress) you're working in a harsher landscape. If an intervention still works under those conditions, where the biology is already strained and the inflammatory load is high, it's a strong signal that the effect is robust and generalizable. The Sudan trials (this one and the two that follows) are stress tests. They show that Acacia works not just in metabolic health but in metabolic

106

dysfunction, where it's needed most.

The 2015 Khartoum study also drives home the *adherence-as-efficacy-multiplier* theme. Patients in resource-limited settings face barriers that wealthier populations don't such as cost, access, literacy, and competing health priorities. An intervention that requires daily commitment only succeeds if it's simple, affordable, and doesn't add burden. Gum arabic, locally sourced and sold in Sudanese markets as a traditional remedy, checked all those boxes. Patients could dissolve it in tea or water at home, it cost pennies per day, and it didn't cause the gastrointestinal distress that would make them stop. The fact that lipid benefits appeared over twelve weeks (enough time for the liver's cholesterol metabolism to fully respond) with 110 out of 120 patients completing the study, proves that adherence held. This is the real-world test of cardiovascular intervention.

Khartoum again, 2018. This time, the study is a full randomized, placebo-controlled trial, the gold standard. Rasha Babiker and colleagues enroll patients with type 2 diabetes in a randomized, double-blind, placebo-controlled trial and randomly assigned them to 30 g/day of Gum arabic (Hashab gum from Acacia Senegal) or 5 g/day of pectin placebo for 12 weeks [4]. This is a population at extremely high cardiovascular risk due to the metabolic trifecta of hyperglycemia, dyslipidemia, and chronic inflammation. The trial has two primary endpoints: *Visceral Adiposity Index* and *blood pressure*. Let's define VAI briefly, because it's a calculated composite that matters deeply for cardiovascular prognosis.

The Visceral Adiposity Index combines waist circumference, body-mass index, triglycerides, and HDL-cholesterol into a single score that estimates the burden of *visceral fat* (the deep abdominal fat that wraps around organs and secretes inflammatory molecules). High VAI predicts cardiovascular events better than BMI alone, because visceral fat is metabolically toxic in ways that subcutaneous fat isn't. It drives insulin resistance, produces pro-inflammatory cytokines, and contributes to atherogenic dyslipidemia (high triglycerides, low HDL, small dense LDL particles). Lowering VAI is a therapeutic win. The Babiker trial found significant reductions in visceral adiposity index (−23.7%), modest decreases in BMI (−2%), and a significant within-group fall in systolic blood pressure (−7.6%) with Hashab gum vs the placebo group (2.7%) [4].

How does a fiber lower blood pressure? The mechanisms are indirect and powerful but not explored in these studies. We point possibly to Short-chain fatty acids, especially acetate, that modulate the renin-angiotensin-aldosterone system (RAAS), the hormonal cascade that controls blood volume and vascular tone. Propionate may improve endothelial function by enhancing nitric-oxide production, which relaxes blood vessels. A tighter gut barrier (supported by butyrate-fed colonocytes and bifidobacterium-associated barrier proteins) means less endotoxin leaking into circulation, less systemic inflammation, and less pressure on the endothelium to stay constricted and reactive. The result is a gentler vascular environment with lower pressure, less inflammation, and quieter risk.

Khartoum, 2019. Lamis Kaddam and colleagues turn to an even more challenging population: patients with *sickle-cell disease*. Sickle-cell is a genetic blood disorder where red blood cells deform under low oxygen, causing pain, organ damage, and *chronic hemolysis* (red-cell breakdown). Hemolysis drives oxidative stress and chronic inflammation, which in turn accelerates atherosclerosis and dyslipidemia. Sickle-cell patients often have elevated triglycerides at younger ages than the general population, and they're at high risk of cardiovascular events. This is a special-population stress test of the highest order. If Gum arabic (Hashab gum from Acacia Senegal) can ameliorate dyslipidemia in people whose biology is under constant oxidative and inflammatory assault, it can work anywhere.

The Kaddam trial gave sickle-cell patients Hashab gum daily for twelve weeks and tracked lipid profiles and oxidative stress markers (hydrogen peroxide). The results mirrored the prior Sudan studies whereby total cholesterol, LDL, and triglycerides dropped significantly, and the oxidative stress marker hydrogen peroxide decreased [5]. The lipid response was robust despite the metabolic chaos of chronic hemolysis, a testament to Hashab's ability to modulate the liver's lipid machinery even when the system is under siege.

This study completes the stress-test trifecta with dyslipidemia in otherwise healthy adults (2015), metabolic syndrome and diabetes (2018), and now an inflammatory hematologic disease (2019). Across all three, Hashab gum delivered. The pattern is clear and proves Hashab's effect on cholesterol, triglycerides, and inflammation. This is not the story of fragile flowers that wilt under real-world conditions. These results are durable, generalizable, and reproducible in populations with inflammation and oxidative stress. This is the kind of evidence that makes people trust an intervention.

Jordon, 2023. We shift from clinical trials to molecular mechanism.

Rasha M. Hussien, working with hyperlipidemic mice, asks a question that bridges correlation and causation: *Can we see Acacia gum changing the regulatory machinery that governs cholesterol transport and inflammatory tone at the genetic level?*

Let's teach *microRNAs* briefly, because they're the conceptual frame. MicroRNAs (miRNAs) are tiny snippets of RNA, about twenty-two nucleotides long, that don't code for proteins but instead regulate which proteins get made. Think of them as molecular Post-it notes stuck on messenger RNAs (mRNAs). When a miRNA binds to an mRNA, it can block translation or mark the mRNA for degradation, effectively silencing that gene. Two miRNAs are particularly relevant to cardiovascular biology: *miR-33* and *miR-155*. MiR-33 regulates cholesterol efflux (the process by which cells export excess cholesterol to HDL particles for reverse transport to the liver) and fatty-acid oxidation. MiR-155 modulates inflammatory signaling, affecting macrophage polarization and cytokine production. Tweaking these miRNAs can shift how cells handle cholesterol and how the immune system responds to atherogenic stimuli.

Hussien's experiment gave hyperlipidemic mice Acacia gum (GA) daily in addition to a western diet (WD) for several weeks and then measured hepatic expression of miR-33 and miR-155, alongside serum lipids. The Acacia-fed mice showed upregulation of both microRNAs in the GA + WD group compared to the WD alone group. The GA+WD group showed significant mitigation of hyperlipidemia with decreased blood total cholesterol and triglyceride levels with no weight effect [6]. The hepatic tissue showed better lipid-handling capacity and reduced hepatic TNF-α and improved liver histology. This is mechanistic evidence, not a human clinical endpoint, but it fills a crucial gap. It shows that Acacia's effects aren't just downstream consequences of bile-acid binding and SCFA signaling; they extend into the nucleus, into gene regulation, into the fine-tuning of how liver cells process and export lipids.

Here's where we introduce the *correlation-to-causation ladder*, because it clarifies why this sequence of studies is persuasive. At the bottom of the ladder is correlation where we showed lipids drop in people taking Acacia gum (Delhi, Stanford, Sudan trials). One rung up is mechanistic plausibility where we have coherent stories about bile-acid pull and SCFA signaling that explain *how* lipids might drop. Another rung is dose-response and consistency where we monitor the effect across doses, populations, and study designs. At the top is direct mechanistic proof showing that Acacia gum changes hepatic gene expression, enzyme activity, and cholesterol synthesis in controlled models. The Hussien miRNA study climbs that ladder. It's not a replacement for human trials, but it's the molecular Rosetta stone that translates human lipid drops into cellular cause and effect.

One more thread before we close. The liver isn't an island, and lipid metabolism isn't separate from glucose metabolism. The same propionate that dials down HMG-CoA reductase also modulates hepatic gluconeogenesis, the process by which the liver makes new glucose. The same bile-acid signaling that shifts cholesterol also activates farnesoid X receptor (FXR) and G-protein-coupled bile-acid receptor 1 (TGR5), pathways that regulate insulin secretion, glucose uptake, and incretin hormones like GLP-1. The same calmer inflammatory tone (lower CRP, lower TNF-alpha) that protects arteries also improves insulin sensitivity in muscle and fat. Cardiovascular and glycemic health aren't parallel tracks; they're the same track, and Acacia gum's prebiotic spillover affects both.

The next chapter will unpack the glycemic story in full. Discovering how Acacia flattens postprandial glucose spikes, improves fasting insulin, and supports HbA1c reductions in people with prediabetes and type 2 diabetes. You'll see why the same fiber that became the heart's quiet ally also became the metabolism's steadying hand. The cardiovascular chapter and the glycemic chapter aren't separate stories; they're two angles on the same revolution of a clear, gentle prebiotic that teaches the body to regulate itself better, one cup of tea at a time. That's where we're headed next.

References:

1. Sharma, Rakesh D. "Hypocholesterolemic Effect of Gum Acacia in Men." Nutrition Research, vol. 5, 1985, pp. 1321–1326

2. Mee, K. A., and D. L. Gee. "Apple Fiber and Gum Arabic Lowers Total and Low-Density Lipoprotein Cholesterol Levels in Men with Mild Hypercholesterolemia." Journal of the American Dietetic Association, vol. 97, no. 4, 1997, pp. 422-24

3. Mohamed, Rima E., Mohammed O. Gadour, and Ishag Adam. "The Lowering Effect of Gum Arabic on Hyperlipidemia in Sudanese Patients." Frontiers in Physiology, vol. 6, 2015, article 160.

4. Babiker, Rasha, et al. "Effect of Gum Arabic (Acacia senegal) Supplementation on Visceral Adiposity Index (VAI) and Blood Pressure in Patients with Type 2 Diabetes Mellitus as Indicators of Cardiovascular Disease (CVD): A Randomized and Placebo-Controlled Clinical Trial." Lipids in Health and Disease, vol. 17, no. 1, 2018, article 56.

5. Kaddam, Lamis, et al. "Acacia Senegal (Gum Arabic) Supplementation Modulate Lipid Profile and Ameliorated Dyslipidemia among Sickle Cell Anemia Patients." Journal of Lipids, vol. 2019, Article ID 3129461, 2019.

6. Hussein, Rasha M. "Upregulation of miR-33 and miR-155 by Gum Acacia Mitigates Hyperlipidaemia and Inflammation but Not Weight Increase Induced by Western Diet Ingestion in Mice." Archives of Physiology and Biochemistry, vol. 129, no. 4, 2023, pp. 847-53.

CHAPTER 10

How Hashab became a Glycemic Control Contender

$\mathbf{W}$e are moving from the previous chapter after having learned about how Acacia gum steadies lipid metabolism, quiets vascular inflammation, lowers LDL, trims blood pressure, and reduces visceral fat. The mechanisms were clear but complex. Bile-acid sequestration pulls cholesterol from the bloodstream, short-chain fatty acids signal the liver to ease off cholesterol synthesis, and a tighter gut barrier reduces the endotoxin leak that inflames arteries. Importantly, those same mechanisms don't stop at lipids. They cross the aisle into glucose metabolism, the other half of the cardiometabolic story. If you calm the gut's traffic signals every day, does the bloodstream's sugar also stop speeding? Does the liver ease its constant glucose production? Does the pancreas get to take a break? This chapter answers those questions through fifteen years of research, from stable-isotope tracer studies to randomized controlled trials in people with type 2 diabetes that showed *HbA1c* improvements and *adiponectin* rising. Adiponectin being a hormone that whispers "burn fat, spare sugar" to every cell.

Before we begin the journey, let's teach two foundational concepts, because they'll recur throughout this book. First, *endogenous glucose production* (EGP) is what we'll call the "liver glucose faucet". Between meals and overnight, when you're not eating, your blood sugar doesn't crash to zero because your liver is steadily releasing glucose into the bloodstream. It does this by breaking down stored glycogen (*glycogenolysis*) and by making new glucose from amino acids, lactate, and glycerol (*gluconeogenesis*). Think of it as a faucet; when it's wide open, fasting glucose is high. When it's dialed down, fasting glucose normalizes.

People with type 2 diabetes often have a faucet that won't close so their livers keep pouring glucose into the blood even when it's not needed, driving fasting hyperglycemia and making the whole day's glucose control harder. Drugs like metformin work partly by turning that faucet down. However, there are other ways to signal the liver, and one of them is through short-chain fatty acids produced by gut bacteria fermenting fiber.

Second, *acetogenic fibers* are fibers that ferment slowly, deep in the colon, favoring the production of acetate and propionate rather than just quick bursts of hydrogen and CO_2. Hashab gum is a canonical acetogenic fiber because its branched arabinogalactan structure requires cooperative microbial enzyme systems to dismantle, so fermentation happens over twelve to forty-eight hours rather than in the first two hours after ingestion. That slow fermentation feeds bacteria that produce acetate (a two-carbon SCFA) and propionate (a three-carbon SCFA), both of which cross the gut lining, enter the portal vein, and travel to the liver. There, they act as metabolic signals. Propionate inhibits gluconeogenesis (the liver's production of new glucose) by interfering with key enzymes in the pathway. Acetate provides an alternative fuel substrate and modulates insulin signaling. Together, they tell the liver to *ease off the faucet; the gut is sending fuel, and the system is calm.* That signal, repeated every day with every dose of Hashab gum, is the foundation of its glycemic effects.

Now let's watch those effects unfold, study by study, from the first isotope-traced proof that the liver listens, to a 2025 trial showing that adiponectin (the body's "prefer fat over sugar" hormone) rises when you feed the microbes right.

Nantes, France, 2010. A metabolic research ward. Volunteers with metabolic syndrome (the cluster of risks that includes abdominal obesity, high triglycerides, low HDL, elevated blood pressure, and impaired fasting glucose) are enrolled in a controlled feeding study. They're given acetogenic fiber supplements daily, and at the end of the intervention period, they undergo *stable-isotope glucose flux measurements.*

Let's pause to explain that method, because it's how scientists answer the question: *Where is the glucose coming from?* Researchers infuse volunteers with glucose labeled with stable (non-radioactive) isotopes (carbon-13 or deuterium) that can be tracked through the bloodstream. By measuring how much labeled glucose appears and how fast it's cleared, they can calculate two numbers: how much glucose the liver is making (endogenous production) and how much the body is using (peripheral glucose disposal). It's a molecular accounting system, and it reveals whether an intervention is working by reducing production, improving clearance, or both.

Etienne Pouteau and colleagues published their findings in 2010 showing acetogenic fiber supplementation effects. This was a randomized, double-blind, crossover trial, where 21 men with metabolic syndrome consumed 28 g/day of acetogenic fibers (acacia gum plus pectin) or control drinks for 5 weeks to test hepatic and peripheral glucose metabolism under controlled feeding conditions. Researchers combined fasting euglycaemic–hyperinsulinaemic clamps with stable isotope tracers ($[6,6-^2H_2]$glucose for endogenous glucose production ($[^2H_5]$glycerol for lipolysis, and [1-^{13}C]acetate for acetate turnover) to quantify metabolic fluxes mechanistically. Fasting endogenous glucose production fell with fiber (7.9

115

± 1.3 vs 8.6 ± 1.6 $\mu mol \cdot kg^{-1} \cdot min^{-1}$; $P < 0.05$), indicating a selective reduction in hepatic glucose output [1].

Plainly put, the fiber didn't make muscle or fat better at taking up glucose when insulin was present. Instead, it nudged the liver to release less glucose during fasting, as shown by a drop in endogenous glucose production with no change in clamp-measured peripheral insulin sensitivity. In this trial, fasting plasma glucose itself did not change, so the key effect was "turning down the liver faucet" rather than speeding peripheral clearance.

Sudan & China, 2015. A university laboratory studying diabetes models in rats. Abdelkareem Ahmed and colleagues induced alloxan diabetes in rats, which destroys pancreatic beta cells and models insulin deficiency. They then provided 15% Gum arabic in drinking water for eight weeks to one diabetic group, while tracking hepatic enzymes, lipid peroxidation, antioxidant defenses, gene expression, and histology.

Before we report the findings, let's teach the *oxidative-stress quartet*, because these markers will recur and they're the liver's report card. Superoxide dismutase (SOD) and catalase (CAT) are antioxidant enzymes (cellular firefighters) that neutralize reactive oxygen species (ROS) before they damage proteins, lipids, and DNA. Glutathione (GSH) is a small antioxidant molecule that the liver uses to detoxify and to maintain redox balance; low glutathione means the liver is under oxidative siege. Malondialdehyde (MDA) is a byproduct of lipid peroxidation, the process by which ROS attack cell membranes; high MDA means membranes are breaking down.

In diabetes, chronic hyperglycemia generates ROS, overwhelming antioxidant defenses and injuring tissues, especially the liver, which is metabolically hyperactive and vulnerable. When you see SOD, CAT, and GSH rising and MDA falling, you're seeing the liver's defenses restored and the oxidative fire damped.

Ahmed's team found that Gum arabic supplementation significantly lowered liver malondialdehyde, raised glutathione, and increased superoxide dismutase, catalase, and glutathione peroxidase activities. Serum ALT and AST fell, and liver sections showed slight degeneration with Gum arabic versus marked degeneration in untreated diabetics. Gum arabic reduced hepatic oxidative stress and improved antioxidant status in alloxan-diabetic rats [2].

A liver under oxidative stress is a liver that's dysregulated as its insulin signaling is blunted, its gluconeogenesis is overactive, and its capacity to respond to metabolic signals is impaired. Restore the redox balance, and you restore some of that capacity. Second, it aligns with the SCFA story whereby acetate and propionate aren't just metabolic signals; they're also mild antioxidants and anti-inflammatory agents. They reduce oxidative stress directly and indirectly, by lowering systemic inflammation and improving barrier function (less endotoxin leak, less inflammatory cytokine production).

Around that time, Mohammed Babiker and team reported a complementary experiment using a high-fat diet to drive obesity and insulin resistance in mice. This is a common proxy for human type 2 diabetes physiology where excess adiposity and impaired insulin action dominate over beta-cell loss. Gum arabic again improved hepatic oxidative balance by lowering MDA, raising GSH, and boosting antioxidant enzyme activity measures [3].

These were animal studies that were necessary for isolating mechanisms but always one step removed from human relevance. After this, the

117

question was: would the same liver-protective, EGP-modulating effects appear in people with diabetes? The answer came from Khartoum.

Khartoum, Sudan, and Limerick, Ireland, 2017. A collaboration between the University of Khartoum and the University of Limerick conducted a randomized, placebo-controlled, double-blind clinical trial of Gum arabic (Hashab gum from Acacia Senegal) in adults with type 2 diabetes. Patients were on stable oral hypoglycemic therapy; insulin users were excluded by protocol. Participants were randomized to 30 g/day Acacia senegal or 5 g/day placebo (pectin) for twelve weeks. The prespecified glycemic outcomes were fasting plasma glucose and HbA1c, alongside secondary measures of lipid profile and body mass index [4].

Post-prandial excursions are the after-meal glucose spikes. They are the curves that rise sharply after you eat carbohydrates and then fall back toward baseline over two to three hours. Steeper, higher excursions stress the pancreas (which has to secrete more insulin to cover the spike) and damage the endothelium (glucose spikes generate oxidative stress and glycate proteins). *Area under the curve* (AUC) is the mathematical integral of those excursions (the total glucose exposure over time). Flatter curves mean lower AUC, which means gentler demand on the pancreas and less vascular injury. We'll return to these ideas when we hit the 2022 meal-test study, but plant them now.

The 2017 results showed significant within-group reductions in fasting plasma glucose and HbA1c in the Hashab gum arm, while the placebo group did not exhibit comparable improvements in these measures. Lipid profiles improved within the Hashab gum group (LDL-bad cholesterol decreased, HDL-Good cholesterol increased, triglycerides decreased), and BMI declined modestly over twelve weeks. Completion was high (91 of

100 randomized finished), and tolerability appeared acceptable in this short trial, with limited adverse-events reported [4].

Although not specified in this study, let's try to tie this to the mechanisms we've been building. The slow, colonic fermentation of Hashab produces acetate and propionate, which we know from the 2010 French flux study can reduce endogenous glucose production [1]. Those SCFAs also stimulate the release of gut hormones such as GLP-1 (glucagon-like peptide-1) and PYY (peptide YY) from enteroendocrine cells in the distal ileum and colon. GLP-1 enhances insulin secretion from pancreatic beta cells in a glucose-dependent way (meaning it only works when glucose is elevated, reducing hypoglycemia risk), slows gastric emptying (which blunts post-prandial spikes), and may improve beta-cell function over time. PYY also slows gastric emptying and reduces appetite. Both hormones are part of the "ileal brake," the feedback system that moderates nutrient absorption and glucose appearance. The barrier improvements we've documented in earlier chapters (tighter junctions, calmer inflammation, lower endotoxin translocation) reduce the systemic inflammatory load that impairs insulin signaling in muscle and liver. And the hepatic oxidative-stress protection from the 2015–2016 Sudan studies means the liver is better equipped to respond to insulin and modulate gluconeogenesis appropriately [2,3]. All these pathways converge in the 2017 trial's result of better glucose control [4].

Now let's address the elephant in the room which are GLP-1 receptor agonist drugs. Medications like semaglutide and liraglutide have revolutionized diabetes and obesity treatment by pharmacologically raising GLP-1 signaling to supraphysiologic levels, producing dramatic weight loss and glucose reductions. How does Hashab gum compare? The honest answer is that it doesn't compete, it complements. GLP-1 drugs deliver a powerful, acute signal like turning up the volume on a radio. Hashab delivers a gentler, chronic signal like retuning the station so the signal

119

comes in clearer.

The overlap is real as both raise GLP-1. However, Acacia also improves gut-barrier function, reduces endotoxemia, modulates hepatic oxidative stress, raises adiponectin (we'll see this in 2025), and improves lipid profiles. These are pleiotropic effects that a single-target drug doesn't provide. Importantly, Hashab gum is food-grade, taken at home, with no injections, no nausea (a common GLP-1 drug side effect), and no prescription barriers. The positioning is adjunct, not replacement as Hashab gum can reduce the baseline glucose burden and inflammatory load, potentially allowing lower drug doses or delaying disease progression in people who aren't yet on pharmacotherapy. Without clinician oversight, patients shouldn't substitute; but with it, they can layer strategies.

Germany, 2019. A private nutrition-research firm (analyze & realize GmbH) runs a practical, translatable study asking what happens when healthy adults take Acacia gum with a standardized breakfast. Udo Bongartz and colleagues recruit volunteers, serve a fixed test meal, and measure post-prandial glucose and insulin repeatedly over 180 minutes. In a double-blind, controlled, randomized, three-way cross-over study, participants complete three test days: 20 g Acacia gum, 40 g Acacia gum, and no-treatment control, allowing each person to serve as their own control [5].

Before we report the result, let's clarify *with-meal versus between-meal strategies*. Acacia can be used two ways. Taken between meals where for example it's dissolved in morning tea or an afternoon drink as it ferments over the next twelve to twenty-four hours, producing SCFAs that modulate endogenous glucose production and gut-hormone tone. Taken with or just before a meal, it can also exert acute effects such as very mild viscosity

(Acacia doesn't gel, but it does increase solution viscosity slightly at high concentrations), which may slow gastric emptying and carbohydrate absorption. The 2022 meal-test study explores the acute, with-meal strategy.

The study result is that Acacia gum significantly attenuated post-prandial glucose and insulin compared to no treatment. The glucose curve was flatter, the peak was lower, and incremental AUCs over multiple intervals were reduced with both doses. Insulin rose less steeply, with lower peak and AUC at nearly all post-baseline timepoints. The effect was similar at 20 g and 40 g, and tolerability ratings were uniformly "good/very good" in treated arms [5].

This is the grocery-store translation of Acacia's glycemic benefits. You don't need a prescription, a special diet, or meal-replacement shakes. You stir it into what you already eat (yogurt, oatmeal, a smoothie, juice) and the fiber quietly smooths the ride. The mechanism likely involves multiple pathways working in parallel such as slight viscosity slowing the rate at which carbohydrates appear in the bloodstream; incretin signaling (GLP-1/PYY) from the fiber reaching colonic fermentation sites; and possibly some direct interaction with intestinal glucose transporters, though that's less well established. The key takeaway for patients and clinicians is simplicity and adherence. The intervention fits into normal eating patterns, it works meal to meal, and people tolerate it so well that using it daily for months or years is realistic.

Khartoum, Sudan, 2025. Rasha Babiker the same investigator who led the 2017 type 2 diabetes RCT returns with a new question and a new endpoint: *Does long-term Acacia supplementation change adiponectin, the hormone that resets insulin sensitivity and fat metabolism?* She enrolls women with type 2 diabetes in a randomized, double-blind, placebo-controlled trial, giving 30 g/day Gum Acacia or 5 g/day pectin placebo for twelve weeks, and tracks adiponectin, HbA1c, fasting glucose, BMI, and the HbA1c/adiponectin ratio [6].

Let's teach *adiponectin and AMPK*, because they're the system's "prefer fat over sugar" messengers. Adiponectin is a hormone secreted by adipose tissue but paradoxically, it's secreted *less* as you gain fat, especially visceral fat. Lean, metabolically healthy people have high adiponectin; obese, insulin-resistant people have low adiponectin. The hormone improves insulin sensitivity in muscle and liver, promotes fat oxidation (burning fat for energy rather than storing it), reduces hepatic glucose production, and has anti-inflammatory effects. It works partly through activating AMPK (AMP-activated protein kinase-a cellular "fuel gauge" that senses energy status and shifts metabolism toward fat burning), glucose uptake, and mitochondrial biogenesis when activated. Low adiponectin is a risk marker for type 2 diabetes, cardiovascular disease, and metabolic syndrome. Raising adiponectin through weight loss, exercise, or dietary interventions is a therapeutic win.

The 2025 trial found that Gum Acacia supplementation significantly increased serum adiponectin from baseline in women with type 2 diabetes, though between-group differences for adiponectin change were not significant. The HbA1c-to-adiponectin ratio (a composite marker of glycemic control weighted by insulin sensitivity) improved significantly versus placebo, indicating a shift toward better glycemic status relative to adiponectin. BMI decreased modestly but significantly, and fasting glucose and HbA1c fell from baseline which is consistent with a small improvement in glycemia during the intervention period. Tolerability was generally good, with brief early bloating, nausea, or diarrhea that resolved within the first two weeks.

This is your "system rewired" moment. Acacia doesn't yank sugar down with brute force. No sudden hypoglycemia, no metabolic shock. It persuades the system to prefer a calmer road. By feeding beneficial microbes that produce SCFAs. It is associated with modest increases in adiponectin, which nudges AMPK, which tells cells to burn fat and take up glucose more efficiently. The liver eases off gluconeogenesis. The pancreas doesn't have to scream so loudly. The adipose tissue stops hoarding and starts signaling health. It's a slow, cooperative retuning which is the opposite of a drug that overrides physiology. Amazingly, the intervention is gentle and tolerable, patients stick with it long enough for the retuning to take hold.

One more thread before we close, because the diabetes story doesn't end with glucose as it flows directly into the next frontier which is metabolism and satiety. The same SCFAs that modulate hepatic glucose production also modulate appetite and energy intake through gut-hormone signaling. GLP-1 and PYY, released when Hashab's fermentation reaches the distal ileum and colon, don't just improve glucose control; they slow gastric emptying and signal satiety to the brainstem, reducing hunger and food intake.

Adiponectin and AMPK, the metabolic retuning signals we just learned about, also guide fat oxidation and visceral-fat loss (the deep belly fat that drives insulin resistance and cardiovascular risk). When AMPK is activated, cells burn fat preferentially, mitochondria proliferate, and energy efficiency improves. This is the cardiometabolic arc coming full circle as the same prebiotic that lowers LDL and blood pressure in the cardiovascular chapter also raises adiponectin and activates fat-burning pathways in the diabetes chapter, and those pathways lead straight into the satiety and body-composition story.

The next chapter will unpack that story in full and answer how Acacia's slow fermentation drives GLP-1 and PYY release. It will explain how those hormones shape appetite, meal size, and snacking behavior. You will understand how adiponectin and AMPK guide the body toward preferring fat oxidation over glucose dependence; and how all of this translates into practical, day-to-day strategies like when to dose (with meals vs. between meals), how to pair with probiotics (synbiotic logic), and what to expect over weeks and months (the satiety curve isn't instant, but it's durable).

You'll see controlled trials measuring calorie intake, VAS hunger scores, and body composition. You'll see the mechanisms we've touched applied to weight management, metabolic flexibility, and the gut-brain axis. You'll see why Hashab's gentleness, far from being a limitation, is its greatest strength because the body doesn't resist gentle persuasion the way it resists pharmacologic coercion. Afterall, adherence over months and years is what turns a supplement into a lifestyle. That's where we're headed next; the place where prebiotic spillover becomes metabolic freedom, one calm conversation between gut and brain at a time.

References:

1. Pouteau, Etienne, et al. "Acetogenic Fibers Reduce Fasting Glucose Turnover but Not Peripheral Insulin Resistance in Metabolic Syndrome Patients." Clinical Nutrition, vol. 29, no. 6, 2010, pp. 801–807

2. Ahmed, Abdelkareem A., et al. "Gum Arabic Extracts Protect Against Hepatic Oxidative Stress in Alloxan Induced Diabetes in Rats." Pathophysiology, vol. 22, no. 4, 2015, pp. 189–94

3. Babiker, Mohammed E. A., et al. "Effect of Gum Arabic on Oxidative Stress Markers in the Liver of High Fat Diet Induced Obesity in Mice." Gums and Stabilisers for the Food Industry 18, Royal Society of Chemistry, 2016

4. Babiker, Rasha, et al. "Metabolic Effects of Gum Arabic (Acacia senegal) in Patients with Type 2 Diabetes Mellitus (T2DM): Randomized, Placebo Controlled, Double Blind Trial." Functional Foods in Health and Disease, vol. 7, no. 3, 2017, pp. 219–231

5. Bongartz, Udo, Constantin Erlenbeck, and Irene Wohlfahrt. "The Effect of Gum Acacia on Post-Prandial Glucose and Insulin Levels in Healthy Subjects: A Randomized Controlled Cross-Over Study." Food and Nutrition Sciences, vol. 13, 2022, pp. 424–438

6. Babiker, Rasha, et al. "Gum Acacia Supplementation Improves Adiponectin Levels and HbA1c/Adiponectin Ratio in Women with Type 2 Diabetes: A Randomized Controlled Trial." Functional Foods in Health and Disease, vol. 15, no. 3, 2025, pp. 176–190

CHAPTER 11

METABOLISM AND SATIETY

How Hashab Became a Convenient Weight Management
Solution

The morning routine has become automatic. A tablespoon of clear powder dissolved in tea, a sip, a swallow, and the day begins. No thickness to fight through, no aftertaste to grimace at, no bloating to manage an hour later. Just tea, just breakfast, just the ordinary rhythm of a Tuesday. However, somewhere deep in the colon, over the next twelve hours, something quietly extraordinary is unfolding. The arabinogalactan molecules are being dismantled, slowly and cooperatively, by probiotics and their partners. Short-chain fatty acids (acetate, propionate, butyrate) are diffusing into the bloodstream, traveling through the portal vein to the liver, and crossing the blood-brain barrier to reach the hypothalamus. In the distal ileum and colon, specialized cells sense the rising SCFA concentration and respond by secreting hormones into circulation. These hormones travel upstream to the brainstem and the stomach, where they whisper a message that will shape the rest of the day: You've had enough. The system is calm. No need to hunt for more.

We left the previous chapter with a promise. We watched Acacia gum quiet the sugar spikes by flattening post-prandial glucose curves, raising adiponectin, and improving HbA1c through mechanisms that centered on the liver's glucose faucet, hepatic oxidative protection, and SCFA-driven insulin sensitization. Amazingly, those same SCFAs that modulate hepatic

126

gluconeogenesis also modulate appetite. The same gut hormones (GLP-1 and PYY) that improve glucose control by slowing gastric emptying and enhancing insulin secretion also reduce hunger and food intake. The same adiponectin that activates AMPK and shifts cells toward fat oxidation also changes where the body stores incoming calories, favoring muscle glycogen and subcutaneous depots over the dangerous visceral fat.

Glycemic control and weight management aren't parallel tracks; they're the same track viewed from different angles. Today we're shifting the lens to ask a bolder question: Can the same slow, gentle fermentation that teaches the liver to ease off glucose production also teach hunger to whisper instead of shout? Can it change how much people eat by shifting the reasons from willpower and deprivation to genuine satiety and metabolic calm? This chapter answers that question through a decade of research; from methodology studies that cracked the satiety-measurement problem to randomized trials showing body-fat reductions to molecular studies revealing that Acacia gum rewires the stress-hormone micro-machinery that parks fat in the belly and keeps it there.

Before we begin, let's teach two foundational concepts, because they'll frame everything that follows. First, the distinction between *satiety* and *compensation*. Satiety is the feeling of fullness during and after eating. It's the sensation that you've had enough and can stop. It's easy to measure in the lab by giving people a preload (a drink or snack containing the test ingredient), wait thirty to sixty minutes, then offer them a meal and measure how much they eat. If they eat less after the preload than after a control, you've demonstrated a satiety effect. However, here's the catch as some interventions produce satiety in the moment but trigger unconscious compensation later.

The person eats less at lunch because they feel full but then eats more at dinner or snacks more heavily in the evening. By the end of the day, total

127

calorie intake is unchanged. Real, meaningful satiety is the kind that sticks and reduces intake at the next meal without triggering rebound hunger hours later. Measuring that requires sophisticated study designs that track multiple meals and snacks over a full day or longer, accounting for both immediate and delayed responses. It's the difference between a temporary brake and a recalibrated appetite thermostat. Second, let's introduce *GLP-1 and PYY*, the gut-brain satiety messengers, because they're the mechanistic bridge between fiber fermentation and hunger regulation.

The beauty of this system is that it's not pharmacologic coercion; it's physiological communication. The gut is telling the brain, in the body's own language, that fuel has arrived, the system is satisfied, and there's no need to keep hunting for calories. When people lose weight through this pathway, they're not battling with hunger; they're experiencing genuine satiety, the kind the body respects and sustains.

Now let's watch these concepts come to life, study by study, from a Dutch sensory lab measuring fullness that sticks, to a 2022 paper showing that Acacia gum changes which genes get turned on when precursor cells decide whether to become fat cells.

The Netherlands and UK, 2011. A nutrition-research laboratory at a contract research organization. Volunteers arrive in the morning, having fasted overnight, and are randomly assigned to receive one of several preloads: drinks of water containing different doses of Gum arabic (EmulGold or PreVitae), with plain water as the control. After drinking the preload, participants rate their hunger, fullness, and desire to eat on visual analog scales which are usually 100-mm lines that capture subjective appetite over time. Three hours later, they are given a standardized 'eat-as-much-as-you-like' test meal and told to eat until comfortably full.

Researchers weigh the plates before and after, calculating exactly how many calories each person consumed. The study doesn't stop there. In the second study, a second test meal 3 hours after the first allowed the team to see whether people 'made up' for earlier calorie reductions at the next meal.

Wim Calame and colleagues published their findings in 2011, and the paper revealed something unusual. It didn't just report results; it taught other researchers how to measure satiety properly. Let's explain why this methodological rigor matters. Many early fiber-satiety studies used thick gels or high-viscosity preparations (psyllium mixed into pudding, guar gum swelling in the stomach) where the mechanism was partly mechanical with the fiber physically filled the stomach, activating stretch receptors that signal fullness.

Those studies could get away with simpler designs because the effect was large and immediate. However, low-viscosity fibers like Acacia gum don't gel, don't swell dramatically, and don't fill the stomach mechanically. Their satiety effects are subtler, slower, and more endocrine-mediated with GLP-1 and PYY released hours later when fermentation reaches the distal gut. To detect those effects, you need sensitive methods, you need to control for palatability (if the preload tastes bad, people might eat less out of disgust, not satiety), and crucially, you need to measure compensation.

The Calame study evaluated Gum arabic-containing blends for effects on satiety ratings and intake at the next meal, explicitly assessing compensation at a second meal a few hours later using standardized procedures. The results showed that Gum arabic significantly decreases caloric intake 3 hours after consumption. It also showed that consumption of Gum arabic increases the subjective rating of feeling satiated. The study demonstrated that Gum arabic could have an important role in body weight management. Gum arabic's slower fermentation may moderate kinetics,

129

but direct hormone measures were not reported, and mechanistic causation remained inferential in context [1].

The 2011 paper became a methodological reference point, cited by satiety researchers worldwide as the template for testing non-viscous fibers. More importantly for our story, it established the design principles we'll see recur like measuring compensation, controlling palatability, and testing fibers at doses people can actually tolerate daily.

Khartoum, Sudan, 2011. Rasha Babiker and colleagues conducted a randomized, double-blind, placebo-controlled trial testing whether Gum arabic alters body composition in free-living women. They enrolled healthy female students and randomized them to Gum arabic at thirty grams daily in two divided doses or a placebo of one gram pectin daily. Body mass index and body-fat percentage were tracked over six weeks using seven-site skinfolds with Jackson–Pollock equations and the Siri formula. The trial was rigorously double-blind and placebo-controlled.

Subcutaneous fat sits just under the skin. It's the padding you can pinch on your hips, thighs, buttocks, and arms. It's metabolically relatively inert meaning it stores energy without causing much trouble. Visceral fat, by contrast, wraps around your internal organs (the liver, intestines, pancreas, kidneys) and is metabolically toxic. It secretes inflammatory cytokines (TNF-alpha, IL-6), free fatty acids that flood the liver and drive insulin resistance, and adipokines that dysregulate appetite and energy balance.

High visceral fat predicts type 2 diabetes, cardiovascular disease, fatty liver, and even certain cancers, independent of total body weight. A lean person with high visceral fat is at higher risk than an overweight person who has less visceral fat. When body composition changes, what matters most is where the fat comes from. Losing five kilograms of visceral fat changes your metabolic future; losing five kilograms of subcutaneous fat changes your jeans size. Both matter, but one matters more.

The Babiker trial reported significant within-group reductions after Gum arabic intake, demonstrating decreases in BMI and body-fat percentage with the intervention. Compared with the placebo group, which showed increased body-fat percentage and a nonsignificant trend toward higher BMI, the Gum arabic group improved meaningfully over six weeks. Average body weight in the intervention group fell by about one kilogram over the study, aligning with the magnitude implied by the BMI change reported. All 120 randomized participants completed the six-week trial. Gastrointestinal complaints were common in the first week (oral viscous sensation, mild diarrhea, and nausea) but subsided. Body-fat percentage was estimated from skinfolds, the study inferred fat loss from validated anthropometric equations.

The mechanism? At this point in 2012, the pieces were partially known but not yet fully assembled and not reported in this study. The satiety pathway was plausible and supported. The metabolic improvements (better insulin sensitivity, lower inflammatory tone, improved lipid profiles) would reduce the metabolic drive to store fat. Additionally, there was a third, deeper mechanism that wouldn't be proven until 2015 [3] and it was that Acacia gum was changing the hormonal signals that reduce visceral fat through enzyme expression.

Nyala, Sudan, 2015. A laboratory at the University of Nyala studying obesity and metabolic disease in mice. Abdelkareem Ahmed and colleagues are testing whether Gum arabic can reduce visceral adiposity and, if so, through what molecular pathway. They maintain mice on standard chow and administer Gum arabic in drinking water to the treatment group, while controls receive water without Gum arabic. After several weeks, they collect tissues and quantify visceral fat-pad weights and assess 11β-HSD1 gene expression in liver and muscle by qPCR [3].

Before we report the findings, let's introduce *11β-HSD1*, because it's a molecular lever that most people have never heard of but that quietly determines whether you carry your weight around your organs or under your skin. 11β-HSD1 is an enzyme expressed in liver, muscle, and adipose tissue that converts cortisone (an inactive steroid) into cortisol (the active stress hormone). This local regeneration of cortisol inside tissues amplifies glucocorticoid signaling without requiring higher circulating cortisol levels. Why does this matter? Because cortisol, when active inside fat cells, drives several processes that worsen obesity. It promotes fat storage (lipogenesis), especially in visceral depots and it impairs insulin signaling which worsens glucose control. It also favors the differentiation of precursor cells into new fat cells (adipogenesis). People and animals with high 11β-HSD1 activity tend to accumulate visceral fat even without eating more calories, because the enzyme creates a local cortisol "hot zone" that tells fat cells to hoard and multiply. Conversely, inhibiting 11β-HSD1 (either with drugs or through dietary interventions) can shift fat distribution away from visceral depots, improving metabolic health even if total weight doesn't change dramatically.

The Ahmed study found that Gum arabic supplementation significantly reduced visceral adipose tissue mass and down-regulated 11β-HSD1 mRNA in liver and muscle. Body weight changed modestly, but the decline in visceral fat was clear relative to controls. 11β-HSD1 mRNA levels dropped, indicating reduced expression of the enzyme that regenerates active glucocorticoids within tissues. Subcutaneous fat measurements were not the focus, while the visceral depot was explicitly reduced. The liver and muscle findings mattered because these are key metabolic organs implicated in systemic insulin resistance physiology [3]. Let's translate this for a general reader. By dialing down the local stress signal inside tissues, Acacia gum impacts where incoming calories settle away from the organs by reducing visceral fat. This isn't about eating less (though the decreased satiety effects help with that too); it's about changing the body's default instructions for what to do with the energy it receives. It's a deeper intervention than calorie restriction alone, because it addresses the hormonal logic that makes visceral fat so tenacious and so harmful

The 11β-HSD1 story would deepen over the next five years, as Ahmed's group and collaborators in Italy dug into the broader glucocorticoid axis. However, the 2015 paper was the proof-of-concept that Gum arabic doesn't just reduce total fat; it reduces the dangerous fat, through a hormonal pathway that most weight-loss interventions never touch.

Minnesota, 2018-2020. The University of Minnesota. Joanne Slavin (a figure in dietary fiber science) and her colleagues conduct a randomized, double-blind, three-way crossover trial to test Acacia gum in human feeding conditions. The trial feeds orange juice with 0, 20, or 40 g acacia plus a bagel and cream cheese on separate days, then records appetite on visual analog scales and post-prandial glucose at repeated time points. The goal is to answer two questions simultaneously: *Does Acacia gum increase satiety? and Does Acacia gum blunt the glucose spike after a meal?* Both questions matter for weight management, because satiety determines how much you eat next, and glucose spikes determine insulin secretion, which drives fat storage.

The Slavin 2021 trial found increased satiety ratings and significantly lower actual blood glucose at 30 minutes for the 20g dose compared to control, with high overall tolerability but more bloating and flatulence at

40 g compared with control. Appetite scores (hunger, desire to eat, prospective food consumption) were significantly lower at select timepoints (15, 30, 240 minutes) following Acacia gum consumption compared to control. Post-prandial glucose showed a lower value at 30 minutes, without significant AUC differences overall. Critically, gastrointestinal symptoms (bloating, flatulence, rumbling at 40 g versus control) were generally low overall. Participants rated the Acacia-supplemented orange juice as similar to control in acceptability overall. This is how gentle, colonic fermentation often feels. Full without much bloat, satisfied without a texture tax, glucose steadier without an insulin rollercoaster.

Let's connect the dots back to the 2011 methodology study and forward to the hormone story. The 2011 Calame paper taught us that Acacia-containing blends can produce satiety without triggering compensation, showing the effect sticks across multiple meals [1]. Now, in 2019, we're seeing that same effect in a different lab, with different foods, in American participants rather than Dutch ones, confirming reproducibility and generalizability. The glucose-lowering accompanies the satiety naturally, because we assume both effects are mediated by overlapping pathways: GLP-1 slows gastric emptying (which blunts glucose spikes) and suppresses appetite (which reduces intake); PYY reinforces both; and the improved insulin sensitivity from better barrier function and lower inflammation means the pancreas doesn't have to work as hard to clear the glucose that does appear. Satiety and glycemic control aren't separate benefits that happen to coincide; they're two faces of the same metabolic calm.

Nyala, Sudan, and Italy, 2020. A collaboration between Ahmed's group in Sudan and researchers in Italy studying stress-hormone metabolism.

134

Building on the 2015 finding that Acacia gum down-regulates 11β-HSD1, the team asks a broader question: *Does Acacia gum modulate the entire glucocorticoid axis during chronic dietary supplementation?* They design a mouse study measuring plasma corticosterone alongside hepatic and muscular expression of glucocorticoid-metabolizing enzymes and receptors, focusing on 11β-HSD1, 11β-HSD2, and the glucocorticoid and mineralocorticoid receptors, rather than steroidogenic enzyme synthesis pathways [5].

Let's briefly teach *corticosterone*, because it's the readout. In rodents, corticosterone plays the same role that cortisol plays in humans: it's the primary glucocorticoid hormone, secreted by the adrenal glands in response to stress, and it regulates glucose metabolism, fat distribution, immune function, and appetite. Chronically elevated corticosterone (whether from external stress, obesity, or dysregulated HPA-axis feedback) drives visceral fat accumulation, insulin resistance, increased appetite (especially for palatable, energy-dense foods), and muscle wasting. It's part of why chronic stress makes people gain weight, particularly around the middle. Lowering corticosterone, or dampening its tissue-level effects, is therapeutic for obesity and metabolic syndrome.

The 2020 study found that Gum arabic supplementation reduced circulating corticosterone and altered hepatic and muscular gene expression thereby lowering 11β-HSD1, raising hepatic 11β-HSD2, and decreasing hepatic GR mRNA. They demonstrated modulation of glucocorticoid metabolism and signaling in key tissues rather than only a single enzyme. This was broader confirmation of the 2015 story. Acacia gum isn't just tweaking one enzyme in one tissue; it may dampen the stress-hormone axis. In Layman terms, the study concluded that the supplementation of Gum arabic reduced food intake, body weight, VAT, plasma lipids profile and plasma CORT concentration which were associated with modification of hepatic 11β-HSD1, 11β-HSD2 and GR mRNA expression. [5].

Although the mechanism was not defined in the study; it likely involves SCFAs signaling through receptors in the hypothalamus and adipose tissue, altering HPA-axis tone and local glucocorticoid sensitivity. The net effect is a quieter stress signal, less hormonal drive to hoard visceral fat, and better insulin signaling in liver and muscle.

This reframes Gum arabic not as "just fiber" or "just a prebiotic," but as a metabolic tone modulator. It's a substance that changes the baseline hormonal conversation between gut, brain, adrenals, and fat tissue. That's a deeper intervention than simply blocking calories or revving metabolism. It's teaching the system to prefer a calmer, less hoardy state, which makes weight loss easier and weight maintenance more durable because the body isn't fighting you with stress hormones and hunger signals.

Malaysia, 2020. Researchers at Malaysian universities are asking a crucial translational question: *Will an already-dysbiotic, obesity-phenotype microbiome still respond to Acacia Senegal (Hashab gum), or does fiber efficacy collapse when the microbial community is skewed [6]?* This matters because some fibers (particularly those that require specific degrading species) fail to ferment properly in obese individuals whose microbiota lack key taxa. If Hashab only works in lean, healthy people with diverse microbiomes, its public-health value is limited. However, if it works even in dysbiotic, obese-phenotype communities, it becomes a tool for the populations that needs it most.

Let's explain *microbiome compatibility in obesity* briefly. Obesity is associated with shifts in gut microbial composition. Lower diversity means reduced abundance of certain beneficial groups (like some bifidobacteria),

136

and enrichment of taxa associated with energy harvest and low-grade inflammation. Some fibers that work beautifully in lean individuals ferment poorly or incompletely in obese microbiomes because the necessary degrading species are absent or suppressed. This creates a Catch-22 with the people who need prebiotic intervention the most are the ones least likely to respond. The question is whether Hashab gum, with its complex arabinogalactan structure requiring cooperative degradation, can still be fermented by the pared-down, stressed microbial communities typical of obese individuals.

The Malaysian team took fecal samples from obese individuals, inoculated them into pH-controlled anaerobic batch-fermentation systems (in vitro colon models), added Hashab gum, and tracked short-chain fatty acids and microbial shifts over time. The result was reassuring, showing obese-phenotype microbiota still fermented Hashab gum efficiently, significantly increasing Bifidobacterium and not promoting growth of the Clostridium histolyticum group, with measurable modulation of acetate and propionate under controlled pH, while butyrate remained essentially unchanged. The SCFA profiles were reported within the obese-donor system without a lean comparator, so similarity to lean-microbiota fermentations cannot be concluded from these data. This supports broad applicability in principle as obese microbiota retain functional capacity to utilize Hashab gum. If Hashab works in dysbiotic, obese-phenotype inocula, then satiety- and metabolic-relevant SCFA production may be achievable across body-weight categories [6].

Khartoum, Sudan, 2021. Ahmed's group returns with another piece of the obesity puzzle, this time focused on inflammatory tone. We've already learned from earlier chapters that chronic low-grade inflammation (elevated TNF-alpha, IL-6, reduced IL-10) impairs leptin and insulin signaling, creating a vicious cycle where the body can't properly sense satiety or regulate energy balance. In obesity, adipose tissue becomes infiltrated with macrophages and secretes pro-inflammatory cytokines, and the gut barrier often becomes leaky, allowing bacterial endotoxins to enter circulation and amplify systemic inflammation. Improving inflammatory tone (shifting cytokines toward anti-inflammatory profiles) can restore some leptin sensitivity and improve appetite regulation, making satiety signals work properly again.

The 2021 study fed mice a high-fat, obesogenic diet with or without Gum arabic supplementation and tracked plasma cytokines [7]. The result paralleled the earlier inflammation-chapter finding showing Gum arabic shifted the cytokine profile toward anti-inflammatory, with increased IL-10 (the regulatory, "off-switch" cytokine) and reduced TNF-alpha (a master pro-inflammatory signal). The shift was accompanied by lower fasting blood glucose and lipids, but the key takeaway for our satiety story is that a calmer inflammatory background allows leptin (the satiety hormone secreted by fat cells) to reach the brain and do its job. When inflammation is high, the brain becomes leptin-resistant; leptin levels are elevated but the signal doesn't register, so the brain thinks the body is starving even when fat stores are ample, driving continued hunger and fat accumulation. Calm the inflammation, and leptin sensitivity improves, restoring the feedback loop that should naturally suppress appetite when energy stores are sufficient.

From this study we can infer the mechanism for why Acacia gum's satiety effects are durable and don't trigger the metabolic backlash (slowed metabolism, increased hunger) that often derails calorie-restriction diets. By improving inflammatory tone through barrier support and SCFA signaling, Acacia gum keeps the brain's appetite-regulation machinery functional, so hunger naturally recalibrates downward rather than rebounding upward.

Al Ain, United Arab Emirates, 2018. A university setting serving a population at high risk of metabolic syndrome with the cluster of risks that includes abdominal obesity, elevated triglycerides, low HDL cholesterol, high blood pressure, and impaired fasting glucose. Amjad Jarrar and colleagues conduct a randomized, placebo-controlled trial enrolling adults at risk of metabolic syndrome to assess cardiometabolic and gastrointestinal outcomes over twelve weeks. An intervention window to test whether Gum arabic (Hashab gum from Acacia Senegal) improves cardiometabolic risk factors safely. The trial tests Hashab gum supplementation (twenty grams per day) versus placebo over twelve weeks, with endpoints spanning cardiometabolic risk factors (glucose, blood pressure, lipids, anthropometry) alongside validated gastrointestinal symptom questionnaires [8].

The setting matters, because this is a real-world stress test. These aren't healthy volunteers recruited from university campuses; they're young to middle-aged adults dealing with the consequences of years of western-style diets, sedentary work, and genetic predispositions to metabolic dysfunction. They're the people who abandon fiber supplements at the first sign of gas or bloating, who've tried and failed multiple diet interventions, and who need something that fits invisibly into daily life without adding burden. If Hashab gum works here (if it can move risk markers and maintain adherence in this population) it's a genuine therapeutic tool, not just an academic curiosity.

The trial delivered positive results across multiple domains including reduced blood pressure, lower fasting glucose, decreased appetite scores, and improved self-reported bloating and bowel-movement quality in the intervention group. Participants in the Hashab gum group reported improved gastrointestinal comfort, less bloating and improved bowel movements without the increased complaints seen with fermentable fibers. Waist circumference did not change significantly, and fat-free mass decreased slightly [8].

Khartoum, Sudan, 2022. Ahmed and colleagues take the final mechanistic step, asking not just how much fat is stored but whether the genes that promote the formation of new fat cells are being turned up or down. Fat gain can happen through two pathways: existing fat cells enlarging (hypertrophy) or new fat cells forming from precursor cells (hyperplasia via adipogenesis). *Hyperplasia* is particularly insidious because once a fat cell is created, it's permanent. It can shrink when you lose weight, but it doesn't disappear, and it's ready to refill at the first opportunity, contributing to weight regain. Limiting adipogenesis (reducing the formation of new fat cells) can make weight loss more durable by preventing the expansion of the fat-cell pool that drives regain [9].

The researchers fed mice either a normal diet, a high-fat diet, or a high-fat diet containing 10% Gum arabic and then examine gene expression in the liver, focusing on C/EBP-α and 11β-HSD1. Let's introduce this molecule, because it's the master switch for turning precursor cells into fat cells. C/EBP-alpha is a transcription factor (a protein that binds to DNA and turns genes on or off) and it governs the entire adipogenic program. When C/EBP-alpha is highly active, precursor cells (preadipocytes) differentiate into mature, lipid-storing adipocytes, expanding the body's capacity to store fat. When C/EBP-alpha is suppressed, differentiation slows, fewer new fat cells form, and weight gain is blunted even on a high-fat diet. Drugs and dietary interventions that down-regulate C/EBP-alpha are of intense interest in obesity research because they target the root cause of fat-tissue expansion [9].

The 2022 study found that Gum arabic supplementation down-regulated hepatic C/EBP-α expression and significantly limited weight gain in mice on a high-fat diet. The treated mice received the same high-fat diet with added Gum arabic and gained less weight than high-fat controls. The reduction in visceral adipose tissue mass indicated decreased adiposity. This is genomic-level evidence that Gum arabic may reduce the body's drive to store fat under high-fat feeding conditions. It supports the idea that signals observed in human trials have a a biological foundation in liver and stress-hormone–related gene regulation, while acknowledging species and design differences that limit direct extrapolation [9].

Let's tie this back to adherence one more time. The C/EBP-alpha effect doesn't happen overnight. Changes like this probably require weeks of consistent exposure to fermentation products (SCFAs), gut-hormone signals, and calmer inflammatory tone for gene expression to shift and for the cellular decisions about adipogenesis to change. A fiber that people take for two weeks and then abandon because it causes gas or tastes bad will never deliver this genomic nudge. Importantly, a fiber that's invisible, tasteless, and comfortable (that people can take daily for months without thinking about it) gives this deeper mechanism time to work. When adherence is easy, biology has time to change.

Here's the take-home line: Acacia doesn't bully appetite; it tutors it with steady SCFAs, quieter stress enzymes, turned down stress-hormone–related enzymes and dialed down gene signals that normally promote new fat-cell formation.

You dissolve a tablespoon into your morning routine, and over weeks the body learns a different conversation with GLP-1 and PYY saying "you've had enough", 11β-HSD1 dialing down so visceral fat stops hoarding,

C/EBP-α suppressed so the gene program that normally encourages new fat-cell formation is dialed down, and inflammatory tone calm enough that leptin can finally reach the brain and say "we're fine, no need to hunt". Weight loss becomes not a battle of will against biology, but biology quietly choosing a healthier equilibrium because the signals have changed. Taken together, these findings suggest that Hashab gum could be part of a more gentle, biologically aligned strategy for weight management.

Here's the honest comparison to alternatives, stated respectfully but clearly. Fast-fermenting fibers and thick gels can produce early fullness, but they provoke gas, bloating, or texture issues that crater adherence. Hashab's low-viscosity, slow-colonic path yields comfort that keeps people on board for months, which is the only timeline where the deeper mechanisms (enzyme suppression, adipogenesis control) have time to work. On the other hand, "Calorie blockers," appetite stimulants, and thermogenic supplements may swing the scale short-term, but they don't fix the visceral-fat biology (11β-HSD1, stress-axis dysregulation) or adipogenic machinery (C/EBP-alpha) that makes regain inevitable; Hashab gum does, gently and sustainably.

Lastly, because the satiety story connects seamlessly to the next frontier. The same slow, colonic fermentation that produces GLP-1 and PYY also bathes colonocytes (the epithelial cells lining the colon) in butyrate, the short-chain fatty acid that serves as their primary energy source and a potent regulator of cell growth and differentiation. Butyrate has profound effects on colonocyte biology as it promotes normal cell turnover, suppresses hyperproliferation (the runaway cell division that seeds polyps and tumors), induces apoptosis in damaged or pre-cancerous cells, and modulates the expression of genes involved in DNA repair and cell-cycle control. These are anti-cancer effects, and they're direct consequences of the fermentation we've been describing throughout this chapter.

The same SCFA wave that quiets hunger also protects DNA. The same barrier improvements (tighter junctions, calmer inflammation, lower endotoxin translocation) that support metabolic health also reduce the chronic inflammatory signals that promote carcinogenesis. The same microbial shifts (more bifidobacteria, fewer pathobionts) that improve glucose control also reduce the production of genotoxic secondary bile acids and other microbial metabolites implicated in colorectal cancer. Additionally, the glucocorticoid-axis calming we documented in the 2020 Sudan-Italy study (lower corticosterone, suppressed 11β-HSD1) reduces oxidative stress throughout the body, protecting cellular machinery from the kind of damage that accumulates into mutations. The next chapter will unpack this cell-protection story.

References:

1. Calame, Wim, et al. "Evaluation of Satiety Enhancement, Including Compensation, by Blends of Gum Arabic: A Methodological Approach." Appetite, vol. 57, no. 2, 2011, pp. 358–364.

2. Babiker, Rasha, et al. "Effects of Gum Arabic Ingestion on Body Mass Index and Body Fat Percentage in Healthy Adult Females: Two-Arm Randomized, Placebo Controlled, Double-Blind Trial." Nutrition Journal, vol. 11, no. 1, 2012, p. 111.

3. Ahmed, Abdelkareem A., et al. "Gum arabic decreased visceral adipose tissue associated with down-regulation of 11β-hydroxysteroid dehydrogenase type I in liver and muscle of mice." Bioactive Carbohydrates and Dietary Fibre, vol. 6, no. 1, 2015, pp. 31–36.

4. Larson, Riley, et al. "Acacia Gum Is Well Tolerated While Increasing Satiety and Lowering Peak Blood Glucose Response in Healthy Human Subjects." Nutrients, vol. 13, no. 2, 2021, p. 618.

5. Ahmed, Abdelkareem A., et al. "Gum Arabic Modifies Glucocorticoid Metabolic Enzymes Gene Associated with Decreased Plasma Corticosterone Levels in Mice." Biomedical Journal of Scientific & Technical Research, vol. 31, no. 1, 2020, pp. 23917–23924

6. Ahallil, Hammad, Mohamad Yusof Maskat, Aminah Abdullah, and Shahrul Razid Sarbini. "The Effect of Acacia senegal as Potential Prebiotic on Obese Gut Microbiota Using In Vitro Batch Culture Fermentation." Food Research, vol. 4, no. 3, 2020, pp. 814–822,

7. Ahmed, Abdelkareem A., et al. "Gum Arabic Modifies Anti-Inflammatory Cytokine in Mice Fed with High Fat Diet Induced Obesity." Bioactive Carbohydrates and Dietary Fibre, vol. 25, 2021, p. 100258

8. Jarrar, Amjad H., et al. "The Effect of Gum Arabic (Acacia senegal) on Cardiovascular Risk Factors and Gastrointestinal Symptoms in Adults at Risk of Metabolic Syndrome: A Randomized Clinical Trial." Nutrients, vol. 13, no. 1, 2021, p. 194.

9. Ahmed, Abdelkareem A., et al. "Inhibition of Obesity Through Alterations of C/EBP-α Gene Expression by Gum Arabic in Mice with a High-Fat Feed Diet." Carbohydrate Polymer Technologies and Applications, vol. 4, 2022, p. 100231

CHAPTER 12

CANCER AND OXIDATIVE STRESS

How Hashab acts as an antioxidant and Helps Fight Cancer

In every cell in the mitochondria where energy is made. In the membranes that keep the cell's contents organized. In the nucleus where DNA is transcribed and repaired, there's a constant low-grade war between oxidative stress and antioxidant defense. Reactive oxygen species (superoxide, hydrogen peroxide, hydroxyl radicals) are generated as unavoidable byproducts of normal metabolism, and they're amplified by external stressors such as chemotherapy drugs, radiation, environmental toxins, chronic inflammation, and the contrast dyes used in medical imaging. Left unchecked, these free radicals burn through cellular machinery, oxidizing lipids in membranes, damaging proteins, and breaking DNA strands in ways that accumulate into mutations and, eventually, into cancer.

Previously, in the metabolism and satiety chapter, we watched Hashab gum teach appetite by modulating gut hormones and stress-hormone axes. Today we're asking a bolder question: What if a prebiotic could help the body resist the oxidative storms that oncology, cardiology, and even routine medical imaging throw at it? This chapter tells that story, from early studies in the oncology ward showing that Hashab gum protects hearts from chemotherapy damage to recent work showing it shields DNA from contrast-medium injury. The research always returns to the same idea that Hashab gum doesn't fight oxidative fire by dumping chemical foam; it

145

funds the firehouse, keeps the hydrants pressurized, and teaches the defense systems to respond faster and smarter.

Before we begin the journey through the research, let's teach two foundational concepts that frame the entire chapter. First, imagine the cell as a city under intermittent siege. The *glutathione battery* is the power grid that keeps the lights on and the defense systems running. Glutathione (GSH) is a small molecule made of three amino acids, and it exists in two forms: reduced (GSH, the charged battery) and oxidized (GSSG, the depleted battery). When free radicals attack, GSH donates electrons to neutralize them, sacrificing itself and becoming GSSG in the process.

The cell has enzymes that recharge GSSG back into GSH, but this recharging requires energy and raw materials. When the oxidative load is overwhelming, such as during chemotherapy, liver injury, and chronic inflammation, the glutathione pool becomes depleted. The battery runs down, and the city goes dark. Alongside glutathione are the *antioxidant triad*: three enzymes that form the front-line firefighting crew. Superoxide dismutase (SOD) converts superoxide radicals into hydrogen peroxide, a less reactive but still dangerous molecule. Catalase (CAT) breaks hydrogen peroxide into water and oxygen, harmless end products. Glutathione peroxidase (GPx) does the same job as catalase but uses glutathione as the electron donor, linking the enzyme crew to the battery system. When these three enzymes are functioning well and glutathione reserves are high, the cell can weather oxidative storms without permanent damage. When they're depleted or overwhelmed, membranes break down, proteins denature, and DNA accumulates the kind of damage that seeds cancer.

Second, there's a molecular see-saw that determines whether the cell leans toward defense or inflammation. On one side sits *Nrf2* (nuclear factor erythroid 2-related factor 2), a transcription factor that, when activated, migrates to the nucleus and turns on hundreds of genes encoding antioxidant enzymes, detoxification proteins, and repair machinery. Think of Nrf2 as the mayor who, sensing danger, orders the fire department to hire more firefighters, the power company to build more generators, and the repair crews to work double shifts. On the other side sits *NF-κB* (nuclear factor kappa-light-chain-enhancer of activated B cells), a transcription factor that, when activated, turns on genes encoding inflammatory cytokines like TNF-alpha and IL-6, immune-cell recruiting signals, and molecules that amplify the inflammatory cascade. NF-κB is the mayor who, sensing invasion, declares martial law and floods the streets with soldiers which is a necessary response to acute threats but a disaster if it becomes chronic.

Health is the state where the see-saw tilts toward Nrf2. When antioxidant defenses are upregulated, inflammation is kept in check, and the system stays resilient. Disease (cancer, cardiovascular disease, neurodegeneration) is the state where the see-saw tilts toward NF-κB where chronic inflammation overwhelms antioxidant capacity, oxidative damage accumulates, and tissues spiral toward dysfunction. The question for any intervention claiming to protect against oxidative stress is: *Which side of the see-saw does it favor?*

Now let's watch Acacia gum tip that see-saw, study by study, from a 2002 mouse model of chemotherapy cardiotoxicity to a 2024 phytochemical analysis revealing what's in the molecular cup.

Riyadh, Saudi Arabia, 2002. King Saud University, College of Pharmacy. Adel Abd-Allah and colleagues investigated whether "Arabic gum" could protect the heart from doxorubicin's oxidative cardiotoxicity. Doxorubicin treats cancer but also generates reactive oxygen species that damage cardiac tissue. Let's explain the mechanism briefly, because it's the archetype for understanding oxidative injury. Doxorubicin works partly by intercalating into DNA and blocking replication, which stops rapidly dividing cancer cells. However, it also undergoes *redox cycling* in the mitochondria of heart cells. The drug accepts an electron from mitochondrial enzymes, becomes a radical, transfers that electron to oxygen, and generates superoxide and hydrogen peroxide. This happens over and over, turning each doxorubicin molecule into a tiny superoxide generator.

Heart muscle, which is rich in mitochondria and beats constantly, is exquisitely vulnerable. Cardiomyocytes accumulate oxidative damage through lipid peroxidation in their membranes, protein oxidation in their contractile machinery, and mitochondrial dysfunction that impairs energy production resulting in dose-dependent heart failure. Oncologists call this *cardiotoxicity*, and it limits how much doxorubicin they can give, sometimes forcing them to stop treatment before the cancer is fully controlled. The therapeutic index is narrow with enough to kill the tumor, not so much that it kills the heart. Any intervention that could widen that window (protecting the heart without shielding the tumor) would be profoundly valuable.

The team administered a single intraperitoneal dose of doxorubicin (15 mg/kg) to mice, gave Arabic gum orally for five days before and 72 hours after dosing, and assessed injury at 72 hours. They measured serum creatine kinase and cardiac malondialdehyde as key biochemical markers of cardiac injury. They showed Arabic gum significantly lowered creatine kinase and malondialdehyde versus doxorubicin alone, and demonstrated superoxide scavenging in enzymatic and non-enzymatic systems [1].

Let's translate this for a general reader. The drug was still present in the animals, but the heart's oxidative burden was reduced. By scavenging superoxide and limiting lipid peroxidation, Arabic gum lessened membrane damage and leakage of muscle enzymes into blood. The data show reduced oxidative injury footprints. The heart thus retained more biochemical integrity while doxorubicin was still present [1].

This was an animal study, published before the microbiome revolution, so the investigators didn't measure SCFAs or microbial shifts. The pattern fit what we now understand. Slow fermentation of Hashab gum in the colon produces acetate, propionate, and butyrate, which enter circulation and have systemic anti-inflammatory and antioxidant effects. These effects are mostly indirect (SCFAs influence redox balance and immune signaling) rather than simple direct radical scavenging. The 2002 doxorubicin study opened the curiosity that if a food-grade prebiotic could support cardiac antioxidant defenses under chemotherapy, it belonged in the conversation about supportive cancer care, not just as a gut-health supplement.

Riyadh again, 2003. The same university, a year later. Ayman Gamal El-Din and colleagues turn their attention from the heart to the liver, from chemotherapy to the most common cause of acute liver failure in the developed world which is acetaminophen overdose. Let's explain the mechanism briefly, because it's the canonical model for understanding how glutathione depletion leads to tissue death. At therapeutic doses, acetaminophen (paracetamol, Tylenol) is safe; the liver conjugates it with sulfate and glucuronic acid, and it's excreted harmlessly. However, at high doses, those conjugation pathways saturate, and the liver shifts to a backup pathway where cytochrome P450 enzymes oxidize acetaminophen into a highly reactive metabolite called NAPQI (N-acetyl-p-benzoquinone imine). NAPQI is a vicious electrophile because it grabs electrons from anything nearby, oxidizing proteins and lipids indiscriminately. Normally, glutathione neutralizes NAPQI before it can do damage, donating electrons and forming a harmless conjugate. However, in overdose, glutathione is consumed faster than it can be regenerated. The battery dies. NAPQI runs wild, covalently binding to liver proteins, triggering oxidative cascades, and causing massive hepatocyte necrosis. Blood transaminases (ALT and AST enzymes that leak out of dying liver cells) spike into the thousands. Without treatment (the antidote is N-acetylcysteine, which replenishes glutathione), the liver fails, and the patient dies.

The researchers pretreated mice with oral "Arabic gum" (10% solution) for five days, administered intraperitoneal acetaminophen at a hepatotoxic dose, and assessed biochemical injury markers within hours. The Arabic gum treated mice had significantly lower transaminases and reduced hepatic malondialdehyde, indicating less hepatocellular leakage and lipid peroxidation. However, hepatic glutathione fell after acetaminophen and was not preserved by Arabic gum, and antioxidant enzyme activities were not reported. Serum nitrate plus nitrite, elevated by acetaminophen, were significantly reduced by pretreatment, consistent with mitigation of nitrosative stress. The protective effect mirrored the cardiac study in spirit. Arabic gum tempered oxidative and nitrosative injury footprints under a defined toxic insult [2].

The mechanism? The investigators concluded that hepatoprotection likely reflects attenuation of oxidative and nitrosative stress. What is demonstrated is a shift in redox burden with lower ALT/AST, lower MDA, and lower nitrate/nitrite when mice are pretreated with Arabic gum before acetaminophen. In plain terms, the drug insult was still present, but the liver leaked fewer enzymes and showed fewer chemical signs of lipid peroxidation and reactive nitrogen species formation. Arabic gum helped the organ maintain biochemical integrity under acetaminophen stress, consistent with reduced oxidative injury.

By 2003, the pattern was visible: two organs, two different toxins, same result. Hashab gum reduces biochemical markers of oxidative tissue damage. However, the field was slow to connect the dots, because Gum arabic was still categorized as an emulsifier, a texture agent, a boring industrial ingredient. That changed when a team in Argentina decided to write a review that would reframe the conversation.

Argentina, 2012. Universidad Nacional de Tucumán and INQUINOA-CONICET, a chemistry and photochemistry research institute. Mariana Montenegro and colleagues publish a review titled "Gum Arabic: More Than an Edible Emulsifier," and the title is the thesis. For decades, food scientists had focused on Acacia gum's functional properties of viscosity, film-forming, emulsion stability, encapsulation of flavors and oils.

Montenegro's team synthesized a different story researching how Gum arabic's arabinogalactan-protein structure, with its uronic-acid-rich polysaccharide backbone and covalently attached protein moieties, makes it a biological actor, not just a physical one. The uronic acids carry negative charges that catalyze free-radical reactions, reducing the Fenton chemistry that turns hydrogen peroxide into the devastating hydroxyl radical. The branched polysaccharide can form protective films around cells and around encapsulated bioactives, slowing oxidation and improving delivery. The AGP conjugates may directly scavenge certain radicals and when fermented, the produced SCFAs have anti-inflammatory effects that reduce the secondary oxidative stress generated by chronic immune activation [3].

This wasn't new data, it was a reframing, a synthesis that gave industry formulators and academic researchers permission to think of Acacia gum as nutritional armor rather than just a texture aid. The review cited older studies, placed them alongside emerging microbiome science and materials-chemistry insights. It argued that Gum arabic belonged in the conversation about functional foods, nutraceuticals, and supportive care in oxidative-stress diseases. It was published as a book chapter in an InTech open-access volume read by formulators, oncology nutritionists, and bioactives researchers. These are the people who decide what goes into next-generation supplements and medical foods.

The 2012 review was the conceptual hinge. After this, Gum arabic was no longer just "that thing that keeps soda syrup from separating". It was now a redox modulator, a delivery platform, and a prebiotic with systemic reach.

Nyala, **Sudan, 2016**. University of Nyala, a research group we've met several times in earlier chapters studying metabolic disease and obesity. Abdelkareem Ahmed and colleagues are asking whether Gum arabic's (Hashab gum from Acacia Senegal) antioxidant effects extend to endocrine organs. They fed female mice different diets, including a high-fat diet with 10% Hashab gum added, and then examined ovarian tissue measuring antioxidant enzyme activities, lipid peroxidation, and gene expression for oxidative-stress pathways [4].

The result is Hashab Gum improved antioxidant status in the ovary and modulated the expression of genes involved in oxidative-stress responses. This is where we first see evidence that Hashab gum boosts classical antioxidant enzymes in the ovary. The genes that shifted were reported as oxidative stress–related targets alongside higher antioxidant enzyme activities, consistent with enhanced redox defenses in ovarian tissue under dietary stress. When antioxidant defenses rise, downstream inflammatory signaling can diminish, yet specific pathways were not included here [4].

Why does the ovary matter? Because it's an organ under constant oxidative

152

stress (ovulation itself is an inflammatory, ROS-generating event) and because ovarian oxidative damage is implicated in infertility, premature aging of oocytes, and ovarian cancer. Showing that Hashab gum improves ovarian redox status under diet-induced metabolic stress suggests that the spillover effects of gut-microbiome modulation and SCFA production can reach endocrine tissues, though this paper did not measure SCFAs directly. This is the systems-level story showing Hashab gum isn't a targeted therapy for one organ; it's a rising tide that lifts multiple boats by calming inflammation and funding antioxidant defenses everywhere [4].

Khartoum, Sudan, 2017. We move from mice to humans, and from controlled lab toxins to a disease that bathes the body in oxidative stress: sickle cell anemia. Lamis Kaddam and colleagues at Alneelain University conducted what they describe as a Phase II trial in patients with sickle cell disease, testing whether daily Gum arabic (Hashab gum from Acacia Senegal) could improve their antioxidant status [5].

In sickle cell anemia, a single amino-acid change in hemoglobin makes red cells prone to "sickling" in low-oxygen conditions. Sickled cells become rigid, block small vessels (causing pain and organ damage), and break apart, releasing free hemoglobin and iron into the circulation. Free hemoglobin and iron strongly promote reactive oxygen species, including hydroxyl radicals. Patients live under chronic oxidative pressure whereby antioxidant defenses are chronically taxed, oxidative damage accumulates, and inflammatory activity is often elevated. It is one of the clearest human examples of long-term oxidative stress, which makes it a useful real-world test of any putative antioxidant intervention.

In this study, forty-seven patients with homozygous sickle cell anemia (HbSS), aged 5–42 years, were recruited from outpatient hematology clinics. All were in steady-state (no recent transfusions or hospitalizations for crisis). They received 30 g per day of Hashab gum powder (from *"Acacia senegal"*) dissolved in water each morning for 12 weeks. Total antioxidant capacity (TAC), malondialdehyde (MDA), and hydrogen peroxide (H_2O_2) were measured before and after supplementation, and complete blood counts were also obtained. Not every participant completed the full 12 weeks at the target dose (some received Hashab gum for 9–10 weeks) but their last available measurements were included as post-treatment values [5].

The biochemical signal was strong. After Hashab gum intake, TAC increased significantly ($P < 0.001$), while MDA and H_2O_2 (both markers of oxidative stress) fell significantly ($P < 0.05$ and $P < 0.005$, respectively). No control group was included, so the study is pre–post rather than randomized, and it was not designed to formally evaluate pain crises, hemolysis markers, or long-term clinical outcomes. Nonetheless, in a cohort known to have high oxidative load, Hashab gum shifted the redox balance toward higher antioxidant capacity and lower oxidative damage markers over the treatment period [5].

As a result, this 2017 trial functions as a biochemical proof-of-concept bridge from animal toxicology models to human disease. Previous work in rodents had shown that Hashab gum reduces oxidative damage in heart, liver, and kidney under toxic stress. Here we see that its antioxidant effects extend to people with a chronically oxidant-heavy condition. The study does not prove fewer crises or better survival, but it does support the idea that Hashab gum is more than a gut-only prebiotic. Hashab gum behaves as a systemic redox modulator, raising the antioxidant "ceiling" and lowering the oxidative "floor" in a disease where both are badly skewed. In the broader picture of Hashab gum research, this oxidative improvement complements anti-inflammatory findings from other settings, reinforcing the concept that calmer inflammation and stronger antioxidant defenses work together to reduce cumulative tissue damage in oxidative-stress–driven diseases.

Nanjing, China, 2018. Nanjing Agricultural University. Mohammed Hamid and colleagues are testing a hypothesis with profound practical implications: *Can you pair Gum arabic with another protective agent like selenium-enriched yeast and get synergistic benefits that exceed either alone* [6]?

Let's introduce the concept of *adjunctive synergy*. It's the idea that combining agents with complementary mechanisms can amplify protection. Selenium is an essential trace element and a cofactor for glutathione peroxidase, one of the antioxidant triad enzymes. Selenium deficiency impairs GPx activity, leaving cells vulnerable to hydrogen peroxide. Selenium supplementation, especially in bioavailable forms like selenium yeast (where selenium is organically incorporated into yeast proteins), boosts GPx and improves antioxidant capacity. However, selenium alone doesn't address inflammation, barrier function, or the microbial production of SCFAs. Gum arabic does all of those, but it doesn't provide selenium. Pairing them could deliver both the enzymatic boost (selenium $\rightarrow$ GPx) and the systemic modulation (acacia $\rightarrow$ SCFAs $\rightarrow$ Nrf2 tilt, NF-κB quieting, barrier support).

The researchers induced chronic liver injury in rats using carbon tetrachloride (a classic hepatotoxin that generates free radicals and drives fibrosis) and treated animals with selenium yeast, Gum arabic, the combination, or neither. The combination outperformed either agent alone with better preservation of antioxidant enzymes, lower oxidative damage, and critically less collagen deposition and fibrosis (the scarring that turns chronic liver injury into cirrhosis). The synergy was real, and the

155

mechanism was plausible. Selenium fed the enzymatic machinery (GPx), while Gum arabic reduced the inflammatory drive (NF-κB cytokines, immune-cell recruitment) that perpetuates injury and fibrosis. Gum arabic's film-forming properties may also have improved selenium's bioavailability or tissue distribution, though the study didn't prove that mechanistically [6].

This reframes Gum arabic as a platform ingredient which is something that not only has its own benefits but amplifies partners, making it ideal for combination strategies in supportive oncology nutrition, where patients often need multiple micronutrients (selenium, zinc, vitamin D, omega-3s) but struggle with polypharmacy and pill burden. A single, well-tolerated prebiotic that enhances delivery and efficacy of co-supplements is profoundly practical. More research on synergy in a later chapter.

Kuala Lumpur, Malaysia, 2018. A brief technical aside, but an important one for understanding where the field was heading. Ahmed A. M. Elnour, Mohamed E. S. Mirghani, and colleagues at the International Islamic University Malaysia optimized ultrasonic-assisted extraction conditions for Gum arabic, showing that carefully controlled ultrasound (time, temperature, and power) can increase the yield of phenolic compounds and boost measurable antioxidant activity in gum extracts.

This matters because it hints at what we discuss later. Acacia isn't just a big polysaccharide. It also contains trace phenolics, minerals, and other small bioactive molecules that may contribute to its biological effects [7]. Optimizing how these compounds are extracted (for lab studies or for standardized products) improves reproducibility and can maximize potential health benefits. This work contributed to the growing methodological toolkit for extracting and characterizing antioxidant and phytochemical components from Gum arabic, helping frame later efforts to study its smaller bioactive molecules in more detail.

Kuala Lumpur, Malaysia, 2020. A Malaysian nanotechnology and food-science team. Abdelkader Hassani and colleagues publish a paper that represents the modern frontier of using Gum arabic not just as an active ingredient but as a bio-carrier for other actives. They create gallic-acid nanoparticles stabilized by Gum arabic. These are essentially nano-sized assemblies of gallic acid (a potent polyphenol with strong radical scavenging activity) associated with Gum arabic's arabinogalactan-protein matrix [8].

Let's explain why this matters. Gallic acid has impressive antioxidant activity in test systems, but it has low bioavailability and is rapidly cleared. Encapsulating or stabilizing it in nanoparticles can improve dispersion, protect it from degradation, modulate release, and enhance cellular uptake. The problem has always been that making nanoparticles requires a stabilizer to prevent aggregation. Synthetic surfactants work but can raise toxicity concerns. Gum arabic, with its amphiphilic AGP structure (hydrophilic polysaccharide with hydrophobic protein regions), is a natural emulsifier and stabilizer that is food-grade and biocompatible.

The Malaysian team showed that Gum-arabic-stabilized gallic-acid nanoparticles displayed stronger radical-scavenging activity than free gallic acid and demonstrated selective cytotoxicity and uptake in cancer cell lines with low toxicity in normal cells. The nanoparticles were stable with sizes ranging approximately from 35 to 250 nm and exhibited pH-dependent release behavior. This is a modern reason Gum arabic appears in high-performance health formulations. It acts as a gentle nano-carrier, delivering polyphenols and vitamins more effectively than crude mixtures..

The oxidative-protection and delivery-platform stories converge as Gum arabic can both enhance antioxidant performance of cargo and provide a biocompatible carrier to improve targeting and cellular effects in vitro [8].

Remarkably, this study also gives us a chance to highlight some of the modern and even futuristic nano-technological uses of Hashab gum, where it offers both powerful synergy (more on that later) and effective function as a dual carrier.

Menoufia, Egypt, 2021. Menoufia University, Zoology Department.

Islam El-Garawani and colleagues are conducting a study with direct translational relevance by testing whether Arabic gum (Hashab gum and Acacia Senegal) can protect against the oxidative and genotoxic stress caused by radiographic contrast media. Let's teach *contrast-induced oxidative and genotoxic stress*, because it's the bridge to the next chapter and it's an underappreciated source of iatrogenic (medically caused) injury. Iodinated contrast agents (used in CT scans, angiograms, and other imaging procedures) are generally safe, but they generate reactive oxygen species in tissues, particularly in the kidneys, where they're concentrated during excretion. The ROS damage tubular epithelial cells, causing oxidative stress, inflammation, and in some cases acute kidney injury and the damage isn't just local.

Contrast agents cause systemic oxidative stress and *genotoxicity* (DNA damage measurable by specific assays). Let's define those assays, because they're the gold standard for detecting the kind of cellular injury that seeds cancer. The *comet assay* measuring DNA strand breaks process: 1-embed cells in gel, 2-lyse them gently to release DNA, 3-apply an electric field; damaged DNA migrates out of the nucleus, forming a "comet tail" visible under fluorescence microscopy with longer tails meaning more breaks.

Micronuclei are small fragments of chromosomes or whole chromosomes that get left behind during cell division when DNA damage is severe. Soaring micronuclei in bone-marrow or blood cells is a biomarker of chromosomal instability and cancer risk. *8-OHdG* (8-hydroxy-2'-deoxyguanosine) is an oxidized form of a DNA base, guanine, and its presence in urine or tissue is a direct readout of oxidative DNA damage. All three assays tell you the same story. When oxidative stress overwhelms repair systems, the genome takes hits that could eventually become mutations.

The Egyptian study gave rats ioxitalamate (a common iodinated contrast agent) and co-treated one group with Hashab gum. They then measured comet-assay DNA damage in leukocytes, chromosomal aberrations and mitotic index in bone marrow, DNA fragmentation in kidney tissue, and standard oxidative-stress markers in kidney (MDA, nitric oxide, catalase, and glutathione), along with serum urea and creatinine.
The study concluded that Hashab Gum reduced multiple measures of DNA damage and improved antioxidant defenses [9]. Comet damage scores were lower, chromosomal aberrations and DNA fragmentation decreased, MDA and nitric oxide levels dropped, and catalase and glutathione levels were higher than with contrast alone.

This is real genome protection, the kind of effect that, sustained over years, reduces cancer risk. It's clinically meaningful because millions of people undergo contrast-enhanced imaging annually. A safe, well-tolerated daily supplement that reduces the genotoxic burden of medical imaging might, if similar effects occur in humans, contribute to lowering lifetime cancer risk, particularly in patients who require repeated imaging [9].

This study is also an explicit handoff to the next chapter. Contrast-induced nephrotoxicity (kidney injury from imaging agents) is a major clinical problem, especially in patients with pre-existing kidney disease or diabetes. The mechanisms overlap completely with the oxidative-protection story we've been telling. ROS generation, glutathione depletion, lipid peroxidation, inflammatory amplification, and tubular damage. If Hashab gum protects DNA and antioxidant systems from contrast-medium stress, the same mechanisms should protect the kidneys, where contrast is concentrated and where oxidative injury translates into acute and chronic renal dysfunction. The 2021 genotoxicity paper plants the flag placing Hashab gum as a candidate for preventing contrast-induced kidney injury.

Kuwait, 2022. A physiology team investigated one of the most clinically relevant oxidative injuries (myocardial ischemia-reperfusion) using isolated Langendorff-perfused Wistar rat hearts. Let's define *ischemia-reperfusion (I/R) injury*, because it's the oxidative paradox at the heart of cardiology, surgery, and oncology. Ischemia occurs when blood flow to an organ is blocked during a heart attack, during surgery when vessels are clamped, during a stroke, or when a chemotherapy port causes a local thrombosis. Tissues starve for oxygen, metabolism shifts to anaerobic pathways, and cellular machinery starts to fail. However, the real damage often happens during *reperfusion*, when blood flow is restored.

The sudden reintroduction of oxygen causes a massive spike in reactive oxygen species. Mitochondria, damaged by ischemia, leak electrons directly onto oxygen, generating superoxide. Xanthine oxidase (an enzyme that normally produces uric acid) shifts during ischemia and upon reperfusion spews out superoxide and hydrogen peroxide. Neutrophils, recruited by inflammatory signals, arrive and release more ROS. The antioxidant systems, depleted during ischemia, are overwhelmed. Membranes peroxidize, proteins denature, calcium floods into cells causing contractile failure, and cells undergo necrosis or apoptosis. Cardiologists call this "reperfusion injury" and it can account for up to half of the final infarct size after a heart attack. Preventing or limiting I/R injury is a major therapeutic target.

In this study, hearts were assigned to sham, I/R control, GA-only sham, or GA pretreatment protocols for 4 weeks, 2 weeks, or 2 hours before isolation. A separate group received GA only at the onset of reperfusion. Hemodynamics (developed pressure, LVEDP, coronary flow, coronary vascular resistance) were continuously computed, infarct size quantified by TTC staining, and cardiomyocyte injury tracked via CK and LDH in effluent. Oxidative and inflammatory indices were assessed as total oxidant, antioxidant status, SOD in heart tissue, cytokines (TNF α, IL-1β, IL-6, IL-10), total oxidants in heart tissue and coronary effluent. Gum arabic pretreatment for 4 or 2 weeks, and even a single IV dose 2 hours prior, significantly improved left-ventricular and coronary dynamics, reduced infarct size, and lowered CK/LDH versus untreated I/R controls. These regimens decreased pro-inflammatory cytokines (TNF-α, IL-1β, IL-6), increased IL-10, reduced total oxidants, and increased SOD, consistent with dual anti-inflammatory and antioxidant protection [10]. By contrast, adding GA only at reperfusion failed to confer hemodynamic or biochemical protection, underscoring the importance of exposure before ischemia or early pre-ischemic priming. This pattern aligns with an integrated defense demonstrating less oxidative burden, more antioxidant capacity, and a cytokine milieu shifted toward resolution during reperfusion. Taken together, GA pretreatment preserved function and limited necrosis in this I/R model while modulating canonical inflammatory signals [10].

Let's tie this back to the 2002 doxorubicin cardiotoxicity study. Different decade, different lab, different insult (I/R versus chemotherapy), but the same underlying pattern. The broader implication is continuity with earlier cardiotoxic-stress paradigms. When myocardium faces overwhelming oxidative and inflammatory stress, prior GA exposure helps maintain defensive capacity and blunts injury propagation. The mechanistic readouts here were SOD, total oxidants, and cytokines rather than glutathione or catalase. Importantly, the directional effects support an antioxidant and anti-inflammatory framework. When cardiac tissue faces overwhelming oxidative stress, Gum arabic helps it maintain defensive capacity. Such findings nominate Gum arabic as a candidate adjunct for preconditioning contexts where predictable ischemic insults occur, pending translational validation in vivo.

In short, Gum arabic priming quieted reperfusion's storm and improved core injury metrics in isolated rat hearts. The 2022 I/R study is the bookend to the 2002 oncology doorway; twenty years of evidence converging on one conclusion: Acacia funds the Antioxidant firehouse [10,1].

Ouargla, Algeria, 2024. École Normale Supérieure, a phytochemistry and natural-products research group. Khirani Safia and colleagues publish a comprehensive analysis of the phytochemical composition and biological activities of aqueous Gum arabic extracts (Hashab gum from Acacia Senegal). This is the "what's in the brew?" moment, the chemical accounting that explains why Hashab's effects are broader than you'd predict from the polysaccharide alone. They report qualitative phytochemical classes in the aqueous extract revealing saponins, flavonoids, tannins, and alkaloids, with anthocyanins absent. They also confirm antioxidant activity using a DPPH radical-scavenging assay, alongside antibacterial and anti-inflammatory tests [11].

Let's teach *phytochemical co-constituents* briefly. Beyond the big arabinogalactan-protein structure that defines Hashab gum, aqueous extracts (the kind used in most animal and human studies) contain a suite of minor compounds that co-extract. These aren't the primary actives, but they color the edges. Phenolics are direct radical scavengers and can modulate signaling pathways. Qualitative screening in this work reported saponins, flavonoids, tannins, and alkaloids alongside measurable DPPH antioxidant activity. The trace contributions aren't high enough to meet daily-value recommendations, but they can add to bioactivity detected in antioxidant and anti-inflammatory assays. The 2024 phytochemical profile legitimizes the "more than fiber" claim without over-promising. Within Hashab, the polysaccharide is the platform (it ferments, produces SCFAs, supports the barrier, modulates immunity) and the phytochemicals add redox capacity to the whole [11].

This is also a reminder that identity and purity matter. Authentic Hashab gum aka Acacia senegal gum (which as we stated before is not a scientific name anymore because the name Acacia was stolen by Australian lobbyists detailed in the book "The Acacia heist") has a consistent phytochemical fingerprint. Adulterated or low-grade gums (substituted with other species or over processed) lose these co-constituents and deliver inconsistent bioactivity.

The 2024 Algeria paper, paired with the 2012 Argentina review, closes the compositional loop. We know what's in the cup, and we know it's biologically relevant.

The oxidative-stress story flows seamlessly into the next frontier of kidney protection. Every mechanism we've discussed (glutathione preservation, antioxidant-enzyme support, Nrf2 activation, NF-κB suppression, barrier integrity, DNA shielding) applies with special urgency to the kidneys, where oxidative insults converge from multiple directions. Chemotherapy drugs (cisplatin, doxorubicin, methotrexate) accumulate in kidneys and drive nephrotoxicity through oxidative stress and inflammation. Uremic toxins, which build up when kidney function declines, generate ROS and exacerbate the inflammatory milieu, creating a vicious cycle of kidney damage → toxin retention → more oxidative stress → more damage. Additionally, diabetes, hypertension, and obesity (the leading causes of chronic kidney disease) all involve chronic oxidative stress and inflammatory activation in renal tissue.

We've already seen the protective tools Hashab gum brings. It raises antioxidant capacity (higher GSH, SOD, CAT, as seen in the doxorubicin, acetaminophen, I/R, and contrast studies); it dampens inflammatory cytokines (lower TNF-alpha, higher IL-10, as seen across multiple chapters); it protects DNA from oxidative damage (reduced comet tails and 8-OHdG, as seen in the contrast study); it stabilizes barriers and reduces permeability (mucosal cytoprotection in the ulcer study); and it delivers protective co-factors like selenium without toxicity (as seen in the China liver-fibrosis study).

All these mechanisms are directly relevant to nephroprotection with a microbiome angle that's kidney-specific. When gut bacteria ferment fiber, they consume urea that diffuses from blood into the colon, reducing the nitrogen burden that damaged kidneys struggle to clear and lowering uremic-toxin levels that drive oxidative stress systemically. This was touched on in the diabetes chapter's CKD discussion, and it will be front and center in the kidney chapter.

The next chapter will take us from the molecular redox chemistry we've explored here into the clinical nephrology suite. It will include animal models of contrast-induced injury, drug-induced kidney injury and observational studies in CKD patients. The oxidative-stress story and the kidney story aren't separate; they're the same biology applied to the organ that filters the blood, concentrates toxins, and dies quietly when overwhelmed. Hashab gum, by steadying the redox balance and calming the inflammatory tone before the insult ever reaches the nephron, becomes a first-line defense. That's where we're headed next. It's the place where prebiotic spillover, antioxidant resilience, and microbial nitrogen recycling converge to protect the body's most vulnerable filter, one gentle fermentation at a time.

References:

1. Abd-Allah, Adel R. A., et al. "Protective Effect of Arabic Gum against Cardiotoxicity Induced by Doxorubicin in Mice: A Possible Mechanism of Protection." Journal of Biochemical and Molecular Toxicology, vol. 16, no. 5, 2002, pp. 254–259

2. Gamal el-din, Ayman M., et al. "Protective Effect of Arabic Gum against Acetaminophen-Induced Hepatotoxicity in Mice." Pharmacological Research, vol. 48, no. 6, 2003, pp. 631–635.

3. Montenegro, Mariana A., et al. "Gum Arabic: More Than an Edible Emulsifier." Products and Applications of Biopolymers, edited by InTech, 2012, pp. 1-26

4. Ahmed, Abdelkareem A., et al. "Gum Arabic Supplementation Improved Antioxidant Status and Alters Expression of Oxidative Stress Gene in Ovary of Mice Fed High Fat Diet." Middle East Fertility Society Journal, vol. 21, no. 2, 2016, pp. 101–108.

5. Kaddam, Lamis, et al. "Gum Arabic as Novel Anti-Oxidant Agent in Sickle Cell Anemia, Phase II Trial." BMC Hematology, vol. 17, 2017, p. 4.

6. Hamid, Mohammed E., et al. "The Hepatoprotective Effect of Selenium-Enriched Yeast and Gum Arabic Combination on Carbon Tetrachloride-Induced Chronic Liver Injury in Rats." Journal of Food Science, vol. 83, no. 2, 2018, pp. 525–534.

7. Elnour, Mohamed, et al. "Gum Arabic: An Optimization of Ultrasonic-Assisted Extraction of Antioxidant Activity." Studia Universitatis Babeş-Bolyai Chemia, vol. 63, no. 3, 2018, pp. 95–116

8. Hassani, Abdelkader, et al. "Preparation, Characterization and Therapeutic Properties of Gum Arabic-Stabilized Gallic Acid Nanoparticles." Scientific Reports, vol. 10, no. 1, 2020, p. 17808.

9. El-Garawani, Islam M., et al. "The Ameliorative Role of Acacia senegal Gum against the Oxidative Stress and Genotoxicity Induced by the Radiographic Contrast Medium (Ioxitalamate) in Albino Rats." Antioxidants, vol. 10, no. 2, 2021, p. 221.

10. Gouda, Eman, and Fawzi Babiker. "Gum Arabic Protects the Rat Heart from Ischemia/Reperfusion Injury through Anti-Inflammatory and Antioxidant Pathways." Scientific Reports, vol. 12, 2022, article 17235

11. Khirani, Safia, et al. "The Biological Activities and Phytochemical Investigations of Acacia senegal's Aqueous Extracts of Gum Arabic." Brazilian Applied Science Review, vol. 8, no. 2, 2024, pp. 1–14.

CHAPTER 13

How Hashab helps the Kidney Breath Again

The bridge from yesterday's chapter is direct and urgent. Chemotherapy drugs generate cascades of superoxide radicals in cardiac mitochondria. Iodinated contrast agents spray reactive oxygen through renal tubules during medical imaging. High-fat diets kindle inflammatory fires in hepatocytes. Dysbiotic gut communities leak bacterial endotoxins into the bloodstream, activating immune cells that amplify oxidative damage systemically. Every insult we documented in the cancer and oxidative-stress chapter (pharmacologic, dietary, microbial) shares a common thread: they flood vulnerable tissues with oxidative and nitrosative sparks that overwhelm cellular defenses, break DNA, peroxidize membranes, and trigger the inflammatory amplification that turns acute injury into chronic disease.

The kidneys stand at the confluence of all these storms. They filter one hundred and eighty liters of blood daily, concentrating toxins and wastes in their delicate tubules before excreting them as urine. They see the highest concentrations of chemotherapy metabolites as those drugs are cleared from blood. They face the densest exposure to contrast agents, which accumulate in tubular cells during excretion and generate reactive species that damage the very cells trying to eliminate them. They receive the full burden of uremic toxins (indoxyl sulfate, p-cresyl sulfate, trimethylamine N-oxide) that dysbiotic gut bacteria produce when fermenting protein instead of fiber. These toxins inflame tubular epithelium and accelerate the vicious cycle of kidney damage. Additionally, they also bear the metabolic consequences of diabetes and hypertension, where chronic hyperglycemia and elevated blood pressure grind away at the glomerular filtration barrier and tubular machinery year after year, causing the slow-motion collapse we call chronic kidney disease.

If there were an organ that needed the slow, steady, systems-level protection we've been building across eleven chapters it would be the kidney. Today's kidneys are starving for recharged glutathione batteries, Nrf2-tilted gene programs that upregulate defensive enzymes, calmed NF-κB signaling that prevents inflammatory amplification, tightened gut barriers that reduce endotoxin translocation, and microbiome shifts toward short-chain fatty acid production. This chapter tells the story of how that protection moved from desert wisdom to metabolic ward, from animal crystalluria models to dialysis units, until a substance most people knew only as a soft drink additive quietly and convincingly became the kidney's most reliable natural ally. Not through heroic pharmacologic intervention, not through aggressive calorie restriction or dialysis intensification, but through a gentle recalibration of the gut-renal axis that allows damaged nephrons to function a little longer, a little better, day after day.

The Old Sudanese Hunch the Laboratory Finally Measured

Ask a nurse in Omdurman or Khartoum why Hashab gum powder sits on the shelf next to the prescription medications, and you'll hear an answer that sounds almost mythical until you understand the biochemistry beneath it, "It lightens the blood ". For generations, families caring for relatives with kidney disease have given them a daily spoonful of Hashab gum dissolved in water or tea. The phrase "lightening the blood" is a local term describing patients feeling less nauseated, their appetites improved, their fatigue eased slightly, and when blood was drawn, the urea nitrogen numbers edged downward in ways that the medications alone couldn't fully explain.

This wasn't superstition. It was empirical observation passed through generations, the kind of pattern recognition that precedes mechanism by centuries. Only later did the metabolic-ward nitrogen-balance studies, the histology slides showing preserved tubular architecture, the microbiome sequencing revealing shifts away from uremic-toxin producers, and the inflammatory-marker panels showing dropping C-reactive protein finally explain what those nurses and families had sensed. When you feed the colon the right fermentable substrate you create a second nitrogen-excretion pathway that shares the burden with failing kidneys. You shift gut bacterial metabolism away from *proteolysis* that generates vascular toxins and toward *saccharolysis* that produces anti-inflammatory short-chain fatty acids. You dampen the oxidative and nitrosative fires that burn through tubular cells. You quiet the cytokine storms that recruit immune cells into the kidney interstitium and drive the fibrosis that turns reversible injury into permanent scarring. You preserve the cellular machinery (the ion pumps, the mitochondria, the DNA-repair systems) that keeps nephrons filtering blood and reabsorbing what the body needs to keep, even when those nephrons are damaged and struggling.

This chapter follows that clinical hunch from folklore to formal evidence. From a tightly controlled metabolic ward in Philadelphia in the mid-1990s where every gram of dietary nitrogen was accounted for, through animal facilities in Muscat where researchers used crystal-induced kidney injury to dissect molecular mechanisms. We will explore clinics in Baghdad where affordability and tolerability determine whether interventions could scale beyond academic centers, through diabetic-nephropathy models in Germany where the metabolic-renal connection became visible, and finally into dialysis units in Khartoum where patients living with relentless oxidative stress and inflammation showed measurable improvements in antioxidant capacity and cardiovascular risk markers.

The arc spans three decades, four continents, and arrives at one persistent, reproducible finding. When you give people or animals with damaged kidneys a daily dose of Hashab gum (fifteen to thirty grams dissolved in beverages or mixed into foods) their kidneys work better. Not miraculously, not completely, but measurably, reproducibly, and safely, in ways that matter for quality of life and survival. Blood urea nitrogen drops. Serum creatinine stabilizes or declines. Inflammatory markers cool. Oxidative-damage biomarkers improve. Fibrosis slows. Filtration holds on longer. Albuminuria (the protein leak through damaged glomeruli that predicts cardiovascular events) decreases. Critically, patients tolerate the intervention well enough to keep taking it for months or years, which is the only timeline on which these biochemical shifts translate into preserved kidney function.

This is the story of how Hashab gum moved from food additive to renal ally, not by overpowering physiology with pharmacologic force but by re-tuning it at multiple nodes simultaneously, working with the body's own systems rather than against them. It's a story about nitrogen, about oxidation, about inflammation, about microbes, and ultimately about the quiet resilience of tissues when you remove some of the burden they're carrying and give their defensive systems time and fuel to recover.

1996 - The First Clinical Nudge

Philadelphia, Pennsylvania. University of Pennsylvania School of Nursing, a metabolic research unit where precision matters more than comfort and where patients with chronic renal failure agree to follow research-level nutritional monitoring that only strict protocols demand. Donna Zimmaro Bliss and her colleagues are testing an idea that sounds almost too simple. *If damaged kidneys struggle to clear the nitrogen waste that accumulates from dietary protein, and if you can't reduce protein intake much further without risking malnutrition, could you create an alternative excretion route by feeding gut bacteria the right substrate?*

The experimental design was elegant in its rigor. Patients consumed carefully controlled low-protein diets; the standard nephrology approach for slowing disease progression by reducing the nitrogen load that failing kidneys must clear. Every gram of protein, every milligram of nitrogen, was weighed and recorded. Researchers tracked nitrogen like accountants manage money, measuring inputs (dietary protein...) and outputs (urea in urine, nitrogen in stool), and estimating small additional losses through skin and other minor routes with standard formulas. In a healthy person, the equation balances with nitrogen in equals nitrogen out. However, in chronic kidney disease, the primary output route (urea clearance through glomerular filtration) fails progressively. Blood urea nitrogen rises. Patients develop uremic syndrome including nausea, vomiting, confusion, and metabolic poisoning that comes from accumulated waste. The standard interventions are limited including restrict dietary protein (which helps but risks malnutrition), dialyze (which works but requires vascular access, costs, time, and comes with its own complications), or transplant (which requires a donor organ and works beautifully but is available to only a small fraction of patients who need it).

Bliss and her team asked what if we could offload some of that nitrogen burden to the colon? Normally, the colon is a minor player in nitrogen metabolism. Some urea diffuses from blood into the gut lumen (the concentration gradient favors movement from the nitrogen-rich bloodstream into the gut) but without the right conditions, that urea is either reabsorbed or converted to ammonia, which can actually worsen uremia. However, when you provide gut bacteria with fermentable prebiotics (a rich energy source they can metabolize) they grow, and growing bacteria need nitrogen to build their proteins and nucleic acids. That nitrogen can come from either dietary protein or urea diffusing into the colon from the bloodstream. Healthy people with normal kidney function don't rely much on the second route because their kidneys clear urea efficiently as blood urea stays low, so there's not much gradient. However, in kidney disease, blood urea is markedly elevated, the concentration gradient is steep, urea diffuses into the colon in larger quantities, and if bacteria are actively fermenting fiber and need nitrogen for growth, they'll assimilate that urea into their biomass. Those bacteria then leave the body the natural way (in stool) taking the nitrogen with them.

Let's teach this mechanism clearly, because it's the conceptual foundation for everything that follows. *Fecal nitrogen trapping* works like this. You feed patients Hashab Gum, a slowly fermented, highly branched arabinogalactan polysaccharide that only beneficial gut bacteria (probiotics) can metabolize through cooperative enzyme systems. It takes time, typically twelve to twenty-four hours, and happens deep in the colon rather than in the proximal gut. As those probiotics ferment the Hashab, they multiply. Growing bacteria need nitrogen. They pull urea from the bloodstream across the colonic epithelium, incorporate it into their cellular machinery, and when those bacteria are eventually shed into stool and eliminated, the nitrogen leaves with them. You've converted a toxic blood constituent into harmless bacterial protein and excreted it out. The blood urea drops without requiring the kidneys to filter more. The colon has become, functionally, a second excretory organ.

The 1996 Pennsylvania study results felt like a metabolic sleight of hand. Kidney patients supplemented with Gum arabic excreted significantly more nitrogen in their stool compared to the low-protein diet alone, and their blood urea nitrogen levels dropped measurably [1]. The fiber was generally well tolerated, with no increase in stool frequency or diarrhea as about half the patients reported flatulence, mostly in the first two weeks. Patients kept taking it daily for weeks, which allowed the nitrogen-trapping effect to accumulate and blood urea to stabilize at lower levels. This was not a minor metabolic curiosity. It was a dietary strategy that could scale to real patients eating real food in their own kitchens, the kind of intervention nephrologists dream about. Safe, simple, affordable, and effective at lowering serum urea nitrogen and increasing fecal nitrogen excretion in this short trial.

Historically, this study accomplished something crucial. It took a Sudanese clinical tradition (the practice of giving Hashab to kidney patients) and subjected it to the gold standard of metabolic research. It moved Gum arabic from the category of "traditional remedies" (interesting but unproven) to "evidence-based dietary intervention" (mechanistically understood and quantitatively validated). Western nephrologists, trained to be skeptical of folk medicine and demanding controlled trials, now had nitrogen-balance data from a peer-reviewed journal published by a respected academic institution. The conversation could shift from "Does it work?" to "How can we implement this?". It made space for the animal studies that would follow to dissect cellular mechanisms, and it provided clinical justification for eventually testing Acacia in dialysis populations and chronic kidney disease clinics worldwide.

2002 - The Cytoprotection Door Opens

Riyadh, Saudi Arabia. King Saud University College of Pharmacy. If the 1996 Pennsylvania study showed that Gum arabic could help kidneys by redirecting nitrogen waste, the next logical question was whether Arabic gum could protect kidney cells directly when the injury came not from accumulated metabolic waste but from a focused chemical assault. The Saudi researchers chose one of nephrology's canonical toxins called gentamicin (an aminoglycoside antibiotic that saves lives by killing Gram-negative bacteria but damages kidneys by accumulating in the proximal tubular cells that try to reabsorb it).

Let's teach *gentamicin nephrotoxicity* as a clinical problem before discussing the experimental findings, because this injury pattern plays out daily in hospitals worldwide. Gentamicin is cheap, effective, and widely used for serious infections such as sepsis from abdominal sources, hospital-acquired pneumonias, and complicated urinary-tract infections where resistant organisms are suspected. However, unlike antibiotics that are rapidly filtered and excreted, gentamicin lingers. Proximal tubular cells (the workhorses of the nephron that reabsorb most of the filtrate and return water, sodium, glucose, and amino acids to the bloodstream) take up gentamicin through endocytic pathways intended for reclaiming filtered proteins.

Once inside these cells, gentamicin accumulates in lysosomes and mitochondria, where it disrupts protein synthesis, generates reactive oxygen species through mitochondrial electron-transport-chain dysfunction, and triggers apoptotic cascades (the programmed cell death that cells initiate when they sense irreparable damage). Clinically, serum creatinine rises as filtration falls. Blood urea nitrogen climbs. Tubular epithelial cells necrose and slough into the urine. In severe cases, oliguria develops (urine output drops) and acute kidney injury forces temporary dialysis. The therapeutic challenge is brutal as you need to give enough antibiotic to kill the infection, but not so much that you destroy the kidneys. Dosing protocols walk this tightrope by monitoring drug levels and kidney function daily, but injury still occurs, especially in patients who are elderly, dehydrated, or receiving other nephrotoxic drugs simultaneously.

174

The Saudi team designed an animal study to test whether co-treatment with Arabic gum could widen the therapeutic window. They gave rats gentamicin at doses calibrated to produce reliable kidney injury, then assigned one group to receive gentamicin alone and another group to receive gentamicin plus Arabic gum in their drinking water throughout the 8-day exposure period. After eight days (long enough for cumulative nephrotoxicity to manifest) they harvested kidneys and measured the injury markers serum urea and serum creatinine (standard kidney function tests), kidney histology under light microscopy (looking for tubular necrosis and inflammatory infiltrates), oxidative-stress markers (malondialdehyde from lipid peroxidation), and kidney tissue glutathione levels (the rechargeable antioxidant reserve) [2].

The protective effect was clear and consistent with Arabic gum significantly blunting gentamicin nephrotoxicity across every measured dimension. Blood urea and creatinine rose less. Histology showed better-preserved tubular architecture with reduced necrosis. Kidney tissue glutathione levels remained higher in Acacia-treated animals, meaning the antioxidant reserve stayed functional rather than being depleted. Lipid peroxidation (MDA) stayed lower, indicating that cell membranes weren't breaking down as severely. The researchers proposed that the protection came from Arabic gum's ability to inhibit the production of oxygen free radicals and the resulting lipid peroxidation, limiting the oxidative damage that underlies gentamicin's toxic mechanism [2].

Let's translate this for a general reader who doesn't live in the biochemistry weeds. Gentamicin was still present in the kidneys, still generating the oxidative stress that defines its toxicity mechanism. However, in animals receiving Arabic gum, the cellular defense systems didn't collapse under that stress. The glutathione battery (the rechargeable antioxidant reserve) stayed charged rather than depleting. The result was that more tubular cells survived the insult intact, maintaining the filtration and reabsorption

175

functions that define a working nephron. The kidney wasn't invulnerable, but it was more resilient [2].

This 2002 study opened a conceptual door that would frame much of the research to follow. Hashab gum isn't just a nitrogen-management tool working through colonic bacterial metabolism. It's also a *tubular cytoprotector* which is a substance that supports cellular defense systems in the nephron itself, allowing kidney cells to withstand chemical insults that would otherwise kill them. The same antioxidant themes we saw elsewhere (maintaining glutathione and reducing oxidative damage) were now being demonstrated in the kidney model. Later work in other kidney-injury models with Hashab gum and similar compounds examined antioxidant enzymes and signaling pathways such as Nrf2 and NF-κB, but those were not measured in this particular study.

For clinicians, this suggested that Hashab gum might be useful not just for managing chronic kidney disease through nitrogen offloading, but also for preventing acute kidney injury in hospitalized patients receiving nephrotoxic medications such as aminoglycoside antibiotics, chemotherapy regimens (cisplatin, methotrexate), nonsteroidal anti-inflammatory drugs, or iodinated contrast agents for imaging. Every one of those exposures generates oxidative stress that can tip vulnerable patients into acute renal failure. If a food-grade, well-tolerated prebiotic could reduce that risk, it belonged in the preventive toolkit.

2004 - When Resources Are Tight and Tolerance Matters

Baghdad, Iraq. Al-Kadhimiya Teaching Hospital. Aamir Al-Mosawi, a pediatric nephrologist working in a healthcare system strained by international sanctions and conflict, is treating children with end-stage renal disease. Kidney transplantation, which could offer these children decades of additional life, requires donors, surgical teams, immunosuppression protocols, and follow-up care that are beyond reach.

Al-Mosawi tries an intervention inspired by reports of emerging experimental work on Acacia gum and kidney disease. He publishes a brief clinical report summarizing his experience with a small cohort of pediatric ESRD patients. The report is methodologically limited as it's not a randomized trial, there's no control group, the numbers are small, and outcome measurement is mostly observational. However, it conveys something profoundly important that randomized trials sometimes miss; this intervention was feasible. Children tolerated Acacia gum mixed into water or juice. Families could afford it because Acacia gum is relatively inexpensive. The dietary counseling required to implement low-protein feeding plus fiber supplementation was straightforward enough that it could be delivered in short clinic visits by nurses and dietitians who were managing crushing patient loads.

The clinical observations, while anecdotal, suggested benefits with improvements in uremic symptoms (less nausea, better appetite, less fatigue). Two patients completed the study. Both reported improved well-being. Neither became acidotic or uremic, and neither required dialysis during the study period. Both patients maintained urinary creatinine and urea levels not previously achieved without dialysis. In conclusion, dietary supplementation with Acacia gum may help in renal therapy to improve the quality of life and reduce or eliminate the need for dialysis in children with ESRD in some developing countries [3].

This Baghdad vignette matters not because it provides definitive efficacy data (it doesn't) but because it underscores a theme that recurs throughout the entire Hashab gum story. The most elegant mechanism, the most statistically significant result from a perfectly designed double-blind trial, and the most sophisticated molecular understanding is meaningless if the intervention costs more than a patient can pay, causes side effects they can't tolerate, or requires infrastructure that doesn't exist where they live. Hashab gum costs minimally (compared to other pharmaceutical interventions) per day. It dissolves clear in water, changes nothing about taste or texture, and could be stored at room temperature without refrigeration. Children as young as five could take it without complaint. These aren't footnotes to clinical efficacy; they're the determinants of whether efficacy ever reaches real patients.

2010 to 2015 - The Sudanese Omani Decade Mapping Every Lever: Building the Mechanistic Foundation

Muscat, Oman. Sultan Qaboos University, a collaborative research program led by Badreldin Ali that would, over the course of five years, systematically dissect how Hashab gum protects kidneys at the molecular and cellular level. The team needed a reproducible animal model that could mimic chronic kidney disease most patients develop. Not sudden injury from toxins or obstruction, but the slow, progressive decline driven by inflammation, oxidative stress, and fibrosis that characterizes most human CKD. They chose the adenine-induced chronic kidney disease model.

Let's teach this model clearly before walking through the research findings, because understanding the pathophysiology helps make sense of why certain outcomes matter. When rats or mice are fed diets containing excess adenine (one of the purine bases found in DNA and RNA) their metabolism breaks it down and attempts to excrete the byproducts. One of those byproducts is 2,8-dihydroxyadenine, a compound with very low solubility that precipitates as needle-shaped crystals inside renal tubules.

These crystals physically injure tubular epithelial cells as they try to pass through, triggering an inflammatory response. Immune cells infiltrate the kidney interstitium. Tubular cells die by necrosis and apoptosis. Fibroblasts are activated and begin depositing collagen, the scar tissue that replaces functional kidney architecture. Over weeks, the animals develop the full syndrome of chronic kidney disease with rising urea and creatinine (markers of declining filtration), anemia (because damaged kidneys produce less erythropoietin), electrolyte imbalances (potassium and phosphate retention, metabolic acidosis), uremic toxin accumulation, and histological changes that mirror human CKD. It's a robust model that doesn't require surgery, doesn't depend on genetic manipulation, and creates kidney injury through mechanisms (crystal deposition, inflammation, oxidative stress, fibrosis) that are highly relevant to human disease. You can test interventions, measure outcomes biochemically and histologically, and draw mechanistic conclusions about how those interventions work [4].

2010 - Proof of Concept: The first Omani study established that Gum arabic (Hashab gum from Acacia Senegal) supplementation in adenine-induced CKD rats significantly improved renal function as creatinine and urea dropped compared to untreated CKD animals. Kidney histology looked markedly better with less tubular necrosis, less inflammatory infiltrate, and better preservation of normal tubular architecture. Antioxidant enzyme activities (SOD) stayed higher, suggesting that cellular defenses weren't overwhelmed by the oxidative stress that crystals and inflammation generated [4]. The kidneys were still injured (adenine was still forming crystals, inflammation was still present) but the injury was less severe, and in the dimensions that matter for patient outcomes. Better filtration means lower waste accumulation. Less inflammation means slower progression to fibrosis. Preserved tubular architecture means retained reabsorption capacity. This was proof of concept at the systems level. Hashab gum could slow the progression of chronic kidney disease even when the primary insult (crystal injury) was ongoing.

2013 - The Mechanistic Deep Dive: The researchers measured a comprehensive panel of inflammatory, oxidative, and genotoxic markers in adenine CKD rats treated with Gum arabic (Hashab gum from Acacia Senegal). They published their findings in PLOS ONE with full methodological detail and open-access availability. This was the study that turned "Hashab gum helps kidneys" into a mechanistic map that other researchers could build on. Tumor necrosis factor-alpha (TNF-α the master pro-inflammatory cytokine that kicks off cytokine cascades and recruits immune cells) dropped significantly in Hashab-treated animals. Superoxide formation (measured using dihydroethidium fluorescence, showing reactive oxygen species generation in kidney tissue) decreased markedly. DNA double strand breaks (detected by immunohistochemistry for γ-H2AX, the phosphorylated histone marking sites where DNA's backbone has been severed) declined measurably in kidney tissue, meaning the genome was under less assault. Glutathione levels rose and superoxide dismutase activity increased. Histology scores improved on key dimensions with less inflammation, fibrosis, and better glomerular damage scores indicating preserved kidney structure [5].

This wasn't a study saying "Hashab gum helps and we're not sure why". This was a study showing how it helps, pathway by pathway, marker by marker. Less oxidative stress means reactive oxygen species are being neutralized before they damage lipids, proteins, and DNA. Reduced superoxide generation is consistent with better redox balance in kidney cells and less oxidative activation of inflammatory pathways. Quieter inflammatory signaling means TNF-α and related mediators are suppressed, which is consistent with less inflammatory-cell infiltration and less oxidative damage to kidney tissue. Stronger antioxidant defenses means endogenous antioxidant systems such as GSH and SOD are better preserved, and later work suggests pathways like Nrf2 may be involved, although they were not directly measured in this study. Calmer tissue explains that when inflammation is controlled and oxidative damage is limited, fibroblasts don't get activated as aggressively and collagen deposition slows. Additionally, tubular epithelial cells have a chance to repair and regenerate rather than dying and being replaced by scar tissue [5].

The 2013 mechanistic study provided direct evidence that Hashab gum's renal protection operates through suppression of inflammatory cytokines and oxidative stress pathways. By measuring both functional markers (creatinine clearance, proteinuria) and mechanistic markers (TNF-α, superoxide, DNA damage, antioxidant enzymes), the researchers demonstrated that improvement in kidney function correlated with reduction in the molecular drivers of kidney injury. Measuring DNA double strand breaks was particularly important because these are serious genomic lesions that can trigger cell death or mutations. The finding that Hashab gum reduced DNA damage frequency suggested protection at the most fundamental level by preserving the genetic integrity of kidney cells. This reduction in superoxide generation and its downstream damage likely explains why tubular cells survived better, maintained their differentiated functions, and avoided the apoptotic and necrotic pathways that would otherwise deplete the nephron population [5].

2015 - Protecting the Genome: Using the same adenine CKD model, the Omani team measured DNA damage in kidney tissue using the comet assay (the same technique we introduced in the contrast-genotoxicity study from the oxidative-stress chapter) and found that Gum arabic significantly reduced DNA strand breaks (shorter comet tails, indicating less fragmented DNA). They also measured urinary oxidized nucleic acids (8-oxoguanosine and 8-oxoguanine) which are markers of oxidative damage to RNA and DNA bases that are excreted when damaged nucleotides are repaired or degraded [6].

This closed a conceptual loop as Hashab gum isn't just protecting tissues from oxidative and inflammatory injury, it does so in ways that show up as better enzyme levels, cleaner histology, and improved function tests. It's protecting at the deepest level (the integrity of the genetic information itself) reducing the kind of cumulative DNA damage that, over years of chronic inflammation and oxidative stress, seeds the cancers that chronic kidney disease patients develop at rates 2-3x higher than the general population.

The mechanistic explanation connects directly to the previous findings. When you reduce oxidative stress (lower ROS means less hydroxyl-radical attack on DNA bases), reduce nitrosative stress (less peroxynitrite means less strand breakage and base deamination), quiet inflammation (less recruitment of immune cells that would otherwise amplify tissue injury through oxidative burst), and support cellular energy metabolism (better mitochondrial function means more ATP for DNA-repair enzymes to use), you create conditions where DNA-repair systems can keep up with damage rather than falling behind.

Every cell sustains thousands of DNA lesions daily from normal metabolism. What determines whether those lesions accumulate into mutations and cancer is the balance between damage rate and repair capacity. Hashab gum, by reducing the damage rate and supporting the energetic capacity to repair, tips that balance toward genomic stability. The 2015 genotoxicity study showed that the protective effects we'd been documenting in kidneys (better function, calmer inflammation, preserved structure) extend all the way down to the chromosomal level [6].

By the end of 2015, the Omani research program had built a comprehensive mechanistic foundation. The field now understood that Acacia gum works in chronic kidney disease through at least four integrated pathways: (1) fecal nitrogen trapping via colonic bacterial assimilation, reducing uremic waste; (2) antioxidant-enzyme support and glutathione preservation, limiting oxidative damage; (3) anti-inflammatory signaling through SCFA production and NF-κB suppression, reducing cytokine amplification; (4) genotoxic protection, maintaining DNA integrity. Those aren't separate miracles that happen to coincide; they're facets of a single system-level intervention that rebalances gut-kidney-immune crosstalk in ways that slow the progressive loss of nephrons.

2012 - The Diabetes-Kidney Bridge: When Metabolic Disease Meets Renal Failure

Tübingen, Germany. University of Tübingen Department of Physiology, studying diabetic nephropathy which is the leading cause of kidney failure in developed countries and one of the most feared long-term complications of diabetes. Omaima Nasir and colleagues used Akita mice, a genetic model that spontaneously develops insulin deficiency and hyperglycemia, then gave the diabetic Akita mice Gum arabic (Hashab gum from Acacia Senegal) (10% in their drinking water) and followed their kidney function over 1 and 2 weeks, comparing each mouse with its own pre-treatment values.

Diabetic nephropathy deserves a moment of explanation because it illustrates how metabolic disease and kidney disease aren't separate entities but rather two faces of the same underlying pathophysiology. Chronic hyperglycemia (years of elevated blood glucose) damages kidneys through multiple mechanisms working in parallel. Glucose gets into cells through non-insulin-dependent transporters in the kidneys and becomes a substrate for pathways that generate reactive oxygen species. The polyol pathway converts glucose to sorbitol using NADPH (depleting the NADPH that glutathione reductase needs to regenerate reduced glutathione), the hexosamine pathway shunts glucose into inflammatory signaling, and advanced glycation endproducts (AGEs) form when glucose non-enzymatically modifies proteins, creating crosslinked, dysfunctional proteins that activate RAGE receptors and trigger oxidative stress and inflammation.

High glucose also activates protein kinase C isoforms that promote vasoconstriction, increase vascular permeability, and drive extracellular-matrix deposition which is the beginning of fibrosis. The result is progressive damage to both the glomerular filtration barrier (causing it to leak protein into urine) and the tubular reabsorption machinery (impairing the ability to reclaim what's been filtered). Over years, filtration rate declines, albuminuria worsens, blood pressure rises (because the kidney-blood pressure regulatory system is failing), and patients progress toward end-stage renal disease requiring dialysis or transplant.

The challenge in diabetic nephropathy is that it's not just a kidney disease, it's a systemic metabolic disease expressing itself in kidneys. Interventions that only address the kidney (like ACE inhibitors, which reduce glomerular pressure) help but don't fully stop progression. The most effective interventions are those that address both the metabolic dysfunction (glycemic control, insulin sensitization, weight loss) and the kidney injury (blood pressure management, proteinuria reduction).

This is where Hashab gum enters the story with particular elegance, because we already know from the diabetes chapter that it improves glycemic control (has been shown to modestly lower fasting glucose, blunt post-meal glucose peaks, and improve HbA1c and adiponectin in trials). Although the entire exact mechanisms have yet to be clearly mapped out; it's likely through prebiotic mechanisms such as slower intestinal glucose absorption and SCFA-mediated effects on metabolism. If those same mechanisms translate into kidney protection, you've addressed both the upstream metabolic driver and the downstream renal consequence with a single intervention.

The 2012 German study delivered exactly that dual benefit by demonstrating kidney benefits in diabetic mice and added evidence that Hashab gum can also modify how the body handles glucose. Let's teach two clinical endpoints that nephrologists track religiously. *Creatinine clearance* is a surrogate measure of glomerular filtration rate; how many milliliters of blood plasma the kidneys can completely clear of creatinine per minute. It's the fundamental measure of kidney function. When creatinine clearance drops, you're losing filtration capacity, waste accumulates, and you're progressing toward renal failure. *Albuminuria* is the amount of albumin (a protein normally retained in the bloodstream) that appears in urine. Healthy glomeruli are selective filters; they let water, electrolytes, and small molecules through while retaining larger proteins like albumin. When the glomerular basement membrane and podocyte foot processes are damaged (by diabetes, hypertension, inflammatory diseases) albumin leaks through, and the degree of leakage predicts cardiovascular risk (albumin in urine correlates with vascular endothelial dysfunction everywhere, not just in kidneys) and progression of kidney disease. The two measures tell complementary stories. Creatinine clearance tells you about overall filtration capacity; albuminuria tells you about barrier integrity and endothelial health.

Hashab gum improved key kidney outcomes in diabetic mice. In Hashab treated Akita mice, albuminuria (protein loss in urine) fell significantly compared with their own values before treatment. Water and electrolyte handling stabilized which is a secondary but important kidney function that becomes dysregulated in diabetes. Blood pressure decreased significantly, and plasma urea concentrations were reduced along with urinary glucose excretion. The kidneys were still diabetic, still exposed to chronic hyperglycemia but the rate of injury slowed measurably, which in a progressive disease is often the most realistic and valuable goal [7].

For the millions of people with type 2 diabetes who are at risk or already developing diabetic nephropathy, the 2012 Tübingen study suggested that

Hashab gum (already shown to improve HbA1c, fasting glucose, and post-prandial glucose excursions in human trials) could deliver a renal dividend. The same daily tablespoon dissolved in morning tea that helps stabilize blood sugar might also slow the leakage and filtration loss that, left unchecked, leads inexorably toward dialysis [7].

2017 - When CRP Drops Before Chemistry Changes

A Saudi study published in International Journal of Nephrology, brought Gum arabic from animal models back into human patients with chronic kidney disease. Sarra Elamin and colleagues enrolled CKD patients and gave them Gum arabic supplementation for several weeks, measuring inflammatory markers, uremic toxins, and renal function before and after. The headline finding was both surprising and instructive. C-reactive protein (CRP), a key inflammation marker, dropped significantly in the Gum arabic group, even though blood urea nitrogen and indoxyl sulfate (one of the key uremic toxins generated by gut bacteria) didn't change over the short study window [8].

This is an important teaching moment for understanding the *gut-renal axis* at a mechanistic level, because it reveals that uremic-toxin reduction and systemic inflammation are related but separable processes that can improve on different timescales. Let's explain the axis step by step. In chronic kidney disease, the gut becomes a major generator of toxins that worsen the disease and drive cardiovascular complications. Here's how: when glomerular filtration fails, urea accumulates in blood. Some of that urea diffuses down concentration gradients into the gut lumen. If the gut microbiome is dysbiotic, those harmful bacteria will break down dietary protein and the urea they encounter, producing a suite of toxic metabolites. One of these toxins is Indoxyl sulfate derived from bacterial fermentation of tryptophan (tryptophan $\rightarrow$ indole $\rightarrow$ indoxyl sulfate after liver conjugation). Another is P-cresyl sulfate that comes from tyrosine fermentation. Trimethylamine N-oxide (TMAO) comes from choline and carnitine metabolism.

These compounds, normally cleared efficiently by healthy kidneys, accumulate in CKD because filtration is impaired. They're not innocent bystanders; they're biologically active. Indoxyl sulfate promotes endothelial dysfunction, induces oxidative stress in tubular cells, activates profibrotic signaling cascades in the kidney interstitium, and increases cardiovascular calcification. P-cresyl sulfate has similar effects. TMAO promotes atherosclerosis. Together, these uremic toxins create a vicious cycle where kidney disease generates toxins that accelerate kidney disease and cause the cardiovascular events that can kill more CKD patients than kidney failure itself.

Gum arabic interrupts this cycle not by filtering better (it's not a dialysis membrane) but by shifting the gut bacteria away from proteolytic metabolism and toward saccharolytic fermentation. The metabolic output shifts; instead of indole, p-cresol, and ammonia, probiotics produce short-chain fatty acids such as acetate, propionate, and butyrate. Those SCFAs have anti-inflammatory effects rather than pro-inflammatory effects. Acetate and propionate inhibit NF-κB signaling in monocytes and macrophages, reducing cytokine production. Butyrate promotes differentiation of regulatory T cells, which dampen excessive immune responses. SCFAs improve gut-barrier integrity by nourishing colonocytes and strengthening tight junctions, reducing endotoxin (LPS) translocation from gut into blood. All of these effects reduce the systemic inflammation that drives cardiovascular disease, accelerates kidney injury, and makes patients feel tired, nauseous, and unwell.

The 2017 CRP study revealed that this anti-inflammatory effect can manifest *before* uremic toxins drop substantially, because the two processes operate on different timelines and through different mechanisms. Shifting the microbiome toward SCFA production can happen relatively quickly (within days to weeks) as the probiotic community responds to the new substrate availability. Those SCFAs enter circulation and start modulating immune-cell behavior and endothelial function almost immediately. CRP, which has a half-life of about nineteen hours, can drop within days to weeks as cytokine production decreases. However, reducing circulating indoxyl sulfate and p-cresyl sulfate requires not just shifting microbial metabolism but also clearing the accumulated stores of these toxins, which is limited by residual kidney function and can happen more slowly, over weeks to months. So, you can see CRP improvements (a win for cardiovascular risk) before you see chemistry changes (which will follow with longer treatment duration and sustained adherence) [8].

Why does this matter? Because CRP predicts cardiovascular events in CKD patients with remarkable consistency (it's a stronger predictor of heart attacks, strokes, and cardiovascular death than cholesterol in this population) and cardiovascular disease is the leading cause of death in CKD, killing more patients than kidney failure. Lowering CRP through Hashab gum supplementation, even without immediately normalizing every uremic toxin, offers meaningful cardiovascular risk reduction. It also helps explain why patients sometimes report feeling better (less fatigue, better appetite, clearer thinking) before laboratory markers of kidney function have improved substantially. The systemic inflammatory burden has lightened, and that translates into symptom relief.

2018 - When Diabetes Meets CKD Head-On

Muscat and Abu Dhabi, a collaboration between Sultan Qaboos University and UAE University. Mohammed Al Za'abi and colleagues designed a study to test Gum Acacia under what might be the worst-case scenario for any renal intervention. Combine streptozotocin-induced diabetes (chronic hyperglycemia, oxidative stress from glucose metabolism, advanced glycation endproducts damaging proteins) with adenine-induced chronic kidney disease (crystal injury, inflammation, fibrosis). This double-hit model creates animals with overlapping metabolic and structural kidney injuries. This is the kind of multimorbidity that defines most real-world CKD, where patients rarely present with a single clean diagnosis. They usually have a mix of ailments that can include diabetes, hypertension, obesity, recurrent urinary-tract infections requiring nephrotoxic antibiotics, metabolic syndrome and chronic NSAID use for arthritis. If an intervention only works in idealized single-insult laboratory models, it won't translate to the messy complexity of clinical practice.

The study gave rats streptozotocin first to destroy beta cells and induce hyperglycemia, then fed them adenine to superimpose crystalline kidney injury on top of the metabolic injury, creating animals with high blood glucose, high blood urea, both oxidative and nitrosative stress raging, and inflammatory cascades amplifying through multiple pathways. This is the kidney under siege from all directions including metabolic dysregulation generating ROS, crystals physically injuring tubules and triggering immune-cell recruitment, proteolytic gut bacteria producing uremic toxins because kidney clearance is failing, and all of it feeding back to worsen everything else [9].

Gum Acacia supplementation, started at the time of adenine feeding and continued throughout the experimental period, still provided significant protection. Renal injury was clearly ameliorated relative to untreated double-hit animals, with lower protein loss in the urine, better tubular injury markers, improved histology, and lower levels of uremic toxins, even though creatinine and urea remained elevated. Both oxidative stress markers (8-isoprostane and 8-hydroxy-2-deoxyguanosine) and nitrosative

189

stress markers (plasma nitrite and nitrate) decreased. Systemic inflammation cooled: TNF-α, IL-1β, TGF-β1, and adiponectin fell while IL-10 rose, indicating that the cytokine amplification driving disease progression was being damped [9].

The fact that benefits persist even under this combined assault (diabetes plus CKD, metabolic plus structural injury, multiple oxidative pathways active simultaneously) is powerful evidence for robustness. It suggests that Gum Acacia's protective mechanisms aren't narrowly targeted to one injury pathway where they'd fail if a second pathway were activated. Instead, they operate at upstream nodes that influence multiple downstream cascades.

2019 - When Kidneys Fail from Plumbing Problems

Al Ain, UAE University, studying a completely different mechanism of kidney injury called obstructive nephropathy. Fayez Hammad and colleagues used the *unilateral ureteral obstruction* (UUO) model (a surgical intervention where one ureter is ligated, blocking urine drainage from that kidney) to test whether Arabic gum's protective effects extend beyond metabolic and toxin-induced injury to structural, mechanical insults [10].

Let's teach the UUO model and why it matters, because it addresses a clinical reality that's often overlooked in discussions of chronic kidney disease. Kidneys don't just fail from chemistry gone wrong; they fail from anatomy and plumbing gone wrong. Urinary obstruction happens in real life from kidney stones blocking ureters, tumors compressing the urinary tract, benign prostatic hyperplasia obstructing the bladder outlet in aging men, congenital malformations like posterior urethral valves in children, and surgical complications (ureteral injury during abdominal or pelvic surgery, scarring after instrumentation).

When urine can't drain, pressure builds. The renal pelvis and calyces dilate (hydronephrosis). Back-pressure is transmitted to the tubules, compressing them and reducing blood flow. Tubular epithelial cells, stressed by the mechanical distortion and the hypoxia from reduced perfusion, undergo apoptosis. Inflammatory signals are released, recruiting immune cells. Fibroblasts are activated and begin depositing collagen in the interstitium with scar tissues replacing functional kidney parenchyma. If the obstruction is severe and prolonged, the kidney becomes a non-functional, hydronephrotic sac.

The elegance of the UUO model for testing interventions is that it isolates the fibrotic response. You're not dealing with accumulated uremic toxins (blood chemistry stays normal because the opposite kidney compensates) or metabolic abnormalities (no diabetes, no hypertension). The injury is purely mechanical and inflammatory, and the dominant pathology is rapid fibrosis. If an intervention slows fibrosis in UUO, it's acting on the fundamental scarring process that's common to all forms of progressive kidney disease, regardless of what initiated the injury.

The Hammad study ligated one ureter in rats, creating obstruction for 72 hours, then reversed the obstruction by surgically removing the ligature, and measured outcomes in animals that had received Arabic gum supplementation (starting 7 days before obstruction and continuing throughout) versus controls. The key finding was that Arabic gum provided protection during the obstruction phase itself. At 3 days of obstruction, kidneys supplemented with Arabic gum showed significantly less tubular dilatation on histological examination (59.9% versus 82.9%, $p = 0.0003$), lower oxidative stress markers (malondialdehyde decreased 27.2% in treated animals versus a 28.4% increase in controls, $p = 0.002$), and dampened inflammatory and profibrotic cytokine gene expression

(TNF-α: 1.6-fold versus 2.3-fold increase, p = 0.048; TGF-β1: 1.7-fold versus 2.0-fold increase, p = 0.05) [10].

However, when renal function was assessed 6 days after reversal of the obstruction, Arabic gum did not significantly improve functional recovery. Both treated and untreated groups showed persistent impairment: glomerular filtration rate in the previously obstructed kidney remained at only 58-63% of the contralateral kidney with no significant difference between groups, and renal blood flow was similarly reduced to 61-69% with no difference between groups. By this recovery timepoint, the differences in oxidative stress markers and cytokine expression that had been significant during obstruction were no longer apparent [10].

This finding suggests that Arabic gum's protective effect operates primarily by reducing the acute inflammatory and oxidative stress response during active injury, potentially limiting the initial tissue damage that triggers fibrotic pathways. The study demonstrates that Arabic gum can dampen the immediate inflammatory cascade involving TGF-β signaling, which drives fibroblast activation and collagen synthesis. However, the lack of improved functional recovery after obstruction relief indicates that either: (1) the protective effects during the injury phase were not sufficient to translate into better long-term outcomes in this short 6-day recovery window, or (2) additional interventions may be needed during the recovery phase itself to maximize functional restoration [10].

2019 to 2021- Mechanistic Maps

Three additional studies from this period strengthen the mechanistic picture and broaden confidence that Acacia gum's effects in kidney disease are part of a larger pattern of systemic anti-inflammatory and antioxidant protection.

192

Diclofenac Nephrotoxicity, 2019: Faten Shafeek and colleagues at Mansoura University in Egypt tested Gum Acacia against diclofenac-induced kidney injury in rats. Diclofenac is a nonsteroidal anti-inflammatory drug (NSAID) widely used for pain and inflammation, but it's notorious for nephrotoxicity through multiple mechanisms including inhibiting renal prostaglandin synthesis (which reduces renal blood flow and glomerular filtration), generating oxidative stress, and triggering inflammatory and apoptotic cascades in tubular cells. The Mansoura study went beyond measuring just oxidative markers; they quantified specific immune and inflammatory mediators such as monocyte chemoattractant protein-1 (MCP-1), a chemokine that recruits monocytes and macrophages into inflamed tissues; complement receptor-1 (CR1), a regulator of the complement system that can influence complement-mediated tissue injury; and pro-apoptotic pathway markers showing cells initiating programmed death [11].

Gum Acacia significantly improved all of these pathways: it reduced MCP-1 and caspase-3 (and the pro-inflammatory cytokines IL-1β and TNF-α), while increasing IL-10 and CR-1 levels. MCP-1 dropped, meaning less recruitment of inflammatory cells into the kidney. When you reduce the number of macrophages and neutrophils infiltrating injured tissue, you reduce the secondary damage those cells cause through release of reactive oxygen species, proteases, and pro-inflammatory cytokines. CR1 upregulation suggested that Acacia was affecting complement-system activation, part of innate immunity that, when dysregulated, causes bystander injury to healthy tissue. Additionally, pro-apoptotic pathway suppression meant that tubular cells that were stressed but not yet dead were being given a chance to survive and repair rather than initiating the suicide cascade [11].

Let's teach these mechanisms briefly because they show that Gum Acacia's protective reach extends beyond "just" being an antioxidant. MCP-1 is one

193

of the master control signals in inflammation. When tubular cells are injured (by toxins, ischemia, immune attack, whatever) they secrete MCP-1, which diffuses into the interstitium and bloodstream and acts as a homing beacon for monocytes. Those monocytes cross the endothelium, enter the kidney tissue, differentiate into macrophages, and begin releasing tumor necrosis factor-alpha, interleukin-1β, and reactive oxygen species. Those signals activate fibroblasts, which start depositing collagen. If you can lower MCP-1 early, you break the amplification loop so fewer monocytes arrive, less cytokine production occurs, and less fibrosis develops.

That's immunomodulation, not just antioxidant support. The complement system (of which CR1 is part) is ancient innate immunity which is a cascade of proteins that tag pathogens for destruction and create membrane-attack complexes that punch holes in cell membranes. In autoimmune diseases and inflammatory conditions, complement can be activated inappropriately and damage host tissue. Modulating complement activation protects bystander cells. Also, preventing apoptosis, while sometimes undesirable (you want damaged cells to die if they're too injured to repair), is beneficial when it preserves tubular epithelial cells that are stressed but salvageable. Therefore, keeping those nephrons alive means preserving filtration capacity [11].

The 2019 diclofenac study showed that Gum Acacia's toolkit for protecting kidneys includes not just antioxidant enzymes and glutathione, but also immunomodulatory effects on chemokine signaling, complement activation, and cell-survival pathways. This is systems-level resilience, not single-target suppression.

Rheumatoid Arthritis Phase-II Trial, 2021: A small Phase-II trial in Sudan by Ebtihal Kamal and her colleagues tested Gum arabic (Hashab gum from Acacia Senegal) supplementation in rheumatoid arthritis patients and found improvements in systemic inflammatory markers, with secondary benefits to hepatic and renal laboratory profiles even though the kidneys weren't the primary target [12]. These studies are outside the main kidney-disease narrative, but they serve as useful ballast for the argument that Hashab gum's anti-inflammatory effects are generalizable. If it cools inflammation in rheumatoid arthritis (an autoimmune disease), in sickle-cell disease (a hemolytic disorder), in metabolic syndrome, in CKD, and in multiple animal models of inflammatory injury, you're seeing a consistent pattern that transcends any single disease mechanism. That consistency builds clinical confidence that the intervention will translate across a range of inflammatory phenotypes that practicing nephrologists encounter.

2020 - Dialysis Units and the Antioxidant Bank Account. When Every Advantage Matters

Omdurman, Sudan. Alneelain University Medical School, working directly with hemodialysis units in a clinical setting where oxidative stress is highest, cardiovascular risk is most acute, and quality of life often determines whether patients continue treatment or give up. Nour Elkhair Ali and colleagues ran a Phase-II clinical trial on patients with maintenance hemodialysis, giving them Gum arabic (Hashab gum from Acacia Senegal) daily for several months and measuring antioxidant capacity and inflammatory markers [13].

Hemodialysis patients live in a unique and brutal metabolic state. Three times per week, they're connected to machines that remove their blood, pass it through artificial membranes to filter waste, and return it to their bodies. Each session generates oxidative stress through multiple mechanisms. One of the main ones is blood contact with synthetic membranes which activates complement and white blood cells releasing reactive oxygen species. A second oxidative stress mechanism is the repeated cycles of removing blood and returning which creates miniature ischemia-reperfusion events. Additionally, residual kidney disease means that antioxidant systems (kidneys normally produce and activate antioxidants) are impaired and therefore the uremic milieu itself (persistent elevation of toxins despite dialysis) generates ongoing oxidative damage. The result is that hemodialysis patients have chronically low antioxidant capacity, chronically elevated inflammatory markers (CRP, IL-6), and extraordinarily high cardiovascular risk including heart attacks, strokes, and heart failure. These are the leading causes of death, killing more dialysis patients than kidney failure itself.

The trial measured *Total Antioxidant Capacity* (TAC) which is an integrative blood test that captures the net antioxidant reserve. Let's explain TAC briefly, because it's a different kind of measurement than what we've discussed before. Instead of measuring one specific antioxidant (like vitamin C levels) or one specific enzyme (like SOD activity), TAC assays ask: *If I challenge this plasma sample with a standardized oxidative stress (a known amount of free radical generator), how much oxidative damage occurs?* Plasma with high TAC neutralizes most of the challenge and shows little damage; plasma with low TAC is quickly overwhelmed and shows extensive damage. TAC rises when multiple antioxidants and antioxidant enzymes are functioning well (vitamin C, vitamin E, uric acid, albumin, glutathione, SOD, catalase, GPx all contribute) and it falls when the system is depleted. It's like asking "What's in your bank account?" instead of "How much is in your checking account alone?"[13].

In the Omdurman hemodialysis trial, TAC increased significantly in patients taking Hashab gum compared to baseline measurements and CRP also dropped [13]. Both findings are clinically important. Higher TAC means these patients had more antioxidant reserves to weather the oxidative stress that each dialysis session and each uremic day imposes. Lower CRP means reduced systemic inflammation, which translates to lower cardiovascular risk and, plausibly, better long-term outcomes.

Importantly, the finding that matters most for real-world implementation is tolerance. Hemodialysis patients can be on ten to fifteen medications (phosphate binders, blood-pressure pills, erythropoietin for anemia, vitamin D, iron supplements, anticoagulants) and they're dealing with dietary restrictions (low potassium, low phosphate, fluid limits), time commitments (twelve hours per week in the dialysis chair), and the physical and emotional exhaustion of chronic illness. Adding another intervention to that burden, even a beneficial one, will fail if it causes side effects, complicates the regimen, or costs too much. Hashab gum dissolved easily in water, required no dose titration or lab monitoring. In rare cases it caused minor gastrointestinal symptoms that were resolved within two weeks, and cost less per month than a single dose of many renal medications. Adherence was excellent; dropout rates were low. Patients kept taking it for months, which is why TAC and CRP had time to shift [13]. This is the adherence principle that runs through every chapter of this book, and it's worth restating forcefully here: *the most effective intervention in the world is worthless if patients can't or won't use it long enough to derive benefit.*

2020 to 2021 - The Microbiome Finally Takes the Stand. When Metabolomics Meets Next-Generation Sequencing

Two independent research groups, working without coordination, used cutting-edge microbiome sequencing and targeted metabolomics to make the gut-renal axis visible at molecular resolution. These weren't the first studies to suggest that Hashab gum works through the microbiome (that's been implicit throughout) but they were the first to map the precise bacterial shifts and measure the actual short-chain fatty acids in blood, proving the mechanism rather than inferring it.

Qatar, 2020: Maha Al-Asmakh and colleagues at Qatar University analyzed samples from rats with chronic kidney disease induced using the adenine model by collaborators, examining animals supplemented with Gum Acacia(SUPER GUM™ -Modified Hashab Gum) while using next-generation DNA sequencing to profile the gut microbiome (identifying which bacterial species were present and in what proportions) and liquid chromatography-mass spectrometry to measure circulating short-chain fatty acids. The before-and-after picture was definitive.

Bacterial taxa associated with pathogenic processes (especially Proteobacteria, and families such as Verrucomicrobiaceae that expand in CKD) were reduced by Hashab gum treatment, while beneficial groups were partially restored. Beneficial SCFA-producing taxa (especially Lactobacillaceae and other butyrate-producing Firmicutes such as Coprococcus and members of Ruminococcaceae) were depleted in CKD and were partly restored by Hashab gum. This is the fundamental shift from proteolytic to saccharolytic metabolism. When you feed beneficial bacteria highly fermentable prebiotics, those bacteria will gain a competitive advantage and expand, while bacteria that specialize in protein fermentation and produce toxins are outcompeted and decline.

Plasma levels of short-chain fatty acids improved. Propionate was significantly restored in Hashab-treated CKD rats compared to untreated CKD controls, and butyrate showed a similar upward trend, although this was not statistically significant. This is crucial because it proves that microbiome changes aren't just compositional curiosities because they translate into functional metabolic changes that reach systemic circulation. Those SCFAs don't stay in the colon; they're absorbed across the colonic epithelium, enter the portal blood, travel to the liver (where they modulate hepatic metabolism), continue into systemic circulation (where they interact with immune cells, endothelial cells, and kidneys), and even cross the blood-brain barrier (where they influence neuroinflammation and cognition). The SCFAs measured in plasma are the likely mediators linking microbiome shifts in the colon to better kidney outcomes, and their changes support this mechanism, although inflammation wasn't directly measured in this study.

Additionally, renal function improved in parallel with these microbiome and metabolite changes showing lower urea, lower creatinine, better biochemical markers, and reduced pathogenic bacterial abundance. The investigators went beyond simple association. They showed that Hashab gum shifted the microbiome toward fiber-fermenting bacteria, increased circulating SCFAs (especially propionate), and improved biochemical markers of kidney function. They showed correlations between harmful bacterial taxa presence and worse renal markers. This pattern supports a mechanistic chain linking Hashab gum, the microbiome, SCFAs, and kidney protection, even though the anti-inflammatory step itself wasn't directly measured in this experiment [14].

Oman and Qatar, 2021: Arun Lakshmanan, working at Sidra Medicine in Qatar with collaborators including Badreldin Ali's team at Sultan Qaboos University in Oman, replicated and extended the findings using a slightly different CKD model (adenine-induced, but with different dietary protocols and sampling timepoints) using a standard 16S rRNA sequencing pipeline (Illumina MiSeq and QIIME) to analyze the microbiome. The fact that two closely linked research teams, working in different labs but using similar methods, arrived at very similar conclusions strengthens confidence that the findings are robust and not artifacts of one particular experimental setup [15].

Again, Gum Acacia induced prebiotic shifts as it reversed increases in Actinobacteria, Proteobacteria, Tenericutes, and Verrucomicrobia that accumulated in CKD. Again, butyrate production specifically increased, being completely restored to normal levels. Critically, the researchers confirmed that these shifts persisted even under the dysbiotic conditions created by chronic kidney disease [15].

This answers a question we visited in previous chapters but had lingered in the background of this chapter: Does a "sick" microbiome (one that's already been disrupted by uremia, medications, dietary restrictions, and inflammation) still respond to prebiotic fiber, or is it too damaged? Some fibers fail in dysbiotic contexts because they require specific bacterial species to degrade them, and if those species have been wiped out by antibiotics or suppressed by disease-related changes, the fiber just passes through unfermented. Hashab gum's complex, branched arabinogalactan structure requires cooperative degradation by multiple bacterial enzyme systems, which creates functional redundancy. Even if some degrading species are depleted, others can compensate. The 2021 Oman-Qatar study proved that Hashab's fermentation profile is robust enough to work even in the microbial chaos of chronic kidney disease [15].

Let's spell out the gut-renal axis formula one more time, because it's the mechanistic foundation that connects everything from the 1996 nitrogen-balance study through the 2020 dialysis trial and finally to these 2020–2021 microbiome papers: Proteolytic fermentation in the colon → indole, p-cresol, ammonia → liver conjugation → indoxyl sulfate, p-cresyl sulfate accumulate in CKD → damage tubules, inflame vessels, promote fibrosis. Saccharolytic fermentation in the colon → acetate, propionate, butyrate → absorbed into blood → inhibit NF-κB, promote regulatory T cells, improve barrier, provide fuel → reduce systemic inflammation, protect kidneys.

Hashab gum pushes the system from the first pathway to the second. Fewer toxins are made because bacteria are busy fermenting fiber instead of protein. More protective SCFAs are produced because fiber fermentation yields SCFAs as the primary metabolic end product. The net effect is less damage, more protection, slower progression, better outcomes [14, 15].

2022 - Meta-Analysis for Guideline Writers: When Individual Studies Become Weight of Evidence

Khartoum, Sudan. A team led by Selma Abdelrahman Hussein, with collaborators in Sudan and Saudi Arabia, conducted a systematic review and meta-analysis, aggregating data from randomized controlled clinical trials testing Gum arabic in renal failure. Let's explain *meta-analytic confidence* briefly, because it's a different kind of evidence than any single study provides, and it's the currency that guideline panels and formulary committees trade in.

When one study shows that an intervention works, it could be true, it could be chance (statistical noise), or it could be bias (the study was poorly designed, the investigators had conflicts of interest, the patients were selected in ways that favor the intervention). When multiple independent studies in different populations and settings all show the same benefit, confidence rises as the probability that all are false positives due to chance drops dramatically. A meta-analysis systematically searches for all available studies, applies quality criteria to exclude the weakest ones, extracts outcome data in standardized formats, and combines results using statistical methods that weight larger, higher-quality studies more heavily. The output is a pooled effect estimate (an average treatment effect across all studies) with a confidence interval that narrows as more data is added. The larger the pooled sample, the tighter the confidence interval, and the more certain we are that the effect is real and not artifact.

The 2022 Sudan meta-analysis concluded, after screening 574 records: "The efficacy of GA supplementation on the serum creatinine, urea, sodium, and potassium of chronic renal failure (CRF) patients depends on the period of treatment. The longer the period of treatment is applied, the more significant reduction was obtained on serum urea and creatinine but not on sodium and potassium. In addition, the CRF stage of the patient plays a role in the efficacy of intervention where the efficacy of GA treatment in early stages is more significant than the advanced stage. Moreover, the intake of LPD shows obvious enhancement to the prebiotic activity of colon bacteria and subsequently significant reduction in the blood level of creatinine and urea. However, based on the studies collected and used in the present systematic review and meta-analysis, it can be confirmed that GA is effective in the early stages of renal failure more than late stages" [16].

For a progressive disease like CKD, where the goal is to slow decline rather than cure, and where patients live with the disease for years to decades, those incremental benefits compound into meaningful delays in reaching dialysis, fewer cardiovascular events, and better quality of life.

For formulary committees writing institutional guidelines, for hospital pharmacy-and-therapeutics committees deciding whether to stock Gum arabic, for insurance companies considering coverage, and for international nephrology societies updating clinical practice guidelines, the 2022 meta-analysis provided summary evidence. This isn't just one interesting trial in one unusual population; it's a finding supported across multiple contexts, with safety established and mechanisms understood.

2023 & 2024 - The Edges Sharpen: Aflatoxins, Diabetes Refinements, and Pump Protection

As the field matured, researchers continued to test Hashab gum against different nephrotoxic insults and to drill deeper into cellular mechanisms, refining the picture and filling gaps.

Egypt, 2023: Aflatoxicosis: Obeid Shanab and colleagues at South Valley University tested Acacia gum (Hashab gum from Acacia Senegal) against aflatoxin-induced kidney injury. Aflatoxins are mycotoxins produced by Aspergillus species that contaminate stored grains (corn, peanuts, rice) in hot, humid climates, and they're a real-world public-health problem in regions with poor food storage infrastructure. Aflatoxin B1 is hepatotoxic, nephrotoxic, and generates oxidative stress. It also triggers inflammatory and apoptotic pathways in liver and kidney cells. The Egyptian team gave rats aflatoxin B1 to induce kidney injury, supplemented some with Hashab gum (7.5g/kg daily), and measured inflammatory markers (TNF-α, IL-6, iNOS, NF-κB/p65), apoptotic pathway markers (cleaved caspase-3-17/19, cytochrome c), oxidative stress (Nrf2, SOD1), and kidney histology [17].

Hashab gum significantly reduced inflammatory and apoptotic signaling, lowered oxidative stress, and improved histology. This study doesn't break new conceptual ground (we've seen these protective patterns repeatedly across gentamicin, adenine crystals, diclofenac, diabetes, and obstruction) but it extends the applicability to an environmentally relevant toxin. It says: Hashab gum's cytoprotective effects aren't narrowly specific to pharmaceutical nephrotoxins or crystal injury; they extend to naturally occurring environmental toxins, which matters for populations in sub-Saharan Africa, Southeast Asia, and Latin America where aflatoxin exposure is common and kidney disease burden is high.

Egypt, 2024: Diabetic Nephropathy Refinement: Ahmed and colleagues at Beni-Suef University revisited diabetic nephropathy using a nicotinamide-streptozotocin model which is a refinement over straight streptozotocin because nicotinamide partially protects beta cells, creating a diabetes phenotype closer to human type 2 diabetes (some residual insulin secretion, insulin resistance) rather than complete insulin deficiency. Again, Gum arabic improved renal outcomes showing lower urea, lower creatinine, better histology, reduced oxidative stress markers and enhanced antioxidant enzyme activities. The consistency across diabetes models (streptozotocin alone, nicotinamide-STZ, STZ plus adenine) reinforces that Acacia's renal protection isn't model-specific or dependent on one particular method of inducing hyperglycemia. It's robust across the metabolic-injury spectrum [18].

Sudan, 2024: The Pump and the Ultrastructure: Bashir and colleagues, working across King Khalid University (Saudi Arabia), Mansoura University (Egypt), the University of Khartoum (Sudan), and Princess Nourah bint Abdulrahman University (Saudi Arabia) published what may be the most mechanistically satisfying endpoint yet. They measured Na^+/K^+-$ATPase$ activity and gene expression in diabetic rat kidneys treated with Acacia Senegal (Hashab gum), and they used electron microscopy to examine glomerular ultrastructure [19].

Let's teach Na^+/K^+-ATPase clearly, because it's not just another enzyme; it's the engine that powers everything the kidney does beyond filtration. Na^+/K^+-ATPase is an ion transporter embedded in the basolateral membrane (the blood-facing side) of tubular epithelial cells throughout the nephron. It uses ATP (cellular energy) to pump three sodium ions out of the cell into the bloodstream and two potassium ions into the cell from the bloodstream. This creates concentration gradients: low sodium inside the cell, high sodium in the tubular lumen (the urine-forming side). Those gradients are the electrochemical driving force for everything else the nephron does like reabsorbing filtered sodium, water, glucose, amino acids, and bicarbonate from the urine back into blood. Without Na^+/K^+-ATPase running continuously, those gradients collapse, reabsorption fails, and the kidney loses the ability to concentrate urine or regulate electrolyte balance. Patients develop salt wasting, dehydration, metabolic acidosis, and hyperkalemia (the syndrome of renal tubular failure even if glomerular filtration is still occurring).

The 2024 study found that Hashab gum, especially when combined with insulin, improved renal markers (urea, creatinine, creatinine clearance) and oxidative-stress parameters (MDA, SOD, catalase, GSH), and brought Na^+/K^+-ATPase activity closer to normal values, and reduced mRNA expression of the Na^+/K^+-ATPase α-1 subunit, suggesting a return toward normal regulation of the pump. Electron microscopy showed better-preserved glomerular ultrastructure. The basement membrane looked more normal, podocyte foot processes (the interdigitating cellular projections that form the filtration slits) were less effaced, endothelial capillary cells were less damaged, and the overall architecture was less disrupted [19].

This is a deeply satisfying mechanistic close for the kidney chapter, because it connects biochemistry to cellular machinery to tissue structure to organ function. Hashab gum's effects appear to start with reduced oxidative stress and better antioxidant enzyme activity, which then support healthier cell function and structure in the kidney. This molecular reality (appropriately regulated Na^+/K^+-ATPase pumps maintaining gradients) leads to the ultrastructural (intact glomerular basement membrane, preserved podocyte and endothelial cell architecture) to the functional (better creatinine clearance and protein handling, indicating improved overall kidney performance). It's not just that the kidney works better; we can see why it works better, all the way down to the pumps and pores.

The kidney doesn't fail only in aggregate statistics such as rising creatinine, and accumulating urea. It fails in pumps that stop pumping, in membranes that start leaking, in mitochondria that can't make ATP, in DNA that accumulates unrepaired lesions, in cells that choose apoptosis over continued struggle. Hashab gum, by working at all those levels simultaneously helps kidneys keep functioning even when they're under metabolic and inflammatory siege. That's the quiet, cumulative power of a systems-level intervention.

Liver and Pancreas in Conversation with Kidneys

The kidney doesn't fail in isolation, broadcasting distress signals into silence. It fails in conversation with other organs, and two of its most important metabolic partners are the liver and the pancreas. The same short-chain fatty acids that we've watched travel from the colon to the kidneys (acetate, propionate, butyrate) don't stop at the renal tubules. They actually reach the liver first because colonic blood drains through the portal vein directly into hepatic circulation before entering systemic circulation. In the liver, those SCFAs modulate glucose production (propionate directly inhibits gluconeogenesis, the synthesis of new glucose), lipid synthesis (acetate can be converted to acetyl-CoA and used for fatty-acid synthesis, but it also signals satiety pathways that reduce overall lipogenesis), and inflammatory tone (SCFAs suppress Kupffer-cell activation, reducing hepatic cytokine production). Every one of those hepatic effects has kidney implications. Lower glucose means less hyperglycemia-driven oxidative stress in diabetic nephropathy, reduced lipid dysregulation means less oxidized LDL accumulating in renal vessels, and quieter hepatic inflammation means fewer circulating cytokines reaching and damaging kidneys.

The same reduction in systemic uremic toxins and inflammatory mediators that protects tubular cells and glomeruli also eases the burden on pancreatic beta cells (the insulin-secreting cells that burn out under chronic inflammatory stress and lead to diabetes) which then drives diabetic nephropathy in a vicious cycle. Indoxyl sulfate and p-cresyl sulfate, the uremic toxins generated by harmful gut bacteria, don't just damage kidneys; they also impair insulin secretion and promote beta-cell apoptosis. When Hashab gum shifts the microbiome away from producing these toxins, beta cells face less oxidative and inflammatory stress, insulin secretion improves, glycemic control stabilizes, and the metabolic-renal loop becomes virtuous rather than vicious.

This is the *hepato-renal axis* and the *pancreatic-renal axis* emerging into view. Organs don't march toward dysfunction independently; they drag each other down through shared inflammatory pathways, oxidative mediators, and metabolic derangements. When you intervene at the gut level (modulating what bacteria produce, what signals reach the bloodstream, what inflammatory tone bathes every tissue) the benefits radiate to every organ downstream of that portal vein.

Same biology, different organs, one integrated story of how a prebiotic that begins in the colon reverberates through the portal vein to every tissue the blood touches. That's where we're headed next.

References:

1. Bliss, Donna Zimmaro, et al. "Supplementation with Gum Arabic Fiber Increases Fecal Nitrogen Excretion and Lowers Serum Urea Nitrogen Concentration in Chronic Renal Failure Patients Consuming a Low-Protein Diet." American Journal of Clinical Nutrition, vol. 63, no. 3, 1996, pp. 392-98.

2. Al-Majed, Abdulhakeem A., et al. "Protective Effects of Oral Arabic Gum Administration on Gentamicin-Induced Nephrotoxicity in Rats." Pharmacological Research, vol. 46, no. 5, 2002, pp. 445-51

3. Al-Mosawi, Aamir J. "Acacia Gum Supplementation of a Low-Protein Diet in Children with End-Stage Renal Disease." Pediatric Nephrology, vol. 19, no. 10, 2004, pp. 1156-59.

4. Ali, Badreldin H., et al. "Effects of Gum Arabic in Rats with Adenine-Induced Chronic Renal Failure." Experimental Biology and Medicine, vol. 235, no. 3, 2010, pp. 373-82.

5. Ali, Badreldin H., et al. "Effect of Gum Arabic on Oxidative Stress and Inflammation in Adenine-Induced Chronic Renal Failure in Rats." PLOS ONE, vol. 8, no. 2, 2013, p. e55242.

6. Ali, Badreldin H., et al. "Gum Acacia Mitigates Genetic Damage in Adenine-Induced Chronic Renal Failure in Rats." European Journal of Clinical Investigation, vol. 45, no. 12, 2015, pp. 1221-27.

7. Nasir, Omaima, et al. "Effects of Gum Arabic (Acacia senegal) on Renal Function in Diabetic Mice." Kidney and Blood Pressure Research, vol. 35, no. 5, 2012, pp. 365–372.

8. Elamin, Sarra, et al. "Gum Arabic Reduces C-Reactive Protein in Chronic Kidney Disease Patients without Affecting Urea or Indoxyl Sulfate Levels." International Journal of Nephrology, vol. 2017, 2017, Article ID 9501470.

9. Al Za'abi, Mohammed, et al. "Gum Acacia Improves Renal Function and Ameliorates Systemic Inflammation, Oxidative and Nitrosative Stress in Streptozotocin-Induced Diabetes in Rats with Adenine-Induced Chronic Kidney Disease." Cellular Physiology and Biochemistry, vol. 45, no. 6, 2018, pp. 2293-2304.

10. Hammad, Fayez T., et al. "The Effect of Arabic Gum on Renal Function in Reversible Unilateral Ureteric Obstruction." Biomolecules, vol. 9, no. 1, 2019, article 25.

11. Shafeek, Faten, et al. "Gum Acacia Mitigates Diclofenac Nephrotoxicity by Targeting Monocyte Chemoattractant Protein-1, Complement Receptor-1 and Pro-Apoptotic Pathways." Food and

Chemical Toxicology, vol. 129, July 2019, pp. 162-68

12. Kamal, Ebtihal, et al. "Dietary Fibers (Gum Arabic) Supplementation Modulates Hepatic and Renal Profile among Rheumatoid Arthritis Patients, Phase II Trial." Frontiers in Nutrition, vol. 8, 2021, article 552049.

13. Ali, Nour Elkhair, et al. "Gum Arabic (Acacia Senegal) Augmented Total Antioxidant Capacity and Reduced C-Reactive Protein among Haemodialysis Patients in Phase II Trial." International Journal of Nephrology, vol. 2020, 2020, article 7214673

14. Al-Asmakh, Maha, et al. "The Effects of Gum Acacia on the Composition of the Gut Microbiome and Plasma Levels of Short-Chain Fatty Acids in a Rat Model of Chronic Kidney Disease." Frontiers in Pharmacology, vol. 11, 2020, article 569402

15. Lakshmanan, Arun Prasath, et al. "The Influence of the Prebiotic Gum Acacia on the Intestinal Microbiome Composition in Rats with Experimental Chronic Kidney Disease." Biomedicine & Pharmacotherapy, vol. 133, 2021, article 110992

16. Hussein, Selma Abdelrahman, et al. "Efficacy and Safety of Gum Arabic on Renal Failure Patients: Systematic Review and Meta-analysis." Sudan Journal of Medical Sciences, vol. 17, no. 4, 2022, pp. 459–475

17. Shanab, Obeid, et al. "Nephroprotective Effects of Acacia senegal against Aflatoxicosis via Targeting Inflammatory and Apoptotic Signaling Pathways." Ecotoxicology and Environmental Safety, vol. 262, 2023, article 115194

18. Ahmed, Osama M., et al. "Therapeutic Role of Arabic Gum against Nicotinamide/Streptozotocin-Induced Diabetes and Nephropathy in Wistar Rats." Egyptian Pharmaceutical Journal, 2024

19. Bashir, Salah O., et al. "Improvement of Na^+-K^+ ATPase Activity and Gene Expression Associated with Glomerular Ultrastructural Protection in Diabetic Nephropathy by Acacia senegal: Role of Oxidative Stress Disturbances." International Journal of Morphology, vol. 42, no. 1, 2024, pp. 205–15.

CHAPTER 14

The Same Metabolic Tuning examined from another angle

The Organ at the Crossroads

If the kidneys are the body's filtration system, working quietly in the back to remove waste and maintain chemical balance, then the liver is the control tower. It's the metabolic command center where every decision about fuel, storage, detoxification, and defense gets made. Every molecule absorbed from the gut (glucose from breakfast, fatty acids from lunch, fiber fragments, bacterial metabolites, environmental toxins, medication residues) lands here first, carried by blood flowing through the portal vein directly from the intestines into the hepatic circulation before joining the general bloodstream. The control tower sorts what arrives. Glucose gets stored as glycogen or released as needed, fats get packaged into lipoproteins or oxidized for energy, toxins get conjugated and prepared for excretion, nutrients get distributed, and inflammatory signals either get amplified or suppressed depending on the liver's current state.

When the control tower is harried, when oxidative sparks are flying through hepatocytes, when inflammatory cytokines are broadcasting alarm signals, when fat accumulates faster than it can be processed, when toxins arrive faster than detoxification enzymes can handle them; the pancreas sitting nearby in the abdominal cavity bears the metabolic brunt. Lipids linger too long in the bloodstream after meals, bathing pancreatic beta cells in fatty acids that weren't meant to stay elevated for hours. Those beta cells strain to secrete enough insulin to clear the excess glucose and fat, firing repeatedly until their secretory machinery begins to falter. Glucose curves sharpen and stay elevated longer. The feedback loop between liver glucose output, pancreatic insulin secretion, and peripheral insulin sensitivity (the triumvirate that maintains metabolic homeostasis) starts to drift out of tune. What began as a stressed liver becomes prediabetes, then type 2 diabetes, with diabetic complications radiating outward to kidneys, eyes, nerves, and vessels.

The question this chapter answers is both simple and audacious: Can a gentle, food-grade prebiotic bend both the liver and pancreas back toward metabolic steadiness? Can slow colonic fermentation of a branched arabinogalactan polysaccharide, happening deep in the distal colon hours after ingestion, send signals that calm hepatocyte oxidative stress, reduce fat accumulation in liver tissue, dampen inflammatory cascades, preserve pancreatic islet architecture, and ultimately allow these two critical organs to function more smoothly under the chronic metabolic stress of modern life?

The trail of studies spanning twenty-three years, from France to Egypt to Sudan to Brazil, says yes. The reasons are simultaneously mechanical (changing how fat emulsions present to digestive enzymes), metabolic (shifting hepatic fuel handling and inflammatory tone), and microbial (rebalancing the gut ecosystem that feeds signals into the portal vein). What follows is that trail, so you can see how the mechanistic pieces assemble into a coherent picture of liver-pancreas protection.

2001 - The Interface That Explains a Thousand Lunches

Marseille, France. The Centre National de la Recherche Scientifique, where biophysicists and enzymologists study how digestive enzymes work at the molecular level. Before we can understand how Gum arabic might affect fat digestion and downstream metabolic consequences, we need to understand where pancreatic lipase (the enzyme responsible for breaking down dietary triglycerides into fatty acids and glycerol that can be absorbed) does its work.

Here's the key insight that changes how you think about fat digestion. Pancreatic lipase doesn't work in the water phase where most enzymes operate, and it doesn't work in the oil phase where the fat molecules are. It works precisely at the interface; the shimmering boundary where emulsified fat droplets meet the aqueous digestive fluid. Picture a tiny sphere of olive oil suspended in the watery environment of your small intestine, stabilized by bile salts that coat its surface and prevent it from coalescing with other oil droplets. Pancreatic lipase must land on that spherical surface, bind to the lipid substrate right at the oil-water boundary, and perform its catalytic chemistry while one part of the enzyme is touching water and another part is touching oil. The enzyme's activity depends critically on how easily it can access and bind to that interface. This depends on how much surface area is available, how the bile salts and other surfactants are arranged, and what the charge and chemistry of the interface looks like.

Gum arabic's arabinogalactan-protein structure makes it amphiphilic (it has regions that interact with water and regions that interact favorably with hydrophobic molecules. This means it naturally accumulates at oil-water interfaces, exactly where lipase is trying to work. When you consume Gum arabic with a fatty meal, some of those molecules migrate to the surface of emulsified fat droplets, forming a subtle film that doesn't block lipase access completely but changes the geometry, the binding kinetics, and the time the enzyme spends productively attached to its substrate. Think of it as adding a soft bumper to a billiard table as the balls still move and

212

collide, but the angles and velocities shift just enough to change outcomes. Lipase can still dock and work, but the rate and efficiency are modulated. The CNRS team, led by Ali Tiss, Frédéric Carrière and colleagues measured these effects precisely. They used purified pancreatic lipase, controlled oil-water emulsion systems, and biophysical techniques that could track enzyme binding and activity at interfaces. They found that Gum arabic indeed altered lipase interfacial binding under low–bile salt conditions, inhibited its activity. In these lab systems the effects were measurable but modest, and the study did not assess fat absorption in living organisms. In principle, slightly slowing triglyceride breakdown at the droplet surface could flatten post-meal blood-lipid peaks and spread fat absorption over a longer period, potentially reducing the acute lipid load that organs like the liver and pancreatic beta cells experience, but this idea was not tested in this study [1].

This 2001 biophysical finding provided mechanistic insight into how a soluble prebiotic fiber like Gum arabic can interact with digestive enzymes at interfaces. However, connecting this interfacial chemistry directly to organ protection would require additional research. The interfacial film phenomenon could theoretically influence satiety through slower fat digestion, potentially affect post-prandial lipid peaks relevant to cardiovascular considerations, and might reduce lipotoxic exposure to pancreatic beta cells which are the insulin-secreting cells that can be stressed by excess fatty acids [1].

For potential applications, this in-vitro study showed that Gum arabic can alter lipase–substrate interactions at fiber-like concentrations. It established a physical-chemical mechanism rather than purely correlative observations, showing how a low-viscosity soluble fiber could theoretically modulate nutrient processing in ways that might benefit metabolic health.

2017 - The Pancreas Under the Microscope: Islets Given Room to Breathe

Cairo, Egypt. Ain Shams University, where researchers asked whether Arabic gum could protect pancreatic tissue and reduce diabetes-related damage in a mouse model. To understand why this study matters, we need to briefly explain *beta-cell lipotoxicity*; a phenomenon that helps explain why obesity and insulin resistance so often progress to frank diabetes.

Pancreatic beta cells, clustered in the islets of Langerhans scattered throughout the pancreas, have one primary job. Their primary job is to sense glucose levels in the blood and secrete precisely calibrated amounts of insulin to keep those levels stable. They're exquisitely sensitive metabolic sensors, ramping insulin secretion up when you eat and dialing it back down between meals. However, they weren't designed to operate in an environment of chronic nutrient excess with persistently elevated glucose combined with persistently elevated free fatty acids. These are the metabolic signatures of obesity and insulin resistance.

When beta cells are chronically exposed to high concentrations of fatty acids (particularly saturated fats like palmitate), those fats infiltrate the cells and trigger a cascade of problems. Some of these problems include mitochondrial dysfunction that generates excess reactive oxygen species, endoplasmic reticulum stress that activates the unfolded protein response, activated inflammatory signaling, and insulin secretion that becomes impaired even as demand is highest. This is lipotoxicity (cellular poisoning by excess fat) and it's a major mechanism by which obesity transitions from insulin resistance (where the pancreas can still compensate by making more insulin) to type 2 diabetes (where beta cells begin to fail and glucose control is lost).

Anything that reduces the post-meal lipid surge (lowering the height of the

214

fatty-acid peaks that beta cells see after each meal) or that calms the oxidative and inflammatory stress within islet cells, could theoretically preserve beta-cell function and delay or prevent diabetes progression. That's what Doaa Mohamed El-Nagar tested in a low-dose streptozotocin mouse model of type 2 diabetes, where repeated STZ injections partially destroy β-cells and cause persistent hyperglycemia [2].

Mice were divided into groups including diabetic controls receiving no treatment, and diabetic mice given a daily oral dose of Arabic gum (15% w/v) for 12 days. At the end of the experiment, the researchers measured blood glucose levels (the clinical standard), examined pancreatic histology under the microscope, used immunohistochemistry to stain for insulin (which would show whether beta cells were still present and functional), and measured oxidative stress markers and apoptotic markers in pancreatic tissue [2].

The results were visually striking and biochemically clear. Blood glucose levels were significantly lower in the Arabic gum group compared to diabetic controls. When pancreatic sections were examined under the microscope, islet architecture was markedly better preserved in the Acacia-treated animals (the islets were larger, more organized, with less inflammatory infiltrate and less cellular disruption). Insulin immunostaining (which labels β-cells as brown areas under light microscopy) showed stronger, more widespread signal in the Arabic gum group, indicating that more beta cells were alive, intact, and producing insulin. Oxidative stress markers (malondialdehyde immunostaining) were improved, and markers of apoptosis (the programmed cell death that eliminates damaged beta cells permanently) were reduced [2].

Let's translate this for the detailed picture. Type 2 diabetes isn't a switch that flips from normal to diabetic overnight; it's a gradual process where beta-cell mass and function decline over years or decades, first compensating for insulin resistance, then gradually failing under the chronic strain. Anything that slows that decline (preserving more beta cells in a functional state for longer) delays diabetes onset in prediabetic individuals, slows progression in early diabetics, and potentially reduces the need for injectable insulin in established disease. The 2017 Egyptian study suggested that Arabic gum can lower blood glucose and protect islet structure, likely via antioxidant and anti-apoptotic effects.

2019 - The Fatty Liver Era: The First-Pass Proof

Cairo, Egypt. Egypt's National Research Centre, Asmaa Taha is studying non-alcoholic fatty liver disease (NAFLD); the pandemic within the pandemic, affecting roughly a quarter of adults globally and rising in parallel with obesity and metabolic syndrome. NAFLD starts with simple steatosis (fat accumulation in hepatocytes without significant inflammation), can progress to non-alcoholic steatohepatitis (NASH, where inflammation and hepatocyte damage develop), and in a subset of patients continues to fibrosis, cirrhosis, and liver failure or cancer. It's now the leading indication for liver transplantation in many countries, and there's no approved pharmaceutical treatment that consistently reverses it. The standard advice (lose weight, exercise, reduce sugar and alcohol) works but depends entirely on sustained behavior change, which most patients struggle to achieve.

Before diving into the 2019 study, we need to explain concepts (*portal-vein first-pass* and the *gut-liver axis)* that are fundamental to understanding why Gum arabic affects the liver so directly. Unlike most of your circulation, where arteries branch into capillaries in tissues and then veins carry blood back to the heart, the intestines have a unique arrangement. Capillaries in the intestinal wall (where nutrients, bacterial products, and anything else that crosses the gut barrier enter the bloodstream) drain into the portal vein, which carries blood directly to the liver before it reaches the heart or general circulation. This means the liver receives the first, most concentrated dose of whatever the gut produces. When you eat a meal, the spike in glucose, amino acids, and fatty acids hits the liver first. When your gut bacteria ferment prebiotics and produce short-chain fatty acids, those SCFAs travel through the portal vein and reach hepatocytes at concentrations higher than anywhere else in the body. When your gut barrier becomes leaky and allows bacterial lipopolysaccharide (endotoxin) to translocate into blood, the liver sees that inflammatory signal first and strongest.

This anatomical arrangement creates the gut-liver axis where the liver is literally downstream of gut metabolism, and the signals coming through that portal vein (nutrients, microbial metabolites, inflammatory mediators) directly modulate hepatic gene expression, inflammatory tone, lipid metabolism, and glucose production. When gut fermentation shifts toward short-chain fatty acid production (acetate, propionate, butyrate), those SCFAs enter hepatocytes and act as signaling molecules. Propionate directly inhibits gluconeogenesis (the synthesis of new glucose), acetate modulates lipid metabolism, and butyrate has anti-inflammatory effects on Kupffer cells (the liver's resident macrophages). When the microbiome is dysbiotic and producing uremic toxins, inflammatory mediators, or excess endotoxin, the liver bears the brunt of that inflammatory signal. The gut-liver axis means that interventions targeting the microbiome aren't just acting locally in the intestines; they're sending new signals to the liver, potentially changing hepatic function even without direct contact.

The 2019 Egyptian study examined whether Gum arabic supplementation could improve liver status in an experimental NAFLD model while documenting parallel changes in gut bacteria. Eighteen male albino rats with diet-induced fatty liver were given a high fructose–high fat diet, with one group receiving 10% Gum arabic for 5 weeks, while researchers

217

measured total liver fat (Folch extraction), liver histology, and the relative abundance of Bacteroidetes and Firmicutes in fecal samples using real-time PCR [3].

Why did this matter clinically? NAFLD is a disease of metabolic overload and inflammatory tone, both of which are influenced by what's happening in the gut. Most proposed treatments target the liver directly (antioxidants, anti-inflammatory drugs, insulin sensitizers) with mixed results and often significant side effects. The 2019 Egyptian study examined whether Gum arabic supplementation could improve liver status in NAFLD while documenting parallel changes in the gut microbiome [3].

The findings showed hepatoprotective effects showing liver total fat decreased significantly in the Gum arabic group compared to the fatty liver control group, reaching levels comparable to normal controls. Histological analysis revealed marked improvement with far less fatty degeneration visible in hepatocytes. However, microbiome analysis showed only slight, statistically non-significant increases in Bacteroidetes and the Bacteroidetes-to-Firmicutes ratio. The authors concluded that while Gum arabic showed hepatoprotective potential, it "did not have a marked modulating effect on intestinal microbiota and more studies are needed in that area". This suggested the liver benefits might operate through mechanisms beyond simple microbiome modulation [3].

The two main findings of this study might seem counterintuitive given that we were trying to make a case that Gum arabic helps the liver via microbiome changes. However, these findings add further credence and solidifies emerging evidence (discussed later) that suggests Gum arabic works through multiple independent pathways beyond SCFA's. The counter-intuitive result warranted more research into these independent pathways. How did Gum arabic improve those hepatic markers if microbiome changes were not significant according to research results.

218

2020 - The Bridge Line from Kidneys to Hepatocytes

Abha, Saudi Arabia. King Khalid University, Mohammed and colleagues are conducting a study that we'll use for just one paragraph because its primary function in our narrative is to serve as an explicit conceptual bridge. Mohammed and colleagues examined Gum arabic's effects on diabetic kidney disease in streptozotocin-treated rats, showing antioxidant effects and partial protection of kidney structure with Gum arabic alone, and near-normal renal function and histology when Gum arabic was combined with insulin. These effects included improved glycemic control and lipid profile, better renal oxidative-stress markers, and reduced (though not completely prevented) glomerular and tubular damage [4].

The kidney chapter documented it in nephrons; this chapter is documenting it in hepatocytes, Kupffer cells, hepatic stellate cells, and pancreatic islets. One metabolic network, one intervention, multiple organ benefits explored across different experimental systems. We move forward now to studies specifically targeting liver and pancreas pathology.

2021 - Lightning Strikes, and the Liver Stays Standing: Acute Injury Protection

Nyala, Sudan, University of Nyala in collaboration with Nanjing Agricultural University in China. They wanted to test whether Gum arabic's protective benefits extend beyond slow metabolic problems (fatty liver, diabetes) to fulminant hepatotoxicity; the kind of injury that kills hepatocytes rapidly and requires immediate cellular defense. They chose carbon tetrachloride (CCl_4), the classic experimental hepatotoxin. Let's teach CCl_4 as a concept because it will appear again in the fibrosis study and it's worth understanding why researchers use it. Carbon tetrachloride is a "laboratory lightning bolt"; a chemical that, when metabolized by liver enzymes (particularly cytochrome P450), generates highly reactive free radicals (trichloromethyl radicals) that immediately attack anything nearby. They steal electrons from the fats in cell membranes, starting chain reactions of destruction. They damage proteins by oxidizing amino-acid side chains and they also disrupt cellular integrity. The result is rapid, severe hepatocyte injury whereby cells swell, membranes rupture, organelles fragment, and cells die by necrosis and apoptosis. Inflammatory signals are released and immune cells are recruited. If the exposure is acute and then stopped, the liver can regenerate; if exposure continues, fibrosis develops as stellate cells are activated to wall off the damage. CCl_4 is useful precisely because it's predictable, dose-dependent, and it creates injury through oxidative pathways that mirror many real-world liver insults including acetaminophen overdose, alcohol poisoning, oxygen deprivation during surgery, and viral hepatitis [5].

Before walking through the 2021 study, let's also teach *transaminases as "leak detectors"*. Alanine aminotransferase (ALT) and aspartate aminotransferase (AST) are enzymes that normally work inside hepatocytes, shuttling amino groups around in normal metabolism. When hepatocyte membranes are damaged (by toxins, viruses, ischemia, inflammation) these enzymes leak out into the bloodstream where they can be measured. High ALT and AST in the blood means liver cells are being destroyed right now. When you give an intervention and see ALT/AST drop, it's a direct signal that hepatocyte membranes are staying more intact meaning fewer cells are dying, damage is being contained, and the parenchyma is being rescued. It's one of the most clinically relevant signals in hepatology because it tracks active injury.

The Nyala team gave rats CCl_4 (twice weekly for three weeks) to induce severe liver injury, with some animals receiving Gum arabic supplementation (5% of diet) before and during the toxic exposure. After the injury period, they measured three categories of markers that define whether liver cells are being protected: 1-liver enzymes (ALT and AST), 2-oxidative stress (malondialdehyde from lipid peroxidation, 3-depletion of antioxidant enzymes including SOD and GSH-Px), 4-inflammatory cytokines (TNF-alpha, interleukin-1β, interleukin-6), and 5-apoptotic markers (caspase-3 activation via gene expression and immunohistochemistry). They also examined liver histology under the microscope to see what the tissue looked like [5].

The protective effect was comprehensive and multi-layered. ALT and AST (the leak gauges) dropped significantly in Gum arabic–supplemented animals, meaning fewer hepatocytes were rupturing and spilling their contents. Malondialdehyde (the signature waste product of gut destruction) was markedly reduced, indicating that the free-radical storm unleashed by CCl_4 was being contained before it could propagate through membranes. Tumor necrosis factor-alpha, the master inflammatory cytokine, was suppressed, meaning the inflammatory amplification cycle (where injured cells release signals that recruit immune cells that release more cytokines that injure more cells) was being interrupted. Caspase-3 expression, the executioner enzyme of apoptosis, was lower, meaning cells that were stressed but salvageable were being given a chance to repair rather than initiating programmed death. Importantly, histology told the final story; liver architecture was better preserved, with less necrosis, less inflammatory infiltrate, less hepatocyte swelling and disruption [5].

This is the pattern we've seen repeatedly throughout the book. Oxidative stress, inflammation, and apoptosis are the three horsemen of cellular injury in virtually every organ and disease model. Gum arabic consistently attenuates all three. The 2021 CCl_4 study anchored that pattern specifically in hepatotoxicity; when the liver is hit with an acute chemical insult designed to overwhelm defenses proving Gum arabic provides measurable cellular protection. For clinicians, this kind of data matters because acute liver injury (from acetaminophen overdose, from alcohol binges, from drug reactions, from ischemia during surgery) is a clinical reality where we have limited tools and where even modest improvements in hepatocyte survival translate into better outcomes and fewer liver-failure cases requiring transplantation.

2021 - Not Just Injury Control: Stopping the Scar Builders

Nyala, Sudan. The same research group, now asking a different question:

If Gum arabic protects against acute liver injury, does it also slow chronic liver fibrosis; the progressive scarring that turns reversible injury into irreversible cirrhosis? To understand why this matters, we need to briefly explain the cellular machinery of *hepatic fibrosis*.

When hepatocytes are repeatedly injured (by alcohol, by viruses, by metabolic stress, by toxins) they don't just die and regenerate indefinitely. After repeated injury cycles, *hepatic stellate cells* (normally quiescent cells that store vitamin A and sit quietly in the space between hepatocytes and sinusoidal blood vessels) become activated. Once activated, stellate cells transform into myofibroblasts, proliferating and synthesizing collagen at high rates. This collagen deposition is an attempt to wall off injury and maintain structural integrity, but when it becomes excessive and disorganized, it creates scar tissue that disrupts normal liver architecture, impeding blood flow, and impairing hepatocyte function.

The molecular signals driving stellate-cell activation include transforming growth factor-beta 1 (TGF-β1), the master profibrotic cytokine, and alpha-smooth muscle actin (α-SMA), a marker of myofibroblast differentiation. When you measure TGF-β1 and α-SMA going up in liver tissue, you're watching the scar machine turn on. Chronic fibrosis progresses to cirrhosis (nodular, scarred liver with compromised blood flow and failing synthetic function) which leads to portal hypertension, liver failure, and hepatocellular carcinoma. Stopping or slowing fibrosis is one of the major goals in hepatology because it's the point where reversible disease becomes irreversible [6].

The Nyala group used the same CCl_4 model but now given repeatedly over weeks to induce chronic injury and fibrosis rather than single acute injury. Rats received CCl_4 injections twice per week for 7 weeks, with or without Gum arabic supplementation in their diet. At the end of the experiment, they measured markers of fibrosis: 1-hydroxyproline content in liver tissue (hydroxyproline is an amino acid abundant in collagen, so tissue hydroxyproline is a direct measure of collagen deposition), 2-TGF-β1 and α-SMA expression (the molecular signals driving fibrosis), and 3-Sirius red staining that makes collagen visible under the microscope) [6].

The results demonstrated Gum arabic significantly reduced collagen deposition. Hydroxyproline content was lower in supplemented animals. TGF-β1 and α-SMA expression dropped, indicating that stellate cells were less activated and producing less fibrotic signaling. Histological sections showed less collagen staining, with better-preserved normal lobular architecture [6]. This wasn't just putting out the acute oxidative fire documented in the first 2021 study; this was asking the scar-building machinery to stand down, to reduce the chronic remodeling response that turns hepatitis into cirrhosis.

Why this moves Gum arabic into the chronic-disease lane? Fibrosis is the slope toward cirrhosis, and that slope determines quality of life and survival for patients with chronic liver disease. Current antifibrotic therapies are limited and the most effective intervention is removing the underlying cause (stop drinking, cure hepatitis C, lose weight in NAFLD), which works but requires behavior change or expensive drugs. An adjunct that reduces fibrotic signaling, is safe for long-term use, and is tolerable enough that patients can continuously take it for years, could slow progression for the millions of people living with chronic liver disease who haven't yet reached cirrhosis.

2021 - DNA Calm Across Tissues: When Genome Protection Travels

Fortaleza, Brazil. Federal University of Ceará, Avelino is conducting a study that expands beyond the liver to show that Gum arabic's protective effects operate at the most fundamental level (genomic integrity) and that this protection isn't confined to one organ. Before discussing the study, let's explain *antigenotoxicity* and why it matters for cancer prevention and healthy aging.

Genotoxicity is damage to DNA (strand breaks, base modifications, chromosome breaks) caused by reactive oxygen species, reactive nitrogen species, chemical mutagens, radiation, or failed DNA replication. Cells sustain thousands of DNA lesions daily from normal metabolism. What determines whether those lesions accumulate into mutations, chromosomal aberrations, and eventually cancer is the balance between damage rate and repair capacity. *Antigenotoxic* interventions are those that reduce the damage rate, either by neutralizing the reactive species that attack DNA (antioxidant mechanisms) or by supporting DNA-repair systems. Two standard assays for measuring genotoxicity are the *comet assay* and the *micronucleus test* (which measures chromosome fragments or whole chromosomes that get lost during cell division and form small extra nuclei, indicating chromosome breakage or mitotic failure).

The Brazilian team used a colorectal carcinogenesis model whereby mice were given chemical carcinogens to induce DNA damage and

224

inflammatory stress in the intestinal tract, liver, and bone marrow (where rapidly dividing cells are particularly vulnerable to genotoxic insults). After carcinogen exposure, some animals were supplemented with Gum arabic (2.5% or 5%) via gavage for twelve weeks. At the end of the experiment, tissues were harvested and analyzed for aberrant crypt formation, genotoxicity, and oxidative stress markers in colon, liver, blood, and bone marrow samples.

The findings showed cross-tissue protection. Gum arabic significantly reduced the number of aberrant crypts in treated animals compared to controls. Likewise, there was a decline in colonic, hepatic, and systemic genotoxicity and oxidative stress markers in the GA-treated groups. These results demonstrate systemic protection reaching intestinal mucosa, liver tissue, and bone marrow (indicating protection of rapidly dividing hematopoietic cells) [7].

This study did something conceptually important as it showed that Gum arabic's protective effects aren't narrowly targeted to one organ or one injury mechanism. The same intervention that was protecting hepatocytes from CCl_4 and reducing liver fibrosis in Sudan was protecting intestinal epithelial cells, hepatocytes, and bone marrow cells from genotoxic damage in Brazil. DNA damage, in any tissue, is heavily driven by oxidative stress (reactive species that attack DNA bases and break phosphodiester bonds) and interventions that reduce systemic oxidative tone, support cellular antioxidant defenses, and quiet inflammatory signaling protect genomes wherever DNA is undergoing damage [7].

For liver and pancreas specifically, this matters because these organs face high genotoxic pressure. The liver metabolizes toxins, drugs, and carcinogens, generating reactive intermediates while the pancreas faces oxidative stress from high metabolic activity in islets. Both are sites of cancer development (hepatocellular carcinoma, pancreatic adenocarcinoma) where accumulated DNA damage drives malignant transformation. Keeping DNA calmer (fewer strand breaks today) means lower mutation pressure tomorrow, which over years translates into lower cancer risk. The 2021 Brazilian study demonstrated that Gum arabic's benefits extend to genomic stability, a layer of protection beneath the cellular and tissue-level effects we've been documenting.

2022 - Real-World Toxin: When the Food Chain Strikes the Liver

Ismailia, Egypt. Suez Canal University, Noha Ahmed is testing Arabic gum against a toxin that matters for public health in ways that laboratory chemicals like CCl_4 don't. The public-health challenge is that you can't easily eliminate aflatoxin exposure in regions where climate and storage conditions favor mold growth. The solution requires massive infrastructure investment in improved grain storage, drying, and monitoring. In the meantime, dietary interventions that could reduce the hepatotoxic and carcinogenic effects of the aflatoxin that does get consumed would be enormously valuable. Particularly if those interventions are affordable and culturally acceptable in the populations at highest risk.

The Suez Canal team gave rats aflatoxin B1 to induce liver injury, with some animals receiving Arabic gum supplementation (7.5 g/kg/day). They measured liver enzymes (transaminases), oxidative stress markers (malondialdehyde, glutathione peroxidase activity, total antioxidant capacity, Nrf2 and SOD1 protein expression), inflammatory markers (inducible nitric oxide synthase, tumor necrosis factor-alpha, interleukin-6, NF-κB), and apoptotic markers (caspase-3), alongside histological examination of liver tissue [8].

Arabic gum provided significant protection. Liver enzymes stayed lower, oxidative stress was reduced (less MDA, preserved glutathione peroxidase activity, restored SOD1 and Nrf2 expression, maintained total antioxidant capacity), inflammatory cytokines were suppressed (lower iNOS, TNF-alpha, IL-6, and NF-κB), and apoptosis was dampened (reduced caspase activation). Histology showed better-preserved hepatocyte architecture with less necrosis and inflammatory infiltrate [8].

This wasn't a surprise as we have already seen Arabic gum protect against oxidative, inflammatory, and apoptotic injury from multiple insults. However, it was critically important contextually because it moved the intervention from "useful in lab toxicity models" to "potentially protective against a real-world dietary carcinogen that's killing people". For African and Asian countries with high aflatoxin exposure and limited resources to solve the storage-infrastructure problem, the 2022 AFB1 study suggested a plausible public-health strategy to promote consumption of Arabic gum (which is produced locally in many of these regions, particularly the Sahel) as a daily dietary supplement that could provide some hepatoprotection against unavoidable aflatoxin exposure. It's not a perfect solution (the real solution is preventing contamination) but it's a practical harm-reduction approach while infrastructure improves.

2022 - The Hepato-Renal Loop: When Organ Failures Amplify Each Other

Alexandria, Egypt. Medical Research Institute, Shimaa Antar Fareed is examining a clinical scenario that's devastatingly common but often overlooked in single-organ research. They are researching the bidirectional relationship between kidney and liver disease, where uremia causes hepatic injury. Let's explain the hepato-renal loop clearly because it's the conceptual framework for understanding why interventions that affect both organs matter clinically.

227

When kidneys fail (from diabetes, hypertension, drug toxicity, obstruction, inflammation), they stop clearing uremic toxins (indoxyl sulfate, p-cresyl sulfate, urea, others) and those toxins accumulate in blood, circulating everywhere. The liver, receiving blood continuously, is exposed to high concentrations of these uremic toxins, which generate oxidative stress in hepatocytes, impair mitochondrial function, and trigger inflammatory signaling. Meanwhile, when the liver fails (from cirrhosis, fatty liver disease, hepatitis, toxins), it can't synthesize normal amounts of albumin and clotting factors, can't clear ammonia efficiently (leading to hepatic encephalopathy), and can't maintain proper blood flow through the portal system (leading to portal hypertension and ascites). The altered blood flow patterns and inflammatory environment negatively affect renal blood flow and filtering function. The two organs are in constant communication (kidney disease makes the liver sicker, liver disease makes the kidneys sicker) and the loop can spiral toward combined organ failure where prognosis is grim, and treatment options are limited.

The Egyptian researchers created uremic rats using a two-stage surgical nephrectomy procedure (subtotal nephrectomy in the left kidney, followed by total right nephrectomy one week later) and examined liver status in these animals, with and without Gum arabic supplementation for five weeks. They measured biochemical parameters and performed comprehensive liver histology including light microscopy, electron microscopy, and immunohistochemical studies, asking whether the liver injury by kidney failure could be reduced by an intervention known to reduce uremic-toxin generation and systemic oxidative stress [9].

The result is Gum arabic improved both blood chemistry and tissue structure in kidney-failure rats. Hepatocytes looked healthier under the microscope, with less pathological changes, less inflammatory infiltrate, and better-preserved architecture as confirmed by morphometric measures. Biochemical markers confirmed the histological observation with parameters that were elevated in uremic rats and showed great improvement with GA administration [9].

This study reinforced the interconnected network view we've been building. Gum arabic's effects on one organ create benefits in another because organs are metabolically and biochemically linked. The kidney chapter showed how Acacia reduces uremic-toxin generation by shifting gut bacterial metabolism away from proteolysis and toward saccharolysis. Less indoxyl sulfate and p-cresyl sulfate are made because bacteria are fermenting fiber instead of protein. Those toxins, when reduced systemically, bathe the liver in a less inflammatory milieu. The short-chain fatty acids produced from Gum arabic fermentation travel through the portal vein to the liver, directly reducing hepatic inflammation and oxidative stress. The improved gut barrier (documented in IBD studies) reduces LPS translocation that would activate hepatic Kupffer cells.

All of these mechanisms (microbiome rebalancing, uremic-toxin reduction, SCFA signaling, barrier integrity) work simultaneously, and their effects travel through the bloodstream to every organ. Fix the gut-kidney axis, and the liver breathes easier.

2024 - One Hospital Insult, Two Organs Saved: Dual Protection in Practice

Saudi Arabia in Collaboration with Egypt, Abdalla Abdalla and colleagues are leading a study asking whether Arabic gum (Hashab gum from Acacia Senegal) could protect both kidneys and liver simultaneously when both organs are being injured by the same nephrotoxic and hepatotoxic drug. We introduced gentamicin nephrotoxicity in the kidney chapter (the aminoglycoside antibiotic that accumulates in proximal tubular cells and generates oxidative stress, leading to acute kidney injury) but gentamicin doesn't only hit kidneys. It also causes hepatotoxicity, particularly with prolonged use or high doses, through similar oxidative mechanisms.

Let's frame *dual-organ drug injury* as a clinical problem: hospitals routinely use medications that are necessary for treating serious infections or other conditions but that carry significant organ toxicity. Aminoglycosides for Gram-negative sepsis. NSAIDs for pain and inflammation. Chemotherapy for cancer. Contrast agents for imaging. Clinicians have to balance the therapeutic benefit against the risk of acute kidney injury, hepatotoxicity, or both. If there was a safe, well-tolerated adjunct that could be given alongside these medications to reduce organ injury without interfering with therapeutic efficacy, it could change outcomes as you could use higher doses when needed, treat for longer durations, and use these drugs more safely in vulnerable patients (elderly, diabetic, already compromised renal or hepatic function). That's the promise the 2024 Saudi-Egypt study was testing [10].

The researchers gave mice gentamicin at doses known to cause both nephrotoxicity and hepatotoxicity (80 mg/kg for 15 days), with different groups receiving water extract of Hashab gum (300 mg/kg) either sequentially after gentamicin treatment or co-administered simultaneously with gentamicin. After the treatment period (one month total), they measured kidney function markers (creatinine, blood urea nitrogen), liver function markers (ALT, AST), oxidative stress markers in both organs (malondialdehyde, glutathione, catalase), cytokine levels, and cytokine levels in kidney and liver tissue [10].

The protection was simultaneous and substantial. In Hashab gum-treated animals (both sequential and co-administration groups), kidney markers were significantly better (lower creatinine and urea, with creatinine reaching control levels), liver markers were significantly better (lower

ALT and AST), oxidative stress was reduced in both organs (less MDA, preserved GSH, maintained catalase activity), and cytokine levels improved. The same intervention, given as simple water extract that could be administered as easily as an oral preparation, protected both organs at once [10].

For hospital protocols, this is transformative data. Rather than requiring separate hepatoprotective and nephroprotective agents (each with their own side effects, drug interactions, monitoring requirements, and costs), you could potentially use a single food-grade adjunct. The mechanism explains why dual protection is plausible. Hashab gum's antioxidant support (preserving glutathione, supporting catalase), anti-inflammatory effects, and cellular protection work at a level that's relevant to any cell facing oxidative and inflammatory injury. Whether that cell is a proximal tubular epithelial cell in the kidney or a hepatocyte in the liver. The systemic reduction in oxidative stress and improved antioxidant defenses benefit every organ in the stress field [10].

The 2024 study also reinforced a practical point about formulation as this wasn't a proprietary extract requiring specialized processing. It was Hashab gum dissolved in water and administered orally. That's the same formulation patients can make at home by stirring Hashab gum powder into water. The translatability from research to practice is immediate [10].

2024 - Multimorbidity Is the Rule, Not the Exception: When Liver and Kidneys Fail Together

Cairo, Egypt. Cairo University, Manal Lotfy and colleagues are examining dual-organ toxicity (the combined hepatic and renal damage caused by environmental toxicants) which represents a common clinical scenario since many toxins (pesticides, drugs, heavy metals) injure both organs simultaneously.

The challenge is brutal as patients with cirrhosis develop complications such as ascites (fluid accumulation in the abdomen), variceal bleeding (from high portal pressure), hepatic encephalopathy (confusion from ammonia accumulation), and coagulopathy (impaired clotting from reduced synthesis of clotting factors). All are difficult to manage and require medications (diuretics, lactulose, albumin infusions, blood-pressure management) that themselves can stress the kidneys. When those patients also have CKD, their kidneys struggle to handle the altered hemodynamics, uremic toxins accumulated from reduced clearance, and the medications required to manage cirrhosis complications. Mortality is high, and therapeutic options narrow dramatically as both organs fail because interventions for one can worsen the other.

The Cairo team used an animal model combining liver and kidney injury through chlorpyrifos-methyl (CPM) administration (an organophosphate pesticide causing oxidative damage to both organs) then supplemented some groups with Gum arabic (either 15% w/v in drinking water or 1 g/kg by gavage) for eight weeks while tracking markers of both liver function (ALT, AST, total bilirubin, total protein, albumin) and kidney function (creatinine, urea), alongside oxidative stress markers (MDA, GSH, SOD, catalase) and histopathological indicators of inflammation in both organs [11].

The findings were that Gum arabic improved markers of both liver and kidney function simultaneously. Liver enzymes decreased significantly toward normal levels, kidney markers (creatinine and urea) improved substantially, oxidative stress indices dropped in both organs (reduced MDA, preserved GSH, maintained SOD and catalase), and histology of both liver and kidney tissue showed markedly less severe pathology with reduced necrosis, fibrosis, inflammatory infiltration, and cellular degeneration [11].

This wasn't a complete reversal (both organs showed residual damage from the toxin), but it was meaningful protection. The kind of incremental improvement that demonstrates dual-organ antioxidant and anti-inflammatory efficacy. This study addressed a toxicological reality relevant to clinical medicine. Many patients face combined hepatorenal injury from environmental exposures, medications (NSAIDs, antibiotics, chemotherapy), or metabolic diseases where oxidative stress damages multiple organs. These patients need interventions that are safe enough to use when both organs are vulnerable, simple enough that adherence is realistic, and effective enough to reduce oxidative damage across organ systems. The pesticide model demonstrates proof-of-concept for multi-organ protection through antioxidant mechanisms. The 2024 dual-organ study showed it provides measurable benefit in the scenario where it's most needed.

Coda: Livers That Breathe Easier, Islets That Last Longer

By now the pattern is difficult to miss. A low-viscosity, easily tolerated prebiotic that blends invisibly into water, tea, juice, or yogurt. It doesn't taste like medicine, doesn't require refrigeration, doesn't interact with drugs, costs less per month than most clinical interventions. It gently modulates fat digestion at oil-water interfaces, reducing the acute lipid surges that stress beta cells. It spares pancreatic islet architecture under diabetic metabolic stress, preserving insulin-secreting capacity. It calms hepatocyte oxidative storms in both acute injury and chronic fibrosis, working through the same antioxidant-anti-inflammatory-anti-apoptotic triad across injury models. It reduces DNA damage across tissues, lowering mutation pressure that would otherwise accumulate toward cancer. It operates through the gut-liver axis, sending improved metabolic signals (more SCFAs, fewer uremic toxins, less endotoxin) through the portal vein to retune hepatic metabolism. Importantly, it keeps working when organs fail together, providing bidirectional benefit in the hepato-renal scenarios where therapeutic options narrow and prognosis darkens.

This is not a promise of cure or reversal of end-stage disease. It's a promise of steadier metabolic terrain with fewer oxidative sparks, quieter inflammatory chatter, better-preserved cellular machinery, stronger barriers against the toxins and stresses that modern life imposes. For the fatty liver patient trying to avoid progression to cirrhosis, for the prediabetic patient whose beta cells are straining, for the cirrhotic patient whose kidneys are beginning to falter, for the hospitalized patient receiving nephrotoxic and hepatotoxic medications, that steadier terrain can be the difference between progression and stabilization, between organ failure and preserved function, between transplant list and continued independent life. It's chronic care at its most fundamental. It's not a heroic rescue, but daily support that allows organs to keep functioning a little longer, a little better, under conditions they were never designed to endure indefinitely.

Immunity and Antimicrobial Effects

The story doesn't end with the liver and pancreas. Two live threads from this chapter lead directly into the immune and antimicrobial territory we're heading toward. First, the antigenotoxic and anti-inflammatory profile creates calmer immune training. When DNA damage and inflammatory cytokine levels are lower (in intestinal mucosa, in liver tissue, in bone marrow where immune cells are born) the immune system develops in a less inflammatory milieu. Chronic low-grade inflammation skews immunity toward hyperresponsiveness, drives autoimmune tendencies, and exhausts regulatory mechanisms. The Brazilian study showed that Gum arabic reduces DNA damage across tissues, including bone marrow where hematopoietic stem cells give rise to all immune lineages. The liver studies showed consistently reduced inflammatory cytokines (TNF-alpha, IL-6, iNOS). When the tissues where immune cells develop, patrol, and respond are in a calmer oxidative and inflammatory state, those immune cells train differently and are better able to discriminate threats from normal tissue. They are more capable of resolving inflammation rather than amplifying it. That sets the table perfectly for discussing how Hashab gum affects regulatory T-cell development, mucosal immunity, and inflammatory bowel disease, which your next chapter will cover.

Secondly, the SCFA signals that steadied liver and pancreas also teach immune cells. The same propionate, acetate, and butyrate molecules that traveled through the portal vein to reduce hepatic gluconeogenesis and quiet Kupffer cells don't stop there. They circulate systemically, reaching lymphoid tissues, mucosal-associated immune structures, and even crossing into the brain. Short-chain fatty acids are now recognized as major immunomodulatory signals. Butyrate promotes differentiation of regulatory T cells (Tregs) that suppress excessive immune responses, propionate modulates dendritic-cell function affecting how antigens are presented and whether tolerance or inflammation is induced, and acetate affects neutrophil function and antibody responses.

Your next chapter will document how Gum arabic affects pathogen overgrowth, mucosal barrier function, and immune regulation.

References:

1. Tiss, Ali, et al. "Effects of gum arabic on lipase interfacial binding and activity." Analytical Biochemistry, vol. 294, no. 1, 2001, pp. 36–43
2. El-Nagar, Doaa Mohamed. "Pancrease-protective effects of Arabic gum on diabetic type 2 streptozotocin-induced in albino mice." Research Journal of Pharmaceutical, Biological and Chemical Sciences, vol. 8, no. 1, 2017, pp. 1263–1270
3. Taha, Asmaa Ramadan, Sahar Alokbi, and Hoda Mabrok. "Hepatoprotective Effect of Gum Arabic in Non-Alcoholic Fatty Liver and Potential Modulation of Intestinal Microbiota (FS07-07-19)." Current Developments in Nutrition, vol. 3, suppl. 1, 2019, article nzz040.FS07-07-19.
4. Mohammed, Muataz E., et al. "Preventive Role of Gum Arabic Administration on STZ Induced Diabetic Kidney Disease in Rats; Renal Antioxidant and Histopathological Evidence." International Journal of Morphology, vol. 38, no. 4, 2020, pp. 1003–1009.
5. Hamid, Mohammed, et al. "Protective Effect of Gum Arabic on Liver Oxidative Stress, Inflammation and Apoptosis Induced by CCl4 in vivo." EAS Journal of Nursing and Midwifery, vol. 3, no. 1, Feb. 2021, pp. 27-34,
6. Hamid, Mohammed, et al. "Dietary Gum Arabic Alleviates Carbon Tetrachloride Induced Liver Fibrosis in Wistar Rats." Asian Journal of Research in Animal and Veterinary Sciences, vol. 8, no. 3, 2021, pp. 1-12
7. Avelino, André Luís Nunes, et al. "Antioxidant and Antigenotoxic Actions of Gum Arabic on the Intestinal Mucosa, Liver and Bone Marrow of Swiss Mice Submitted to Colorectal Carcinogenesis." Nutrition and Cancer, vol. 74, no. 3, 2022, pp. 956–964
8. Ahmed, Noha, et al. "Arabic Gum Could Alleviate the Aflatoxin B1-Provoked Hepatic Injury in Rat: The Involvement of Oxidative Stress, Inflammatory, and Apoptotic Pathways." Toxins, vol. 14, no. 9, 2022, article 605.
9. Fareed, Shimaa Antar, et al. "Ameliorating Effect of Gum Arabic on the Liver Tissues of the Uremic Rats; A Biochemical and Histological Study." Tissue and Cell, vol. 77, Aug. 2022, article 101832
10. Sayed, Abdalla Abdalla Abdalla, et al. "Water Extract of Arabic Gum Ameliorates the Gentamicin-Induced Nephrotoxicity, Hepatotoxicity, Oxidative Stress Markers and Cytokine Levels in Mice." South Eastern European Journal of Public Health, vol. 25, suppl. 2, 2024, pp. 2074–2084.
11. Lotfy, Manal Mohamed, et al. "Biochemical Studies on Efficiency of Natural Gum in Chronic Kidney Failure and Liver Cirrhosis in Rats." World's Veterinary Journal, vol. 14, no. 3, 2024, pp. 293–310

CHAPTER 15

The Research Explaining Systematic
Antioxidant & Anti-inflammatory effects

From Background Noise to Clean Signals

Imagine trying to hear a doorbell when the smoke alarm in your house never stops chirping. You know the doorbell's working but the signal gets lost in the constant, grating background noise. Your nervous system, overwhelmed by the false alarm that never resolves, eventually learns to tune everything out. That's our analogy for the innate immunity operating inside a body awash in gut-derived endotoxin and chronic oxidative stress. The microbial threats are real, the danger signals ring clearly, but the immune system's ability to respond precisely and proportionally has been dulled by months or years of inflammatory static. This static is the low-grade but relentless noise created when a leaky gut barrier allows bacterial lipopolysaccharide to translocate into circulation. It's what inevitably happens when dysbiotic microbes produce inflammatory metabolites instead of protective SCFA's, when the liver and kidneys are bathed in uremic toxins and oxidative stress that spills over into immune tissues.

The chapters we've just completed established something foundational for understanding immunity. Hashab gum lowers the background noise through its slow colonic fermentation producing acetate, propionate, and butyrate. Additionally, it does so through the strengthening of intestinal tight junctions that reduce endotoxin translocation. More importantly for this chapter, it does so through systemic reduction of oxidative stress and inflammatory cytokines throughout the liver, kidneys, and bone marrow where immune cells are born. Hashab gum creates what we might call a quieter immunological terrain. The smoke alarm stops chirping. The inflammatory static fades to a manageable hum. In that calmer environment, something remarkable but underappreciated becomes possible. The first responders of innate immunity don't just wake up from their exhausted, desensitized state; they start working better.

Neutrophils and macrophages (the professional immune cells that patrol tissues, recognize danger, and respond within minutes) regain precision, speed, and effectiveness which is lost to chronic inflammatory noise. What follows is the story of how researchers discovered, measured, and validated that Hashab gum's gentle metabolic retuning translates into upgraded immune function at the cellular level. It's a story told through four studies spanning four years and three continents, moving from isolated immune cells in laboratory dishes to blood drawn from human volunteers. The studies will answer mechanistic questions about how cells kill bacteria to practical questions about whether this works in aging immune systems. The studies document improvements in the fundamental maneuvers of innate immunity and they do so in ways that suggest a different philosophy of immune support. Not hyper-stimulation that risks autoimmunity and chronic inflammation, but precision enhancement that works with the body's own signals, amplifying appropriate responses when needed while maintaining the capacity to stand down when threats pass.

2020 - The Day Neutrophils Got Their Webbing Back

Hannover, Germany, in collaboration with Khartoum, Sudan. Before we can understand what the 2020 study discovered, we need to establish who the first responders are and what they actually do when infection threatens.

When bacteria breach a barrier (through a cut in skin, across a weakened intestinal wall, into the lungs via inhaled droplets) the immune system's opening response doesn't come from antibodies (those require days to weeks to develop) or T cells (which need time to be activated and expand).

The opening response comes from *innate immunity*, the ancient evolutionarily conserved defense system that predates adaptive immunity by hundreds of millions of years and that operates on timescales measured in minutes to hours rather than days to weeks. Think of innate immunity as the body's professional first responders. The patrol officers already on duty, constantly surveilling tissues, trained to recognize broad categories of danger (bacterial cell walls, viral nucleic acids, damaged self-cells releasing alarm signals) and respond immediately with a standardized playbook.

The stars of innate immunity are two types of white blood cells called *neutrophils* and *macrophages*. Neutrophils are the most abundant white blood cells in human circulation; billions of them, with lifespans of only hours to days, constantly being produced in bone marrow and patrolling through blood vessels. When infection or injury occurs, neutrophils are chemically summoned to the site within minutes, squeezing through blood-vessel walls and migrating through tissues toward the source of danger signals. Macrophages are longer-lived cells that reside in tissues of the liver (Kupffer cells), lungs (alveolar macrophages), brain (microglia), and throughout the gut lamina propria where they continuously sample their environment. Macrophages are always clearing cellular debris and dead cells during normal maintenance but are also capable of rapid activation when they encounter pathogens.

Healthy innate immunity is about *precision*, deploying the right tactic at the right intensity for the specific threat, then standing down quickly once the threat is cleared. Chronic inflammatory conditions, immunosenescence, metabolic diseases, and the endotoxin-rich environment of gut dysbiosis all tend to impair this precision, leaving neutrophils either hyporesponsive (they don't activate strongly enough when real threats appear) or hyperresponsive (they activate inappropriately, causing collateral damage to healthy tissue). The former leaves you vulnerable to infection; the latter drives chronic inflammatory diseases.

With that foundation, we can understand what the 2020 Hannover-Khartoum collaboration tested and why their findings mattered. Researchers led by Shima Hassan Baien and Nicole de Buhr, working across veterinary medicine and human immunology labs, asked a straightforward question: *Does Gum arabic (Hashab gum from Acacia Senegal) directly affect how innate immune cells function when they encounter bacteria?* They looked beyond the microbiome effects (those were already well-documented), the systemic anti-inflammatory signaling effects (also established), and instead focused on the direct interaction with the immune cells themselves. *Could Hashab gum modulate intracellular killing mechanisms?*

They used granulocytes (the category of white blood cells that includes neutrophils) isolated freshly from human blood and from cattle blood. These cells were exposed to Hashab gum in culture dishes, then challenged with two of the most clinically relevant bacterial pathogens called Staphylococcus aureus (the Gram-positive bacterium responsible for everything from skin infections to pneumonia to sepsis) and Escherichia coli (the Gram-negative gut bacterium that causes urinary tract infections, bloodstream infections, and food poisoning). The researchers measured phagocytosis rates (how many bacteria each neutrophil engulfed), oxidative burst intensity (how much reactive oxygen was generated through intracellular ROS production), and bacterial killing efficiency (counting how many bacteria survived after exposure to the immune cells), alongside direct antibacterial effects of Hashab gum extracts themselves and cell viability (making sure the Hashab gum wasn't just killing the immune cells, which would be a pyrrhic victory) [1].

The results were striking and consistent across measured parameters. Hashab gum exhibited direct antibacterial effects against certain S. aureus and E. coli strains. Phagocytosis increased (more bacteria were engulfed per cell-The intracellular oxidative burst strengthened) and reactive oxygen species production rose within the granulocytes. Critically, these functional improvements translated into the outcome that matters most, which is bacterial survival dropped. Both S. aureus and E. coli were killed more efficiently when neutrophils had been exposed to Hashab gum. The effects were concentration-dependent (higher Hashab gum concentrations produced stronger effects) and occurred without compromising neutrophil viability. This means the immune cells weren't being whipped into suicidal hyperactivation but rather were performing their intracellular killing jobs more effectively [1].

Let's emphasize what made this finding particularly elegant. The enhancement focused on intracellular mechanisms showing increased ROS production leading to more effective phagocytosis and intracellular bacterial killing. Interestingly, no effect was seen on neutrophil extracellular trap (NET) formation, suggesting Hashab's immunomodulatory effects operate specifically through enhancing intracellular antimicrobial pathways rather than extracellular trapping mechanisms. The phrase that captures this is "targeted enhancement of specific immune functions". The neutrophils became more effective at their core intracellular killing job without necessarily engaging all possible antimicrobial mechanisms [1].

Why was this a hinge moment in the Hashab gum's research narrative? The answer is that up to 2020, Hashab gum's reputation lived almost entirely in metabolic and microbiome research. It was a prebiotic that

241

shifted gut bacteria, a viscosity modifier that slowed nutrient absorption, a fermentation substrate that produced helpful short-chain fatty acids, an anti-inflammatory that calmed oxidative stress in tissues. The 2020 innate-immunity study pulled it into a different scientific domain (cellular immunology, direct immune-cell modulation) and showed that whatever Hashab gum does to benefit health, it's not only working through the microbiome or systemic metabolism. It's also directly engaging the immune system's hardware, the cells themselves, enhancing their intracellular antimicrobial capacity in ways that could explain clinical observations about infection resistance and inflammatory control that had been documented but not mechanistically understood [1].

The real-world ripples of this discovery span both human medicine and agricultural veterinary practice. In hospitals, *S. aureus* and *E. coli* are the organisms clinicians battle daily. Skin and soft-tissue infections, surgical-site infections, catheter-associated bloodstream infections, and ventilator-associated pneumonias are to name a few. An intervention that helps neutrophils trap and kill these pathogens more efficiently in the crucial first hours after exposure could mean the difference between an infection that's cleared by the innate immune system alone (no antibiotics needed) and one that establishes itself, requiring antibiotics and sometimes escalating to sepsis. This means fewer antibiotics started "just in case", and shorter courses when antibiotics are truly needed. These micro-decisions, multiplied across thousands of patients, contribute to antimicrobial stewardship and slow the evolution of resistant strains.

The bovine component of the study addresses a parallel challenge in agriculture. Bovine mastitis, the inflammation and infection of dairy cows' udders, is the most economically significant disease in dairy farming globally. It reduces milk production, requires antibiotics (which means milk must be discarded during treatment and for a withdrawal period afterward), and when chronic, forces early culling of productive cows.

Most mastitis cases are caused by *Staphylococcus aureus* and *E. coli*; the same organisms this study used. If Hashab gum supplementation could enhance bovine neutrophil function enough to help cows clear early infections before they establish, or to reduce the severity and duration of mastitis cases, the economic and animal-welfare implications would be substantial. Additionally, because Hashab gum is already a food-grade substance with no withdrawal period required, it could be supplemented routinely without creating the residue concerns that come with preventive antibiotic use.

The mechanistic question the 2020 study raised; how does Hashab gum enhance neutrophil function? would be addressed by the studies that followed. However, we can predict the likely pathways based on what we've learned in previous chapters.

The 2020 study established that Hashab gum affects innate-immunity cells directly and functionally. The next question was: *what molecular changes inside those cells drive the functional improvements?* And *how does Hashab gum enhance neutrophil function?*

2022 - Arming the Cells with Their Own Antibiotics

Port Sudan, Sudan. Red Sea University, where researchers were pursuing a mechanistic hypothesis: *If Gum arabic (Hashab gum from Acacia Senegal) enhances neutrophil and macrophage antimicrobial function, are those cells producing more of their own endogenous antimicrobial molecules?* Before diving into what they found, we need to explain what *cathelicidin* is and why increasing its production is valuable.

Human cells, particularly immune cells and epithelial barriers, produce their own antibiotics; small peptides and proteins that can kill or inhibit bacteria, viruses, fungi, and parasites. These are called *antimicrobial peptides* (AMPs), and they represent the ancient, evolutionarily conserved first line of chemical defense that predates the modern adaptive immune system by hundreds of millions of years. Every animal and plant produces AMPs; even primitive organisms like insects rely heavily on them. They work through mechanisms distinct from conventional antibiotics. Rather than targeting specific bacterial enzymes or metabolic pathways (which bacteria can mutate to evade), most AMPs physically disrupt microbial membranes. They're positively charged molecules that are attracted to the negatively charged surfaces of bacterial membranes. Upon attraction they insert themselves and create pores, causing the microbe to leak and die. Since this mechanism depends on fundamental physical chemistry rather than specific molecular targets, it's much harder for microbes to evolve resistance.

In humans, the most studied and important antimicrobial peptide is *cathelicidin*, also called LL-37 after the 37-amino-acid active form that's cleaved from a larger precursor protein. Think of cathelicidin as a Swiss army knife of innate immunity. Its primary function is punching holes in bacterial membranes and it's particularly effective against Gram-positive bacteria like *Staphylococcus* and *Streptococcus*, though it has activity against Gram-negative bacteria, fungi (including *Candida*), and enveloped viruses as well. Nevertheless, cathelicidin does more than just direct killing. It modulates inflammation and promotes the recruitment and activation of immune cells when appropriate but also limits excessive inflammatory responses that would damage host tissue. It promotes wound healing by supporting epithelial-cell migration and angiogenesis. It neutralizes bacterial endotoxins, blunting the inflammatory cascade that LPS otherwise triggers. Moreover, it's expressed not just by circulating immune cells (neutrophils, macrophages, NK cells) but also by epithelial barriers (skin, respiratory epithelium, gastrointestinal mucosa, urogenital tract) by providing continuous antimicrobial surveillance.

The body tightly regulates cathelicidin production. At baseline, expression is moderate, providing routine barrier defense without wasting resources. When infection or inflammation is detected (through 1-pattern-recognition receptors sensing bacterial products, 2-inflammatory cytokines like IL-1β and TNF-α, 3-vitamin D signaling (which is why vitamin D deficiency impairs immune function)), cathelicidin expression ramps up which increases local antimicrobial activity exactly when and where it's needed. After the threat passes, expression returns to baseline. It's an elegant system where you produce your own antibiotics, regulate them contextually, while avoiding the cost and resistance pressure of continuous external antibiotic use.

That's the conceptual framework for understanding what the 2022 Red Sea University study asked: *Can Hashab gum increase cathelicidin expression in immune cells?* Researchers led by Nagat Siednamohammeddeen supplemented mice with Hashab gum dissolved in drinking water (15% or 30% w/v for 28 days), then isolated peripheral blood mononuclear cells and induced them to differentiate into macrophages in culture (monocytes are circulating precursors that become tissue-resident macrophages when they leave the bloodstream). They measured cathelicidin (CRAMP in mice) transcription using molecular techniques [2].

The result revealed dose-dependent effects whereby Hashab gum supplementation at 15% concentration significantly increased cathelicidin expression in monocyte-derived macrophages (p=0.023), but the 30% concentration did not show significant increase (p=0.055). This suggests an optimal dosing range rather than a simple dose-response relationship. The researchers confirmed that dietary supplementation produces systemic changes in immune-cell gene expression, as the effect was detected in cells isolated from animals after consuming Hashab gum, indicating that the changes persist when those cells are removed from the body and cultured [2].

This finding deepened the mechanistic story in a satisfying way. The 2020 study showed that neutrophils and macrophages function better when exposed to Hashab gum as they grab and zap more effectively. The 2022 cathelicidin study began to explain why they function better at certain concentrations showing they're better armed at the transcriptional level. The cells aren't just performing their existing maneuvers more vigorously; they're upregulating transcription of antimicrobial peptides (molecular weapons) that make those maneuvers lethal to pathogens. Instead of relying solely on the oxidative burst or the acidic, enzyme-filled environment of the phagosome, these cells may be primed to deploy membrane-disrupting peptides that kill through a completely independent mechanism. Redundancy in antimicrobial systems is valuable because pathogens that evade one mechanism (some bacteria have catalase that neutralizes hydrogen peroxide from the oxidative burst, for example) are still vulnerable to others [2].

The historical footnote is worth noting: the same Sudanese research institutions that contributed to the oxidative-stress studies (Alneelein University, Nyala University) and the renal-protection studies (University of Khartoum) we documented earlier are now producing sophisticated cellular immunology, measuring gene expression and molecular mechanisms in immune cells. That continuity (from traditional knowledge about Hashab supporting health, to modern biochemical studies of antioxidant enzymes, to cutting-edge immunology examining antimicrobial peptides) illustrates how research programs mature when they're rooted in clinical observations and sustained by institutions committed to understanding a substance across multiple biological domains. The desert tree that provided gum for thousands of years is now revealing its mechanisms through the tools of 21st-century molecular biology, and the discovery is happening in the same regions where the tree grows and where the clinical intuition about its benefits where first developed.

The 2022 cathelicidin study showed that Hashab gum upregulates transcription of endogenous antimicrobial peptide genes at optimal concentrations. However, immune cells don't operate alone; they respond to signals from other parts of the immune system, tuning intensity depending on the context. The next study will explore how Hashab gum affects that context-dependent response.

2022 - An Amplifier Force of Good

Taichung, Taiwan. Providence University, where immunologists were investigating a more subtle question about immune regulation. *Gum arabic (Hashab gum from Acacia Senegal) clearly enhances innate immunity, but does it do so indiscriminately (always pushing cells toward higher activation, which would risk chronic inflammation and autoimmunity) or does it work synergistically with the body's own activation signals, amplifying appropriate responses while respecting biological contexts?*

To understand what they tested, we need a brief but clear explanation of *macrophage* biology and the concept of polarization. Macrophages aren't a single cell type with one function; they're plastic cells capable of adopting different functional states depending on the signals they receive from their environment. The two extremes of this spectrum are often called M1 and M2, though real macrophages in tissues exist along a continuum rather than in discrete categories.

M1 macrophages are the "fight" phenotype which are classically activated, pro-inflammatory, and microbicidal. They produce high levels of reactive oxygen and nitrogen species (including nitric oxide from inducible nitric oxide synthase, or iNOS), they express high levels of MHC class II molecules and co-stimulatory molecules for presenting antigens to T cells, they secrete pro-inflammatory cytokines like IL-12 and TNF-alpha, and they're optimized for killing intracellular bacteria and tumor cells. Think of M1 as the clean-up crew during an active infection. They are aggressive, powerful, necessary for clearing pathogens, but if sustained too long or activated inappropriately, they can cause significant collateral damage to healthy tissue.

M2 macrophages are the "repair" phenotype which are alternatively activated, anti-inflammatory, pro-resolving. They produce growth factors and extracellular matrix components, they promote angiogenesis and tissue remodeling, they secrete anti-inflammatory cytokines like IL-10, and they're optimized for wound healing and resolution of inflammation. Think of M2 as the construction crew after the fire is out. Responsible for rebuilding, cleaning up debris, and restoring normal tissue architecture.

Healthy immunity requires flexible switching between M1 and M2 states based on context. During active bacterial infection, you want M1-dominated responses to clear the pathogens. Once the infection is controlled, you want a shift toward M2 to repair tissue damage and resolve inflammation. Chronic inflammatory diseases (rheumatoid arthritis, inflammatory bowel disease, atherosclerosis) are characterized by excessive or prolonged M1 polarization meaning the fight continues even after the original threat is gone, causing tissue destruction. Conversely, some tumors exploit M2 polarization, creating an immunosuppressive microenvironment where macrophages promote tumor growth rather than attacking cancer cells.

The signal that most reliably pushes macrophages toward M1 is interferon-gamma (IFN-γ), a cytokine produced primarily by T cells and natural killer cells when they detect intracellular pathogens (viruses, intracellular bacteria, parasites) or tumor cells. IFN-γ is essentially a permission slip or a "go-time" signal. When it's present, it tells macrophages "there's an intracellular threat that requires your full microbicidal capacity; polarize

248

M1 and clear it". In the absence of IFN-γ or in the presence of anti-inflammatory signals like IL-4 or IL-13, macrophages default toward M2 or remain in a quiescent surveillance state.

The Providence University researchers, led by Chia-Yu Lin and Chao-Hsun Yang, designed an experiment to ask: *what happens when you give macrophages both Hashab Gum and IFN-γ?* If Hashab gum were a blunt immune stimulant, it would push macrophages toward M1 activation even in the absence of IFN-γ, creating a hyper-inflammatory baseline. If it were immunosuppressive, it would block IFN-γ's ability to induce M1 polarization. However, if it were a context-dependent modulator (enhancing appropriate responses when activation signals are present) you'd see a synergy where Hashab gum plus IFN-γ would produce stronger M1 polarization than IFN-γ alone, while Hashab gum in the absence of IFN-γ wouldn't create inappropriate inflammation [3].

That's exactly what they found. Macrophages cultured with Hashab gum alone showed modest changes with slightly elevated expression of some activation markers, but nothing approaching a strong M1 phenotype. Macrophages treated with IFN-γ alone showed the expected M1 polarization with increased expression of iNOS (producing nitric oxide as an antimicrobial), elevated production of reactive oxygen species, higher levels of M1-associated cytokines. Interestingly, macrophages treated with both Hashab gum and IFN-γ together showed synergistically enhanced M1 polarization were that the effects were greater than additive, indicating that Hashab gum amplifies the M1 response when the appropriate activation signal (IFN-γ) is present. Critically, this enhanced M1 programming translated into functional outcomes [3].

Let's emphasize why this finding is so important for understanding the kind of immune modulation Hashab gum provides. Many substances marketed as "immune boosters" create indiscriminate activation where they push

249

immune cells toward inflammatory states regardless of context. This, in the short term might help clear infections but in the long-term risks autoimmunity, chronic inflammation, and immune exhaustion. The phenomenon is analogous to constantly running your car engine at high RPM; you'll get where you're going fast, but you'll burn out the engine sooner. Hashab gum appears to do something more nuanced. It doesn't force the system into a particular state but rather enhances the system's responsiveness to appropriate signals. When IFN-γ says "there's an intracellular threat that requires M1 activation," Hashab gum helps macrophages respond more robustly to that signal.

For practical applications, this finding has direct implications for several clinical scenarios. During vaccination, you want robust M1 responses to the vaccine antigens that result in strong antigen presentation, vigorous T-cell activation, and durable immunity. Hashab gum supplementation during vaccine windows could theoretically enhance the M1 programming of antigen-presenting macrophages, improving vaccine immunogenicity without requiring adjuvants that often cause systemic side effects. During acute infections, particularly intracellular infections where IFN-γ production is high (viral infections, tuberculosis, certain parasites), Hashab gum's ability to amplify M1 responsiveness could accelerate pathogen clearance. In cancer immunotherapy, where re-polarizing tumor-associated macrophages from immunosuppressive M2-like states toward anti-tumor M1 states is a therapeutic goal, combining Hashab gum with agents that produce IFN-γ in the tumor microenvironment could enhance macrophage-mediated tumor killing.

The tolerability dimension is crucial here. Since Hashab gum doesn't create sustained, inappropriate immune activation (it amplifies context-appropriate responses but doesn't lock cells into inflammatory states) it can be used chronically, daily, as a background maintenance intervention. When infection occurs and IFN-γ rises, the cells are primed to respond vigorously.

The 2022 Taiwan study established that Hashab gum's immune effects are intelligent as they work with the body's own activation signals rather than forcing the system into a single state. However, all of these findings (enhanced NET formation, increased cathelicidin, synergistic M1 polarization) had been demonstrated in isolated immune cells or in animal studies. The critical question for translation to human medicine remained. Does any of this work in people?

2024 - Proof in People: Older and Younger Leukocytes Work Better

Göttingen, Germany. University Medical Center Göttingen, where researchers conducted the study that came closer to closing the gap. Taking Gum arabic (Hashab gum form Acacia Senegal) from laboratory benches to human volunteers. From cell-culture dishes to circulating blood, from mechanistic questions to functional proof.

Before presenting what they found, we need to frame one more concept: *immunosenescence*, the gradual decline in immune-system function that accompanies aging. As we age (typically beginning in the sixth or seventh decade of life, though the timeline varies considerably based on genetics, lifestyle, and health status) multiple aspects of immunity deteriorate. The thymus, where T cells mature, involutes (shrinks), producing fewer new T cells. Existing T cells become skewed toward memory phenotypes that are less flexible in responding to new antigens. B-cell antibody responses become weaker and less specific. Relevant to our immediate story, innate immunity (particularly neutrophil and macrophage function) declines. In older adults, neutrophils show reduced phagocytic capacity (they engulf fewer bacteria), weakened oxidative burst (they generate less reactive

251

oxygen), impaired chemotaxis (they migrate less efficiently toward infection sites), and delayed NET formation. Macrophages show similar declines with sluggish activation, reduced production of antimicrobial molecules, and delayed/absent M1 polarization even when appropriate activation signals are present. The net result is that infections that a young immune system would clear quickly and efficiently become more severe, longer-lasting, and more likely to progress to sepsis or require hospitalization. Influenza, pneumonia, urinary-tract infections, skin infections; all become more dangerous with age not because the pathogens are different but because the innate immune response is slower and weaker.

The public-health implications are enormous. Older adults account for most hospitalizations of infectious diseases, most antibiotic prescriptions, and most infection-related deaths. Vaccination effectiveness declines with age because of immunosenescence (the body's ability to mount a response to vaccine antigens weakens). The COVID-19 pandemic illustrated this starkly. While children and young adults generally experienced mild disease, older adults faced severe illness and death at rates hundreds of times higher, driven primarily by immunosenescence compounded by inflammatory dysregulation. Interventions that could slow, halt, or partially reverse immunosenescence (restoring some of the functional capacity that innate immune cells lose with age) would be transformative for healthy aging.

The challenge is that most interventions either don't work (antioxidant supplements, immune "boosters" that show no functional improvement in rigorous testing), work but aren't safe for chronic use (aggressive cytokines or immunostimulants that create inflammatory side effects), or work but aren't tolerable enough for the adherence required to see sustained benefit. An intervention that could genuinely restore some first-responder function, safely enough to use daily for years, and tolerable enough that elderly individuals would keep taking it, would address an unmet need in

252

gerontology and geriatric medicine.

The Göttingen team, led by Jana Seele and Roland Nau with first author Christin Freibrodt, recruited healthy volunteers spanning young adulthood to advanced age (the study included participants aged 20-35 years and participants aged 80-93 years) and tested their whole blood ex vivo with Hashab Gum at (20 mg/mL). Blood was drawn from each participant, stimulated with Hashab for 2 hours under standardized conditions, then challenged with Escherichia coli bacteria to measure phagocytosis and intracellular killing; the fundamental functions of innate immunity [4].

The assay measured how many bacterial colony-forming units survived inside white blood cells over defined time periods after gentamicin killed all extracellular bacteria. The assay is quantitative and direct whereby they counted viable intracellular bacteria by lysing blood cells and plating the lysates, allowing precise quantification of both phagocytic uptake and subsequent intracellular bacterial killing [4].

The results answered the translation question definitively. Hashab gum stimulation increased phagocytosis of E. coli by blood leukocytes for both young and older volunteers. The effect size was substantial and meaningful. Phagocytosis increased by 120.8% in young volunteers (p=0.008) and 39.2% in older volunteers (p=0.004) compared to unstimulated controls, the kind of functional boost that, during an actual infection, could determine whether the innate immune system clears the pathogen before it establishes a foothold. Critically, the improvement occurred in both age groups. Older adults' leukocytes, which typically show reduced phagocytic capacity compared to young adults, showed enhanced phagocytosis and intracellular killing after Hashab gum stimulation. Not back to the levels of young adults necessarily, but measurably and significantly better than their own baseline. The intervention didn't erase immunosenescence, but it partially compensated

253

for it, restoring some of the functional capacity that had been reduced [4].

Let's emphasize that this study represents translation from mechanism to function in the species and age groups that matter for application. The 2020 study showed enhanced innate-immune function in isolated granulocytes exposed to Hashab gum in dishes. The 2022 studies showed cathelicidin upregulation and M1-polarization synergy in animal-derived or cultured cells. However, the 2024 study showed that when human blood leukocytes are exposed to Hashab gum ex vivo; their circulating white blood cells function better at the most fundamental tasks of innate immunity: recognizing, engulfing, and killing bacteria [4].

The mechanistic implications build on previous studies demonstrating Hashab gum modulates immune-cell function (enhancing phagocytosis and intracellular killing, upregulating antimicrobial genes), cellular metabolism (supporting the energetic capacity for oxidative burst), and responsiveness. The demonstration that blood leukocytes from both young and especially older adults respond to Hashab stimulation with enhanced bacterial killing capacity provides proof-of-concept for immunomodulatory effects across age groups.

Now we can add one critical sentence about antimicrobial resistance that ties the individual health benefits to population-level public health. Earlier, more efficient pathogen clearance by innate immunity means fewer bacterial infections progress to the point where antibiotic treatment is initiated. Additionally, when treatment is needed, shorter courses suffice because the immune system is doing more of the clearing work. This is precisely the kind of micro-decisions that, multiplied across millions of patients over years, reduce selection pressure for antibiotic resistance and slow the evolution of multi-drug-resistant organisms that threaten to render modern medicine's antibiotic arsenal obsolete.

The 2024 human study didn't just validate the previous findings; it opened clinical doors. For geriatricians managing frail elderly patients where infection is often the precipitating event that cascades into hospitalization, delirium, functional decline, and death; a safe daily supplement that restores some innate-immune function represents a potential primary-prevention strategy. For oncologists treating patients on immunosuppressive chemotherapy or immune-checkpoint inhibitors; Hashab gum's ability to support baseline innate immunity without creating uncontrolled inflammation could reduce infectious complications that delay treatment. For public-health officials designing interventions to reduce antibiotic use and combat resistance; dietary strategies that enhance the body's own clearance mechanisms offer a population-level complement to stewardship policies focused on prescriber behavior.

Oral Health and Dentistry: The Next Front

The story doesn't end with circulating immune cells and systemic infections. There's one anatomical site where everything we've just learned about innate immunity comes together in ways you can see, feel, and measure daily: your mouth. The oral cavity is where barrier immunity meets microbial biofilms, where cathelicidin and other antimicrobial peptides patrol gingival tissues, where neutrophils and macrophages continuously surveil for pathogens, where phagocytosis and NET formation play starring roles in preventing periodontal disease, and where the balance between commensal bacteria and pathogenic species determines whether you develop cavities, gingivitis, periodontitis, or maintain healthy teeth and gums for life.

The same cathelicidin whose expression increased in macrophages in the 2022 Sudanese study is abundantly present in gingival crevicular fluid (the serum-like fluid that bathes the space between tooth and gum) where it

255

provides continuous antimicrobial defense against *Porphyromonas gingivalis*, *Fusobacterium nucleatum*, and other periodontal pathogens. The same neutrophil functions we documented (phagocytosis, oxidative burst, NET formation) are the primary defense against bacterial invasion of the periodontal ligament and alveolar bone. The same M1 macrophage polarization that increases microbicidal capacity systemically also operates in oral tissues, where the balance between M1 (clearing infection) and M2 (resolving inflammation and supporting tissue repair) determines whether periodontal disease progresses or heals.

Everything you just learned about front-line calm and front-line quick applies directly to the environment inside your mouth, where oral health is determined by the same innate-immune mechanisms we've been studying. It's the same biology, the same mechanisms, and the same substance. The immune system doesn't respect anatomical boundaries; it operates as an integrated network. The mouth is simply where that network becomes most visible and most immediately consequential for daily quality of life and long-term health. That's where our story travels next.

References:

1. Baien, Shima Hassan, et al. "Antimicrobial and Immunomodulatory Effect of Gum Arabic on Human and Bovine Granulocytes Against Staphylococcus aureus and Escherichia coli." Frontiers in Immunology, vol. 10, 30 Jan. 2020, article 3119

2. Siednamohammeddeen, Nagat, et al. "The Effect of Gum Arabic Supplementation on Cathelicidin Expression in Monocyte Derived Macrophages in Mice." BMC Complementary Medicine and Therapies, vol. 22, no. 1, 1 June 2022, article 149

3. Lin, Chia-Yu, et al. "Gum Arabic in Combination with IFN-γ Promotes the M1 Polarization in Macrophage." International Journal of Biological Macromolecules, vol. 209, pt. A, 2022, pp. 506–512.

4. Freibrodt, Christin, et al. "Gum Arabic Increases Phagocytosis of Escherichia coli by Blood Leukocytes of Young and Old Healthy Volunteers." Antibiotics, vol. 13, no. 6, 24 May 2024, article 482

CHAPTER 16

ORAL HEALTH AND ANTI-MICORBIAL
HEALING

Hashab signals to your Mouth

Where Immunity Becomes Visible

In the last chapter, Hashab gum didn't "boost immunity" like a bullhorn blaring indiscriminate activation signals. Instead, it tightened the choreography. Neutrophils grabbed bacteria more efficiently through enhanced phagocytosis. Deployed neutrophils acted with better precision, armed themselves with higher cathelicidin expression, and responded to activation signals like interferon-gamma. The improvements were functional, measurable, and intelligent.

Unlike systemic inflammation in the liver or oxidative stress in the kidneys (processes you can't see or feel directly and that require blood tests to monitor) oral health is immediate and unavoidable. You see your gums in the mirror every morning. You feel sensitivity when cold water hits exposed dentin. You taste the metallic tinge of gingival bleeding. You smell the morning breath that reflects overnight bacterial metabolism. You experience the pain of mucositis ulcers that make eating agonizing. The mouth is the one anatomical site where the abstract concepts we've been building throughout this book (barrier integrity, microbial ecology, inflammatory tone, innate immune function, oxidative stress, wound healing) become tangible, daily, undeniable experiences.

258

Additionally, the mouth is where modern dentistry has developed a peculiar dependence on interventions that work but that patients can't or won't sustain. Chlorhexidine mouthwash is the gold standard antiseptic (it reduces plaque, kills cariogenic bacteria, and improves gingival inflammation in every controlled trial) but it stains teeth brown, creates persistent taste disturbances (dysgeusia) that make food unpleasant for hours, causes mucosal irritation in many users, and disrupts the oral microbiome so thoroughly that beneficial commensals are eliminated alongside pathogens. It's a powerful medicine for short-term, dentist-supervised use after periodontal surgery or during acute infection. However, it's intolerable for long-term use and that presents challenges for disease prevention rather than just treating after development.

Fluoride is extraordinarily effective at strengthening enamel and preventing caries, but fluorosis concerns limit dosing in children. Additionally, systemic absorption raises questions about endocrine effects, and a vocal minority of patients refuse it entirely on philosophical or safety grounds. High-dose topical fluoride varnishes work beautifully but require professional application, limiting frequency and access.

What dentistry has needed (but rarely found) is interventions that patients will actually use consistently for months and years while working through mechanisms sophisticated enough to address the complex, multi-factorial nature of oral disease. Interventions that don't just kill bacteria but modulate biofilm ecology, support remineralization, calm inflammation, and promote healing. They must be safe and pleasant enough to integrate seamlessly into daily life rather than feeling like medical treatments requiring willpower and endurance.

What follows is the story of how Hashab gum crossed from food science and metabolic medicine into the frontline of dentistry and why its unique combination of tolerability, multi-pathway mechanisms, and platform chemistry has positioned it as something genuinely different in oral care. This isn't a story of miraculous cures or dental silver bullets. It's a story of how shifting the terrain produces outcomes that look unremarkable in any single metric but that accumulate into clinically meaningful, sustainable oral health over years and decades. It's the dental embodiment of how modest everyday effects turn into transformative lifetime outcomes.

I. The Enamel Seesaw Tips Back Toward Repair - Osaka, Japan, 2008

Before we can understand what the first modern dental study of Gum arabic discovered, we need to establish how tooth decay actually happens and why "remineralization" isn't just a marketing buzzword but a real, measurable biological process that determines whether teeth survive or fail.

Think of dental enamel as a mineral city. It's a crystalline metropolis of hydroxyapatite, the calcium-phosphate mineral that makes enamel the hardest substance in the human body. This city is constantly under attack and constantly under repair. The attack comes from acids; when bacteria in dental plaque (primarily *Streptococcus mutans*) ferment dietary sugars, they produce lactic acid and other organic acids that drop the pH at the tooth surface below 5.5, the critical threshold where hydroxyapatite begins to dissolve. This is *demineralization*; the mineral bricks of the enamel city are being dissolved away, creating microscopic porosity that, if it continues unchecked, progresses through the enamel into the underlying dentin and eventually forms a frank cavity requiring drilling and filling.

However, demineralization isn't the only process happening. The city has repair crews constantly at work. This is *remineralization*, the process by which dissolved calcium and phosphate ions are redeposited into the enamel crystal lattice, rebuilding the mineral structure and reversing early decay before it becomes irreversible. The repair crew's supplies come primarily from saliva, which is supersaturated with calcium and phosphate ions and contains buffers (bicarbonate, phosphate) that neutralize acid and raise pH back above the critical threshold. Saliva also contains proteins (statherin, proline-rich proteins, mucins) that form a protective film on tooth surfaces and help organize mineral deposition. When you're healthy, when your saliva is flowing normally, when you're not constantly bathing your teeth in sugar or acid, remineralization keeps pace with demineralization and your enamel stays intact.

The *enamel seesaw* is the balance between these two processes. demineralization on one side, remineralization on the other. Caries develop when the seesaw tips toward demineralization due to frequent sugar exposure, consumption of acidic beverages, inadequate saliva flow (from medications, disease, or aging), and poor oral hygiene allowing thick bacterial plaque to produce acid continuously. Prevention and early treatment involve tipping the seesaw back toward remineralization which is reducing acid attacks (less sugar, better plaque control), supporting saliva (hydration, xylitol, pilocarpine in severe xerostomia cases), and delivering materials that strengthen the repair process. With fluoride accepted as being the most proven remineralization substance, as it substitutes into hydroxyapatite to form fluorapatite, which is more acid-resistant and remineralizes more readily than native enamel.

Materials that can tip the seesaw toward remineralization do so through several mechanisms. They can buffer pH, keeping the tooth surface above the critical threshold so demineralization slows or stops. They can deliver calcium and phosphate ions directly to the tooth surface thereby increasing the supersaturation that drives mineral deposition. They can stabilize calcium-phosphate clusters in solutions, preventing them from precipitating prematurely in saliva and ensuring they reach the tooth surface where they're needed. Finally, they can modify the surface chemistry of enamel, creating conditions that favor mineral recrystallization.

There's one more concept we need before diving into the first study: the *acquired enamel pellicle* (AEP). Within minutes of cleaning your teeth, salivary proteins and glycoproteins adsorb onto the enamel surface, forming an ultra-thin film (typically 10 to 1,000 nanometers thick) that acts as a biological interface between the tooth and the oral environment. Think of the pellicle as a protective tarp the tooth throws over itself. It's not a passive barrier; it's a dynamic, organized structure that modulates bacterial adhesion (some bacteria stick preferentially to pellicle rather than naked enamel, which is why even freshly cleaned teeth begin accumulating plaque immediately), regulates mineral exchange (the pellicle is permeable to calcium and phosphate, allowing remineralization while partially buffering acid challenges), and serves as a reservoir for antimicrobial peptides and enzymes from saliva. The quality, composition, and stability of the pellicle matter enormously for oral health whereby a well-formed, properly hydrated pellicle protects enamel better. On the other hand, a dysregulated or poorly hydrated pellicle allows more bacterial attachment and acid penetration.

That's the conceptual foundation. Now we can understand what the Osaka University Graduate School of Dentistry team discovered when they tested Gum arabic's effects on enamel. Researchers led by T. Onishi created artificial caries-like lesions in extracted human third molars. This induced demineralization produced early decay that mimics what happens in mouths when acid attacks overwhelm repair. Following incubation in demineralization solution, they then exposed these lesioned teeth to solutions containing Gum arabic at 10 mg/ml, sodium fluoride at 1000 ppm (the standard remineralizing agent), or distilled water (negative control), then subjected them to demineralization-remineralization cycles designed to simulate the daily rhythm of acid attacks and recovery periods. Before and after the cycling protocol, they obtained contact microradiographs of each sample and calculated mineral distribution quantities to assess remineralization [1].

The results showed genuine remineralization, not just cosmetic effects. Teeth treated with Gum arabic solutions showed remineralization ratios similar to those treated with sodium fluoride, the established clinical standard. Both the Gum arabic and fluoride groups demonstrated significantly greater remineralization ratios compared to the distilled water controls, indicating that the mineral structure was being rebuilt through calcium and phosphate redeposition [1].

The proposed mechanism connected to Gum arabic's mineral content is that Gum arabic contains calcium ions (Ca^{2+}), which could contribute directly to the remineralization process by providing bioavailable calcium for incorporation into the hydroxyapatite crystal lattice. The calcium present in Gum arabic may help maintain supersaturation with respect to tooth mineral in the microenvironment around the lesion, shifting the equilibrium from net demineralization toward net remineralization. Additional mechanisms relate to Gum arabic's polysaccharide structure (such as film formation, stabilization of mineral precursors, or pH buffering) remain to be fully elucidated but the calcium content provides a straightforward biochemical explanation for the observed remineralizing activity.

Why did this 2008 study matter? It moved Gum arabic from "texture agent in foods" to "bioactive dental material with remineralizing capacity comparable to fluoride". This means it could participate in the biological processes determining whether teeth survive or decay, not just a passive filler or thickener in oral care formulations. It was a rigorous, controlled demonstration that Gum arabic drives genuine remineralization measurable by standard dental research methods (contact microradiography and quantitative mineral distribution analysis), achieving effects similar to the clinical standard (1000 ppm fluoride). Critically, it did so using a natural, widely consumed food ingredient, suggesting that dietary or supplemental Gum arabic intake might contribute to caries prevention through systemic or topical remineralizing effects.

II. From Plaque Load to Plaque Behavior: The Antibacterial Turn

Cairo, Egypt 2020. The laboratory antibacterial work established mechanism. Now came the clinical validation in human mouths with plaque, gingivitis, and the messy reality of daily oral hygiene.

Before presenting this landmark trial, we need to address chlorhexidine's clinical dominance and limitations. Chlorhexidine gluconate is dentistry's gold-standard antiseptic mouthwash as it's prescribed routinely after periodontal surgery, recommended for high-caries-risk patients, and used in intensive-care units to prevent ventilator-associated pneumonia. It works brilliantly and throughout every controlled trial spanning five decades, chlorhexidine reduces plaque scores, suppresses pathogens, and improves gingival inflammation indices. Its mechanism is straightforward as it's a cationic antiseptic that binds to bacterial cell walls and mammalian mucosal surfaces, disrupting membranes and killing broadly across bacterial species. However, therein lies the problem for daily, long-term use as chlorhexidine's antiseptic power comes with a cost that patients hate.

Chlorhexidine causes brown staining of teeth from chromogenic reaction products when chlorhexidine interacts with dietary polyphenols like tannins in tea and coffee. The staining is extrinsic and can be removed by professional cleaning, but it's unsightly and requires repeated dental hygiene visits. It creates persistent dysgeusia which is taste disturbance where food tastes metallic, bitter, or simply wrong for hours after rinsing, which destroys quality of life and adherence. It can cause mucosal desquamation (sloughing of the oral mucosa, experienced as rough patches inside the cheeks) and burning sensations that many patients find intolerable. Other effects reported is its broad-spectrum killing eliminates beneficial commensals along with pathogens, disrupting the oral microbiome in ways that may have long-term consequences that we're only beginning to understand (similar to how broad-spectrum antibiotics disrupt the gut microbiome and create dysbiosis that leads to other complications).

So, chlorhexidine is brilliant for short-term, dentist-supervised use. It's effective two weeks after periodontal surgery, during acute necrotizing gingivitis, before and after oral surgery when infection risk is high. However, for the daily months-to-years use, patient adherence collapses. Most people abandon chlorhexidine within days to weeks because it makes their teeth brown and their food taste like metal.

The 2020 trial, led by Dina Kamal and colleagues at Cairo University, with one collaborating researcher from Heidelberg University, was designed as a pragmatic, head-to-head comparison. Take patients at high risk for caries (63 participants categorized using the CAMBRA caries-risk model), randomize them to a Hashab gum-based natural mouthwash versus licorice extract mouthwash versus chlorhexidine (active comparator), and follow them for twelve months measuring the outcomes that matter clinically; DMF scores (counting decayed, missing, and filled teeth at baseline, 3, 6, 9, and 12 months), salivary Streptococcus mutans and Lactobacillus acidophilus counts (culturing saliva samples to quantify cariogenic bacteria), and patient-reported oral side effects [2].

The results were striking and reversed conventional expectations. The Gum arabic–based natural rinse achieved superior long-term caries-prevention and antibacterial effects compared to chlorhexidine. After 12 months, chlorhexidine showed higher DMF scores (more caries development) than both natural mouthwashes (p=0.003 overall; p<0.05 pairwise), with no significant difference between Gum arabic and licorice. For antibacterial activity, all mouthwashes showed significant effects through 6 months over time with no between-group differences. However, after 9 and 12 months, Gum arabic and licorice maintained significant reductions in bacterial counts (p<0.001), while chlorhexidine showed a significant increase in S. mutans and L. acidophilus, consistent with reduced effectiveness and interpreted by the authors as resistance (p<0.001). The tolerability profile diverged because Gum arabic rinse showed no oral side effects [2].

The positioning that emerged was clear and practice-changing demonstrating that Gum arabic–based rinses offered very good long-term efficacy with no reported side effects. That adherence advantage combined with maintained antibacterial efficacy and lower caries incidence transforms clinical outcomes over time. A rinse that patients use for a year without side effects while preventing bacterial resistance produces dramatically better outcomes than a rinse that causes side effects, promotes bacterial resistance, and results in more cavities [2].

The 2020 RCT elevated Gum arabic into the category of oral-care interventions for long-term caries prevention, challenging chlorhexidine's dominance. It wasn't just laboratory promise anymore; it was head-to-head comparison over 12 months showing superior clinical outcomes (lower DMF scores, sustained antibacterial activity without resistance, zero side effects) compared to dentistry's traditional reference standard [2].

III. Quorum Quenching & Smarter Plaque Management

Ras Al-Khaimah, United Arab Emirates, 2024. The review capstone by

Nada T. Hashim, Rasha Babiker, and colleagues at RAK Medical and Health Sciences University, synthesized the accumulating evidence about Gum arabic's quorum-quenching properties and positioned it as a next-generation strategy for periodontal disease management.

The review described the AI-2/LuxS quorum-sensing system and outlined plausible ways Gum arabic could interfere with bacterial communication. It discussed Gum arabic or its components might hinder autoinducer synthesis, compete at receptors, or promote signal degradation, thereby destabilizing biofilm behavior.

The review's clinical framing aligned with a conservative interpretation. Gum arabic is not presented as a broad-spectrum antiseptic that eradicates the oral microbiome. Instead, the authors propose that quorum-quenching approaches could temper biofilm virulence and organization while allowing commensal communities that support pH balance, resource competition, and gingival innate defenses to persist. The emphasis is potential modulation rather than wholesale killing (an adjunctive philosophy paralleling precision over aggression) pending further GA-specific mechanistic work and controlled clinical trials.

The periodontal implications are important because periodontal disease is linked to systemic health. Periodontal pathogens such as Porphyromonas gingivalis and Fusobacterium nucleatum can enter the bloodstream through inflamed-bleeding gingiva, contributing to systemic inflammatory burden measured by markers like C-reactive protein and interleukin-6. Epidemiological data associate periodontitis with increased risk of cardiovascular disease, diabetes complications, adverse pregnancy outcomes, and respiratory disease. In that context, approaches that lessen biofilm pathogenicity without indiscriminately disrupting commensals are attractive adjuncts within periodontal prevention and therapy as they complement mechanical debridement and conventional chemotherapeutics.

These links underscore the relevance of adjunctive biofilm-modulating strategies.

Quorum-quenching strategies that reduce periodontal biofilm virulence without destroying beneficial commensals (thinning plaque without provoking dysbiosis) offer a complementary direction for prevention and therapy. The 2024 UAE review positions Gum arabic as a potential candidate in this field. A food-grade material with long human use, plausible quorum-quenching actions discussed for AI-2/AHL signaling and cited evidence suggesting improvements in plaque-induced gingivitis when used as an adjunct. Its appeal lies in compatibility with ecological approaches and tolerability that could support regular use, while acknowledging that GA-specific molecular mechanisms need longer, larger clinical trials. Accordingly, the review recommends further characterization of active components and controlled studies before routine periodontal deployment in clinical practice.

IV. Gums That Bleed Less, Mouths That Heal Faster (2022)

Khartoum, Sudan, 2022. The antibacterial and quorum-quenching studies explained how Gum arabic affects biofilm ecology and plaque virulence. However, oral health isn't just about bacteria, it's equally about host response. This includes the inflammatory and immune reactions that determine whether bacterial presence causes disease or remains in balanced commensal coexistence. Let's frame *gingival inflammation* clearly before presenting the clinical trial that measured it.

Bleeding gums, gingival redness, swelling, and tenderness. These aren't simply "too many bacteria" but rather the wrong kind of conversation between the biofilm and the host immune system. In health, the biofilm at the gingival margin (the interface between tooth and gum tissue) is dominated by commensal species that produce short-chain fatty acids, maintain neutral pH, and present molecular patterns that the immune system recognizes as non-threatening. The gingival tissue neutrophils and macrophages clear any bacteria attempting to invade tissue. They produce antimicrobial peptides that suppress pathogen overgrowth and maintain barrier integrity through a healthy epithelium with intact tight junctions. The conversation is quiet and results in bacteria staying in the biofilm, immune cells patrol without activating, inflammation remains minimal, and tissues remain pink and firm.

When biofilm ecology shifts (typically driven by poor oral hygiene allowing plaque to accumulate and mature) pathogenic species like *Porphyromonas gingivalis*, *Tannerella forsythia*, and *Prevotella intermedia* expand. These organisms produce lipopolysaccharide (the same LPS that drives gut-derived endotoxemia we've discussed in previous chapters), proteases that damage epithelial barriers, and other virulence factors that actively provoke inflammatory responses. The immune system ramps up leading to increased neutrophil infiltration, macrophages activation toward pro-inflammatory M1 phenotypes, and elevated secretion of pro-inflammatory cytokines (IL-1β, TNF-α, IL-6, IL-8). This is gingivitis; clinically visible as red, swollen gums that bleed easily when touched with a periodontal probe or toothbrush. If the dysbiotic biofilm persists and the inflammatory response continues, gingivitis progresses to periodontitis where tissue destruction (connective tissue attachment loss, bone resorption) occurs, creating periodontal pockets that harbor even more bacteria in a vicious cycle.

Interventions that calm this inflammation (reducing pro-inflammatory cytokine levels, supporting M2-like "repair and resolution" macrophage phenotypes once infection is controlled, preserving epithelial barrier integrity) can break the cycle and allow healing even when bacterial loads haven't been completely eliminated. This is where Gum arabic's documented effects from the immunity chapter become directly relevant. If Gum arabic enhances cathelicidin production in gingival tissues (the same effect documented in systemic macrophages in Chapter 15), and improves neutrophil phagocytosis of oral pathogens, then it should improve clinical gingivitis outcomes not just through antibacterial effects but through host immune modulation.

Researchers at Khartoum Dental Teaching Hospital conducted a placebo-controlled, double-blinded randomized clinical trial specifically designed to measure both plaque control and inflammatory resolution. 60 adult patients with plaque-induced gingivitis were randomized to receive Gum arabic powder applied twice daily plus standard oral hygiene (full-mouth scaling at baseline) versus placebo powder (microcrystalline cellulose) with the same instructions. The trial ran for 60 days, with examinations at baseline, 30 days, and 60 days to measure Gingival Index, Plaque Index, and collection of gingival crevicular fluid samples for cytokine analysis (measuring IL-1β inflammatory mediator) [4].

The results showed the "periodontal double win" with dual effects on biofilm and host response. Plaque indices (MPS) decreased significantly in the Gum arabic group compared to placebo at both 30 days (0.84±0.25(GA) vs 1.09±0.20(placebo), $p<0.001$) and 60 days (0.88±0.29 vs 1.12±0.23, $p=0.002$), confirming the antibacterial/antibiofilm effects documented in previous studies. Gum arabic powder was reducing plaque accumulation. Gingival inflammation improved significantly. Gingival Index scores (MGS) dropped at 30 days (1.09±0.22 vs 1.20±0.16 for placebo, $p=0.012$), and gingival crevicular fluid IL-1β concentrations fell significantly within the GA group while placebo did not. The intervention group showed significant reduction in GCF IL-1β compared to placebo ($p<0.05$), indicating real resolution of inflammatory signaling, not just cosmetic improvement [4].

This is the signature of an intervention working on both sides of the host-microbe interface whereby reduced plaque (from antibacterial activity and reduced bacterial adherence) produces fewer inflammatory triggers, while simultaneously, local inflammatory mediators are suppressed. GCF IL-1β levels declined significantly only in the Gum arabic group between baseline and 60 days. The result is synergistic with the mechanical plaque control from scaling combined with Gum arabic's ongoing effects on both plaque formation and inflammatory response. Gum arabic produced better clinical outcomes than interventions targeting only bacteria or only inflammation. The observed IL-1β reduction suggests Gum arabic suppresses periodontal inflammation at a profound level by modulating local mediators [4].

Patient tolerance was excellent throughout the trial showing 60-day completion with twice-daily powder application demonstrating feasibility. This matters enormously because gingivitis isn't a one-time acute condition; it's a chronic management challenge where daily intervention prevents progression to periodontitis. Patients need something they'll actually use every day for years. The 2022 Sudanese gingivitis trial validated Gum arabic powder as a daily periodontal hygiene tool that combines plaque control with host-response modulation, offering a natural, cost-effective adjunct to mechanical periodontal therapy [4].

Skin and Wound Healing: The Next Frontier

Everything you just learned to trust in your mouth (film-forming moisture balance creating protective barriers without occlusion, quorum-quenching antibiofilm logic that reduces pathogen virulence without sterilization, anti-inflammatory tone that supports resolution rather than just suppressing acute flares, wound-healing support through moisture retention and growth-factor modulation, and delivery-platform chemistry that stabilizes and enhances other therapeutic actives) is exactly what chronic wounds, burns, diabetic ulcers, and fragile skin desperately need. The oral mucosa was the ideal testing ground where rapid turnover rates mean you can see healing effects in days rather than weeks. The environment is controlled enough for clinical trials while realistic enough to predict real-world performance, and outcomes (pain, function, appearance) are immediately relevant to patients.

The lessons translate directly to dermal wounds, where the challenges are structurally identical even if the tissue architecture differs. Chronic wounds fail to heal because biofilms organize on wound beds and resist clearance. This happens because chronic inflammation persists and prevents progression through normal healing stages. Reasons include moisture balance disruption (too dry and epithelial cells can't migrate; too wet and maceration damages tissue), and repeated infections requiring antibiotics that create resistance and dysbiosis.

The next chapter follows Hashab gum's film-forming chemistry that modifies the acquired enamel pellicle becoming the basis for advanced wound dressings. We're moving from one epithelial surface (oral mucosa) to another (skin), but the biology is continuous and the mechanisms are conserved. Hashab gum's advantages all transfer intact to wound care. That's where our story travels next. From the mouth you see in the mirror every morning to the skin that covers your body. Both, when wounded, endure a race between healing and infection, between repair and chronic inflammation, between restoration and permanent disability.

References:

1. Onishi, T., et al. "Remineralization Effects of Gum Arabic on Caries-Like Enamel Lesions." Archives of Oral Biology, vol. 53, no. 3, Mar. 2008, pp. 257-60

2. Kamal, Dina, et al. "Caries Preventive and Antibacterial Effects of Two Natural Mouthwashes vs Chlorhexidine in High Caries-Risk Patients: A Randomized Clinical Trial." The Journal of Contemporary Dental Practice, vol. 21, no. 12, 1 Dec. 2020

3. Hashim, Nada Tawfig, et al. "Gum Arabic as a Potential Candidate in Quorum Quenching and Treatment of Periodontal Diseases." Frontiers in Oral Health, vol. 5, 7 Oct. 2024, article 1459254

4. Effect of Gum Arabic on Plaque-Induced Gingivitis: A Randomised Clinical Trial." Saudi Dental Journal, vol. 34, no. 6, Sept. 2022, pp. 544-49, PMC9453537

CHAPTER 17

THE WOUND HEALER

The Research that Showed How Hashab Transformed Wounds
from Battlefields into Managed Ecosystems

The Tree's First Lesson

In the Acacia forests of Africa and Asia, Acacia trees endure a harsh
existence of six-month dry seasons, temperatures exceeding 45°C, sandy
soils that hold little water, and constant mechanical stress from wind,
animals, and human harvest. When the tree is wounded (by a goat stripping
bark while browsing, by a scoring knife making incisions to stimulate gum
flow, by a branch breaking in a dust storm, by insect boring) it responds
with what appears to be controlled bleeding. A clear to amber liquid
exudate oozes from the injury site, flowing down the trunk in viscous
streams that gradually solidify as water evaporates in the desert heat.

This exudate is Acacia gum in its raw form. Upon injury, the
Arabinogalactan-proteins dissolve in the tree's cellular fluids, mobilize to
the wound site, forming a protective seal over damaged cambium and
xylem. The gum serves multiple functions for the injured tree. It's a
physical barrier preventing water loss through the wound (critical in an
environment where every drop of moisture is precious), it seals out
pathogenic fungi and bacteria that would otherwise colonize the exposed
tissue and cause rot, it provides a scaffolding matrix for the tree's own
wound-healing processes, and it modulates the oxidative stress and
inflammatory-like responses that plants mount when injured. The tree

274

essentially bandages itself with a breathable, antimicrobial, moisture-retaining film and then, weeks later, produces a harvestable crop of solidified gum nodules that humans have been collecting for 70,000 years.

The people who have lived alongside these trees for generations and harvested Acacia gum as both subsistence income and traditional medicine made a logical leap that predated scientific validation by centuries: *If this substance heals the tree's wounds, might it heal ours?* The same exudate that sealed bark injuries became the traditional treatment for human wounds, burns, and skin conditions. The logic was empirical and straightforward; what works for the living tree wood might work for flesh.

Just as these communities knew (long before biochemistry could explain the mechanisms) that Hashab gum supported kidney function (documented in your renal chapter), they knew it supported wound healing. The knowledge was robust enough to persist, to be used daily, to be taught to children and passed across borders.

I. 2012 - Where Skin Care Is Most Unforgiving: The Pediatric Colostomy Trial

Tehran, Iran, 2012. Before diving into the first clinical validation of Hashab gum for wound and skin protection, we need to establish why peristomal skin care in pediatric patients represents on of the hardest possible test cases. If an intervention works here, it will work almost anywhere.

Peristomal skin is the area immediately surrounding a stoma (surgical opening where intestine or urinary tract is brought through the abdominal wall) faces uniquely brutal conditions. In children with colostomies (most commonly created to manage Hirschsprung disease, imperforate anus, or inflammatory bowel disease), liquid stool containing digestive enzymes continuously contacts the skin whenever the ostomy appliance (the adhesive bag that collects output) leaks or needs changing. The enzymes actively digest proteins (which is exactly what skin is made of) creating chemical burns. The constant moisture macerates the epidermis. The repeated application and removal of adhesive ostomy appliances mechanically strips skin layers. Additionally, the child's movement, growth, and natural activity create shear forces that challenge appliance adhesion, leading to more frequent leaks that exacerbate skin damage.

The result is *peristomal dermatitis*; red, inflamed, sometimes ulcerated skin around the stoma that hurts, itches, makes appliance adhesion difficult (creating a cycle of worsening leaks), and requires urgent intervention. Standard treatments include barrier powders (stoma powder made from various polymers that create a protective film), barrier rings and pastes (to fill uneven skin contours and create a flat surface for appliance adhesion), protective skin wipes (often alcohol-based, which burn damaged skin), and in severe cases, prescription topical medications. However, many of these interventions are uncomfortable (alcohol burns), expensive, require multiple products applied in specific sequences (compliance burden for families), or don't fully solve the moisture-management problem.

With that foundation, we can understand what Mehrdad Hosseinpour, Ali Fazeli, and Masoome Agabeigi tested in Tehran: *Could Hashab gum powder and film, applied to peristomal skin in children with colostomies, reduce dermatitis and improve appliance adherence better than standard barrier products?*

The trial enrolled infants undergoing new colostomy creation, randomized immediately after surgery to a barrier for 4 weeks who were experiencing peristomal skin complications including irritation, redness, breakdown, and frequent appliance leaks requiring emergency changes. The intervention saw nurses apply Acacia Senegal (Hashab gum) barrier onto the inflamed peristomal skin. The control was zinc sulfate ointment [1].

The outcomes measured were clinically relevant and reported for rate/severity of peristomal skin inflammation. The results established Hashab gum's barrier showed lower and less sever inflammation rates ($p=0.05$) [1].

The Tehran study provided proof-of-concept that Hashab gum's properties could address real clinical needs in a population where standard treatments often fall short. For product development teams, the trial lowered the barrier to investigating Hashab gum in other moisture-challenged scenarios. If it works on enzymatically active, continuously wet, mechanically stressed pediatric peristomal skin (arguably the hardest environment for any barrier product) then trials in diabetic ulcers, pressure ulcers, graft sites, and oncology dermatitis became justified. The 2012 study was the first domino as it demonstrated that a food-grade material could compete with purpose-designed medical products in real-world clinical care, opening the door for the wound-healing research program that followed.

II. 2020 - The Simple Cream Pathway: Accessibility Without Complexity

Riyadh, Saudi Arabia, 2020. The Tehran study provided proof of application and now Riyadh sought to go deeper. What happens in places without materials-science labs? What happens at home, where patients need something they can recognize, open, and apply without a tutorial? In many clinics carrying the greatest burden of chronic wounds, the bottleneck isn't theory; it's access. Sometimes the intervention with the largest population impact isn't the one at the cutting edge; it's the one simple and affordable enough to actually reach people.

That is the spirit of the 2020 Riyadh study. A team led by Rasha Saad Suliman took a low-complexity path: formulate a straightforward 5% w/w Acacia gum Arabia preparation using a standard British Pharmacopoeia "Aqueous Cream" process, then ask two practical questions. *Does it show organism-specific antibacterial effects in vitro, and does it help wounds close faster in a well-established animal model* [2]? No designer crosslinks, no embedded drug reservoirs, no advanced release kinetics. Just a familiar cream base with Acacia gum added to the aqueous phase.

They started by checking that the cream behaved like a usable topical. The quality-control readouts were basic and relevant to bedside reality. They included appearance and phase stability (opaque, homogeneous), spreadability (mean diameter ~2.2 ± 0.14 for the acacia cream versus ~2.4 for the blank), and a skin-friendly pH (about 6.21 for acacia cream versus 5.54 for the base). These aren't exhaustive rheological fingerprints, but they answer the immediate practical questions a nurse or caregiver would have. Does it spread, does it stay put, and will it be comfortable on skin [2]?

Antimicrobial testing followed two standard lines of evidence. Disc-diffusion assays were used to screen for visible zones of inhibition, and minimum inhibitory concentrations (MICs) were measured where activity was suggested. The signal turned out to be specific rather than universal. Under the conditions reported, the cream did not produce measurable inhibition halos against several headline pathogens of chronic wounds (*Staphylococcus aureus*, *Escherichia coli*, *Pseudomonas aeruginosa*, and *Streptococcus agalactiae)*. Where it did show activity, the effects were concrete enough to quantify via MICs: about 1.25% for *Proteus* spp. and *Staphylococcus epidermidis*, roughly 1.5–2.5% for *Shigella*, and around 2.5% for *Klebsiella* [2].

278

In other words, the antimicrobial contribution here is targeted rather than blanket sterilization; helpful in nudging a colonized wound's bioburden in the right direction, but not a substitute for debridement, cleansing, or systemic therapy when those are needed.

The in-vivo arm used the standard excision model in adult rats. Four groups were followed with an untreated control, a reference group treated with 0.2 mL of IntraSite gel (a commercial hydrogel), and two acacia-cream groups given 0.2 mL of formulations containing 100 mg/mL or 200 mg/mL. Wounds were traced over time to quantify contraction; histology (hematoxylin–eosin and Masson's trichrome) was performed at day 14, with macroscopic healing described through day 15.

The direction of effect was consistent. Compared with the control, Acacia-treated wounds showed faster area reduction, and the day-14 sections revealed a granulation bed with fewer inflammatory cells and more collagen bundles and capillary profiles, the microscopic hallmarks of a maturing repair phase [2].

What does this combination of results prove? First, a credible, source-constrained claim is that a simply made Acacia cream can exert antibacterial effects against selected organisms and can accelerate healing in a recognized animal model, with histology to match. Second, a translational signal that matters outside of research hospitals. The QC data (spreadability and pH) are not esoteric; they're the exact properties that govern whether a cream is pleasant to use and easy to apply. For home care, community clinics, and low-resource settings, those specifics are not trivial details; they are the difference between adherence and abandonment. It shows that a low-complexity Acacia cream can help under some microbiological and biological conditions; and that alone is meaningful.

Seen in that light, the 2020 paper becomes a bridge between the elegance of hydrogel engineering and the daily work of wound care where resources are limited. The hydrogel platform proves that Acacia gum can be shaped into advanced biomaterials; the cream shows that you don't need an advanced lab to realize a portion of those benefits. A nurse managing pressure injuries at home, a clinician in a district hospital, or a community health worker supporting patients with slow-to-heal ulcers can reasonably prefer a product that is inexpensive, shelf-stable, spreadable, and comfortable. Especially if there is preclinical evidence that it helps wounds progress from inflamed to organized repair [2].

For diabetes care, where impaired healing is common and follow-through is everything, the implication is practical rather than grandiose. A simple Acacia cream won't replace the fundamentals of multidisciplinary wound management, but it might become a useful adjunct. One that patients can actually get, understand, and keep using long enough to matter. If the choice is between a technically superior dressing that never leaves a research pharmacy and a "good-enough" cream that can be made and dispensed widely, the latter often delivers the larger public-health dividend.

III. 2024 - Confronting the Main Villain: Staphylococcus aureus in Real Clinical Isolates

Cairo, Egypt, 2024. We've discussed biofilms and chronic wound pathogens abstractly; now it's time to name the enemy explicitly and test Arabic gum against real-world clinical strains; bacteria isolated from actual infected wounds, carrying the resistance mechanisms and virulence factors that make chronic wound infections so difficult to treat.

Concept Reinforcement: Why Diabetic Wounds Welcome Staphylococcus aureus? *Staphylococcus aureus* dominates chronic wound infections for reasons that reflect the failures of diabetic host defenses.

High glucose concentrations in diabetic wound exudate and tissue provide abundant nutrients for bacterial growth. Diabetic neutrophils show impaired chemotaxis (they're slower to arrive at infection sites), reduced phagocytic capacity (they engulf bacteria less efficiently; exactly what your immunity chapter documented Hashab gum improving), and weakened oxidative burst (they generate less bactericidal reactive oxygen). Diabetic hyperglycemia leads to formation of advanced glycation end products (AGEs) that accumulate in tissue and impair immune function. Microvascular disease reduces blood flow, meaning fewer immune cells reach wounds and antibiotic concentrations achieved by systemic administration are lower.

S. aureus exploits these deficiencies. It adheres avidly to damaged tissue and foreign material (including medical implants and dressing remnants). It forms robust biofilms that resist both immune attack and antibiotics. It produces an arsenal of toxins that kill neutrophils and macrophages (leukocidins, hemolysins). It secretes proteases that degrade antibodies and complement proteins, and increasingly, clinical strains carry methicillin resistance (MRSA) and resistance to multiple antibiotic classes. In diabetic foot ulcers, *S. aureus* (including MRSA) is the most frequently isolated pathogen, and its presence correlates with poor healing outcomes, increased amputation risk, and prolonged hospitalization.

Standard treatment (systemic antibiotics) often fails because antibiotics can't penetrate biofilms effectively, because microvascular disease limits drug delivery to the wound, and because prolonged antibiotic courses (common in chronic wounds) drive resistance. Topical antiseptics (iodophors, silver compounds, honey) can suppress *S. aureus* but often cause tissue toxicity, pain, or allergic reactions that limit sustained use. An intervention that reduces *S. aureus* virulence and biofilm capacity while supporting rather than impairing host immune function and tissue healing would address the therapeutic gap.

281

Deyaa M. Elebiary and colleagues approached the problem where it actually lives; the clinic. Instead of relying on long-domesticated lab strains, they sampled 300 real skin-infection specimens across four Egyptian hospitals and worked with the Staphylococcus aureus they found there, then asked whether Arabic gum could blunt a key virulence lever (lipase) while improving healing in infected burns.

Their pipeline mixed bedside relevance with solid bench methods. Isolates were confirmed and profiled on the VITEK® 2 system (AST GP67), establishing antibiotic susceptibility without disc-diffusion shortcuts. Minimum inhibitory concentrations (MICs) for Arabic gum were determined by microdilution in 96-well plates (1,000→0.98 µg/mL; MIC defined as no growth). Against selected S. aureus isolates the MICs clustered between 3.9 and 31.26 µg/mL, with vancomycin shown alongside for context [3].

In an infected burn model in male rats, animals were randomized to no treatment, mupirocin 2% ointment, or topical Arabic gum. After 14 days, histology in the Arabic-gum group showed thin re-epithelialized epidermis, granulation tissue with proliferating vessels, and increased collagen organization (signs of constructive remodeling) whereas untreated infected burns remained ulcerated and necrotic. Mupirocin-treated skin also re-epithelialized, with notable vascular proliferation. The paper describes both arms but does not claim statistical superiority of one over the other [4].

For chronic wounds where bacterial eradication is often impossible and where management aims for controlling virulent factors rather than achieving sterility; anti-lipase activity that preserves tissue integrity while bacteria persist may be more valuable than aggressive bactericidal activity. The message is pragmatic. When eradication is unrealistic, dialing down S. aureus's tissue-damaging machinery matters. Here, Arabic gum simultaneously (1) reduced lipase at sub-MIC levels (a tactic aligned with

282

anti-virulence therapy) and (2) supported tissue repair in infected burns on histology. It's a dual benefit framed around what front-line teams need most which is less enzymatic injury, and more organized healing.

Closing Summation: Wounds as Ecosystems Wanting to Heal

A century of wound care alternated between extremes: dry and scab (let nature take its course, leading to prolonged healing and worse scars), and antiseptic scorched earth (sterilize everything, often damaging healing cells as collateral). Neither paradigm served chronic wounds well. Diabetic ulcers still average 12–20 weeks to close when they close at all. Pressure ulcers persist through months of expensive care, and infections drive resistance while healing stays stuck.

The Acacia gum wound-care arc tells a different story. *Habitable healing.* From protecting the maceration-prone skin of pediatric ostomies to simple creams that work where sophistication can't reach, to quorum quenching that thins biofilms without sterilization. Hashab gum frames wounds not as sterile battlefields but as ecosystems that want to heal if given the right conditions.

The same mechanism we have seen in kidneys (reduced oxidative load, preserved function under metabolic stress), liver (hepatocyte protection, stellate-cell quieting, antifibrotic signaling), immunity (sharper phagocytosis, higher cathelicidin), and oral health (biofilm thinning, mucosal support, remineralization) now manifests on skin as steady, visible repair. Wounds that were stalled for months begin epithelializing. Biofilms that resisted antibiotics thin enough for debridement and immune clearance to finish the job.

Critically, because Hashab gum is safe enough to use, pleasant enough to tolerate indefinitely, and affordable enough to scale globally, the benefits don't stop after two-week trials. They compound in the real world where adherence determines whether laboratory promise becomes lived experience. The tree's lesson (that the same exudate healing bark in the Sahelian desert can heal skin on human limbs) wasn't metaphor. It was biology and chemistry protecting from harsh environments. Traditional knowledge validated by modern tools, now positioned to address one of medicine's most expensive, most painful, and most neglected challenges.

The next chapter documents fertility support and the organic gift helping humans reproduce in an oxidatively stressed, metabolically challenged modern environment. The biology is continuous; the applications keep expanding.

References:

1. Hosseinpour, Mehrdad, et al. "Efficacy of Acacia senegal for Stoma Care in Children with Colostomy." European Journal of Pediatric Surgery (2012; 22(3): 234–237

2. Suliman, Rasha Saad, et al. "In Vitro Anti-Microbial Activity and Wound Healing Evaluation of Acacia Gum Arabia Aqueous Cream." Natural Products Chemistry & Research, vol. 8, no. 1, 24 Feb. 2020, article 369

3. Elebiary, Deyaa M., et al. "Evaluation of Arabic Gum Antibacterial and Wound Healing Activities Against Staphylococcus aureus Isolates Obtained from Skin Infections." Microbial Biosystems, vol. 9, no. 1, 25 July 2024, pp. 129-38

CHAPTER 18

Hashab Gum helps the Seeds

When Wound Chemistry Meets the Most Vulnerable Cells

The last chapter left us watching wounds heal under Hashab gum's protective influence. The chemistry was consistent across formulations. What made those dressings work (membrane protection, redox buffering, osmotic stability, gentle antimicrobial activity without tissue toxicity) wasn't wound-specific. It was cell-protective chemistry operating at fundamental levels of biology.

In communities across Sudan's gum belt, where *Hashab gum* has been harvested for millennia, traditional knowledge included reproductive applications that paralleled the wound-healing uses. Modern reproductive science is discovering they were right with mechanisms we will try to uncover in this chapter.

What follows is the fertility story with multiple studies spanning 2020 to 2024, from testicular protection during chemotherapy to systems-level effects on the microbiota-gut-brain-gonad axis. By chapter's end, you'll understand why the same intervention that protected hepatocytes from chemotherapy-induced oxidative stress protect testicular tissue from cisplatin, and why the microbiome-modulating effects that improved metabolic parameters reach all the way to the hypothalamic-pituitary-gonadal axis that governs reproduction. The connection between wounds

286

and fertility isn't metaphorical; it's mechanistic, validated, and increasingly translatable into practice.

I. 2020 - The Chemotherapy Crucible: Guarding Spermatogenesis Under Cisplatin's Assault

Cairo, Egypt, 2020. Before understanding what Gum arabic can do for fertility under extreme stress, we need to grasp why chemotherapy (particularly platinum-based agents like cisplatin) devastates reproductive function in ways that wound healing after surgery or radiation doesn't fully capture.

Concept: Why Chemotherapy Causes Infertility Cisplatin saves lives by creating DNA crosslinks in rapidly dividing cancer cells, preventing successful cell division and triggering tumor-cell death. The mechanism is elegantly simple and brutally effective. Platinum binds to DNA bases, creating distortions that block replication and transcription while activating DNA-damage checkpoints that initiate apoptosis. However, cisplatin doesn't distinguish between rapidly dividing cancer cells and rapidly dividing normal cells. This impacts the germline in testes, where millions of new sperm cells begin development daily through a precisely choreographed process called spermatogenesis.

Cisplatin attacks the reproductive system through multiple pathways simultaneously. Cisplatin metabolism generates superoxide and hydroxyl radicals that overwhelm cellular antioxidant defenses (glutathione, superoxide dismutase, catalase). The result is lipid peroxidation of cell membranes (particularly devastating in sperm, whose flagellar membranes are rich in polyunsaturated fatty acids required for membrane fluidity and motility), protein carbonylation that inactivates enzymes, and DNA strand breaks in both somatic cells and germ cells.

The oxidative stress and cellular damage activate NF-κB (nuclear factor kappa B) which is the master transcription factor we've met repeatedly in this book as the amplifier of inflammatory responses. Once activated, NF-κB upregulates pro-inflammatory cytokines (TNF-α, IL-1β, IL-6), chemokines that recruit immune cells, and enzymes (like iNOS) that generate additional reactive nitrogen species. This inflammatory cascade compounds the direct toxic effects of cisplatin.

The combined DNA damage, oxidative stress, and inflammatory signaling activate the apoptotic machinery. This leads to caspase-3, the executioner enzyme that orchestrates programmed cell death. In seminiferous tubules, excessive apoptosis of spermatogenic cells depletes the germ-line pool, creating gaps in spermatogenesis that manifest as oligospermia (low sperm count) or azoospermia (absent sperm) persisting months after chemotherapy ends.

Concept: Apoptosis Versus Autophagy in Testes - Not all cell death is created equal. *Apoptosis* is programmed cell death which is a tidy, energy-requiring process where cells systematically dismantle themselves without spilling inflammatory contents. Some apoptosis in testes is normal and necessary (eliminating cells with DNA errors, maintaining appropriate germ-cell numbers), but excessive apoptosis driven by chemotherapy depletes the stem-cell pool faster than it can regenerate. *Autophagy* is cellular self-eating which is cells breaking down and recycling damaged organelles, misfolded proteins, and other cellular debris to generate energy and building blocks during stress. Moderate autophagy is protective and helps cells survive oxidative challenges, but when autophagy is overwhelmed or dysregulated, it can transition into autophagic cell death. Testicular health requires balanced regulation of both pathways; enough apoptosis to eliminate defective cells, enough autophagy to allow survival through temporary stress, but not so much of either that tissue function collapses.

288

With that foundation, R. A. Azouz and E. I. Hassanen tested whether Gum arabic administration could protect against cisplatin-induced testicular damage in rats. The experimental design used twenty adult male Wistar rats divided into four groups: untreated controls, Gum arabic only (7.5 mg/kg body weight daily in drinking water as reported), cisplatin only (single intraperitoneal dose of 7 mg/kg body weight as reported), and cisplatin plus Gum arabic (pretreatment with Gum arabic). Researchers measured body and testis weights, epididymal sperm analysis (count and motility), blood testosterone levels, testicular oxidative stress markers, DNA damage, histopathological changes, and caspase-3 immunostaining [1].

The results demonstrated Gum arabic provided significant protection. Cisplatin administration caused significant reductions in body and testis weights, sperm count, sperm motility, blood testosterone levels, and testicular antioxidants. Importantly it did so while increasing sperm apoptosis, testicular malondialdehyde levels, DNA damage, histopathological alterations, and caspase-3 immunostaining. Pretreatment with Gum arabic improved all these parameters, demonstrating antioxidant and anti-apoptotic effects against cisplatin testicular toxicity [1].

The 2020 Cairo study added precision to that traditional wisdom, showing exactly *how* protection occurs (oxidative defense, inflammatory modulation, apoptotic regulation). The study also raised a question that would drive subsequent research. If Gum arabic protects testes during chemotherapy (the most extreme, most studied male-fertility threat in modern medicine) does it protect against other, more common oxidative and metabolic stresses that affect fertility in much larger populations? Environmental toxins, metabolic diseases, lifestyle factors? That question would be answered by the studies that followed.

II. 2020 - Gum Arabic Versus a Popular Benchmark

 T aif, Saudi Arabia, 2020. The Cairo cisplatin study established that Gum arabic could protect reproductive function under pharmaceutical assault, but fertility research and clinical practice occur in a crowded marketplace of interventions (herbal supplements, nutraceuticals, pharmaceutical agents, and lifestyle modifications) all claiming reproductive benefits. For clinicians and patients making choices, direct comparisons matter: *How does Gum arabic (Hashab gum from Acacia Senegal) perform against established alternatives when tested side-by-side under identical conditions?*

Omaima Nasir and colleagues at Taif University designed a smart comparative study. Using healthy, untreated Balb/c mice (no induced infertility model), they divided animals into parallel treatment groups and measured the standard panel. The comparison was against *Tribulus terrestris*, a herb with substantial traditional use and modern popularity in men's health supplements, credited with boosting testosterone and supporting erectile function through mechanisms thought to involve luteinizing hormone modulation and nitric oxide effects.

Tribulus terrestris isn't a random comparator as it's arguably the most popular botanical remedy for male fertility and sexual function globally. It has deep roots in Ayurvedic and Traditional Chinese Medicine and substantial presence in Western supplement markets. It also has a research base showing reproductive benefits in some animal and human studies, though with variable results and some concerns about high-dose effects. Putting Hashab gum head-to-head with *Tribulus* creates a meaningful benchmark. If Hashab gum performs comparably or better, it legitimizes Hashab in the fertility space; if it underperforms dramatically, that sets realistic expectations.

The experimental design used 27 adult Balb/c mice (18 females, 9 males) divided into three groups with breeding pairs (one male, two females per group): control receiving tap water, 5% Hashab gum dissolved in drinking water, and 5% aqueous extract of Tribulus terrestris spines. Treatment lasted 21 days while breeding occurred. Researchers measured offspring numbers, testosterone levels via immunoassay, female body weight changes during pregnancy, offspring body weights over two weeks, and histopathological examination of male testicular tissue after sacrifice [2].

Results demonstrated Hashab gum's fertility-enhancing effects demonstrating the number of offspring was higher in the Hashab group compared to both control and Tribulus terrestris groups. Living offspring numbers followed the same pattern, with Hashab gum producing more surviving young. Testosterone levels showed the most striking difference. Hashab gum treatment produced significantly elevated testosterone (1.35 ± 0.04 ng/ml, $P < 0.001$) compared to Tribulus terrestris (0.88 ± 0.09 ng/ml) and control (0.85 ± 0.04 ng/ml). This represented approximately 59% higher testosterone than control and 53% higher than Tribulus terrestris [2].

Histopathological analysis revealed normal seminiferous tubules with increased spermatogenesis in Hashab gum treated males. Sections showed well-organized stratified germinal epithelium, appropriate interstitial spaces, and abundant spermatogonia, primary spermatocytes, and mature sperm. Control and Tribulus terrestris groups showed some degenerated germ cells and wider lumina with fewer spermatocytes [2].

Female body weight during pregnancy showed comparable gains across groups. Offspring body weights at baseline and after two weeks of survival were tracked, with all groups showing growth, though control and Tribulus terrestris offspring gained slightly more weight than Hashab gum offspring; suggesting Hashab gum's effects centered on conception and

291

testosterone rather than post-natal growth parameters [2].

Why this study matters for male fertility research? The study established that Hashab gum, a food-grade substance with established safety, produced measurable fertility outcomes in a head-to-head comparison with an herb traditionally used for sexual function. The superiority in offspring numbers and testosterone elevation over Tribulus terrestris suggested Hashab gum's mechanisms extend beyond simple aphrodisiac effects to actual reproductive enhancement [2].

The researchers attributed Hashab gum's effects to its phytochemical composition: flavonoids, alkaloids, tannins, terpenoids, and saponins. These are all compounds known to reduce oxidative stress, which damages Leydig cells and decreases testosterone production. Saponins specifically function as anti-stress modulators and support penile erection, while flavonoids protect against reactive oxygen species that cause erectile dysfunction [2].

The testosterone elevation proved particularly significant because this steroid hormone, synthesized in testicular Leydig cells plays major roles in erectile function, libido, and spermatogenesis. The substantial increase observed with Hashab gum treatment suggested protection of Leydig cell function rather than mere symptom masking [2].

Unlike pharmaceutical interventions for erectile dysfunction (such as sildenafil citrate) which carry cardiovascular risks including fatal arrhythmias, headache, blurred vision, and muscle pain; Hashab gum's food-grade safety profile presents no such concerns. Its established use as a dietary fiber approved by FDA, FAO, and European Union regulations means long-term consumption poses minimal risk. The study's limitation (using normal fertile mice rather than an infertility model) actually strengthened the interpretation that Hashab gum enhances normal reproductive function rather than merely rescuing impaired fertility.

This suggests applications both for subfertile populations and for optimizing fertility in healthy individuals attempting conception. The comparison with Tribulus terrestris provided clinical context. While Tribulus has decades of traditional use in Chinese medicine, Hashab gum outperformed it. This practical endpoint matters more than intermediate biomarkers for couples seeking fertility care. Hashab's success ultimately extends to achieving pregnancy and live births, not by laboratory values alone.

The researchers noted their findings aligned with previous animal studies showing Hashab gum increased semen parameters and spermatogenesis. Future research directions suggested by this study include dose-response relationships (would higher or lower concentrations optimize effects?), duration studies (does longer supplementation provide additional benefits?), combination protocols (could Hashab gum enhance other fertility interventions?), and human clinical trials measuring both semen parameters and pregnancy rates in couples attempting conception.

The mechanism remains incompletely understood, but the study confirmed that Hashab gum's effects involve testosterone elevation and preservation of testicular histological architecture. Whether these effects result primarily from antioxidant protection, hormonal modulation, or other pathways requires further investigation with direct measurement of oxidative stress markers, inflammatory cytokines, and apoptotic signals.

III. 2020 - Everyday Toxins: When Urban Life Attacks Fertility

Muscat, Oman, and Al Ain, United Arab Emirates, 2020. The

cisplatin study addressed pharmaceutical toxicity; the *Tribulus* comparison established bench-marking. Now the focus shifts to environmental toxicants. The everyday chemical exposures affecting fertility in populations that never face chemotherapy but that breathe polluted air, encounter pesticides, consume processed foods with additives, and engage in lifestyle behaviors (smoking, hookah use, alcohol) that generate oxidative stress and directly damage reproductive tissues.

Concept: Environmental Toxicants in a Fertility Frame - Male fertility isn't just about sperm count and motility; it's about the hormonal milieu that makes spermatogenesis possible. Testosterone synthesis in Leydig cells follows a multi-step enzymatic pathway called *steroidogenesis* where cholesterol enters the mitochondria (rate-limited by StAR protein), gets converted to pregnenolone by side-chain cleavage enzyme (P450scc), then proceeds through a series of hydroxylations and oxidations catalyzed by specific cytochrome P450 enzymes (17α-hydroxylase, 17,20-lyase, 3β-HSD, 17β-HSD) until finally producing testosterone.

This pathway is exquisitely sensitive to oxidative stress because the P450 enzymes are heme-containing proteins that can be inactivated by reactive oxygen species, because the steroidogenic pathway itself generates ROS as a byproduct (particularly during the mitochondrial steps), and because cholesterol transport into mitochondria requires intact membrane function that lipid peroxidation disrupts. When environmental toxicants generate oxidative stress or when they directly inhibit steroidogenic enzymes, testosterone production falls, and spermatogenesis suffers even if germ cells are intact because the hormonal support required for sperm development simply isn't there.

Simultaneously, environmental toxins often contain or generate *reactive carbonyls* which are aldehydes and ketones produced by combustion (smoking, air pollution), present in processed foods, or formed when

294

oxidative stress attacks lipids and proteins. These carbonyls react with proteins through carbonylation, modifying amino-acid side chains and inactivating enzymes, structural proteins, and transport proteins. In testes, protein carbonylation affects both Sertoli-cell function (damaging the support machinery for developing sperm) and the sperm cells themselves.

Concept: Membrane Biophysics Under Lipid Peroxidation - Sperm are unusual cells because they're tiny, they're mostly tail, and that tail is packed with mitochondria and built from a membrane extraordinarily rich in polyunsaturated fatty acids. This membrane composition is necessary for the fluidity required for sperm motility (the whip-like flagellar beating), for the membrane fusion events during fertilization, and for organizing signaling complexes that control capacitation and acrosome reaction. However, polyunsaturated fatty acids are exquisitely vulnerable to lipid peroxidation. One free radical can initiate a chain reaction where peroxyl radicals propagate down the fatty-acid tail, each oxidized lipid generating another radical that attacks a neighboring lipid, creating a cascade that rips through membranes.

Picture lipid bilayers as zippers and each fatty acid tail is a zipper tooth. The membrane works because the zipper teeth align in an organized, fluid structure. Lipid peroxidation is like oxidizing those teeth so they become bent, fragmented, and misaligned. The zipper doesn't close properly. The membrane becomes rigid where it needs to be fluid, leaky where it needs to be sealed. Sperm with peroxidized membranes can't swim properly (flagellar beating requires coordinated membrane flex), can't undergo capacitation (which requires controlled membrane lipid remodeling), and can't fuse with the egg membrane (which requires intact fusion machinery). Oxidative stress literally unzips sperm, leaving them immotile, incapable of fertilization, or if they do fertilize, potentially carrying oxidized DNA into the embryo.

With that mechanistic understanding, we can appreciate what Badreldin H. Ali, Suhail Al-Salam, and colleagues at Sultan Qaboos University in Oman and United Arab Emirates University investigated whether Gum Acacia could protect testes from hookah smoke exposure. The combustion-related environmental toxicity is increasingly common globally, particularly in Middle Eastern and young-adult populations where hookah use is perceived as less harmful than cigarettes despite containing similar or higher concentrations of toxins [3].

The experimental design exposed male C57BL/6 mice to hookah smoke in controlled chambers (30 minutes daily for 30 consecutive days), with parallel groups receiving Gum Acacia supplementation (15% w/v dissolved in drinking water). Four groups were studied: air-exposed controls, hookah smoke only, Acacia gum only, and hookah smoke plus Acacia gum (n=8 per group). Twenty-four hours after the last exposure, researchers measured reproductive hormones, biochemical markers, and testicular histopathology [3].

Researchers measured:
1. Plasma reproductive hormones (testosterone, estradiol, luteinizing hormone, androgen-binding protein, inhibin B)
2. Plasma biochemical markers (alkaline phosphatase, lipopolysaccharide-binding protein, uric acid, lactate dehydrogenase)
3. Testicular homogenate inflammatory cytokines (IL-1β, IL-6, TNF-α, TGF-β1)
4. Oxidative stress markers (malondialdehyde for lipid peroxidation, 8-oxo-2'-deoxyguanosine for DNA damage, cytochrome C, glutathione reductase activity)
5. Nitrosative stress markers (nitrite, nitrate, total nitric oxide), transcription factors (NF-κB, Nrf2)
6. Steroidogenic acute regulatory protein (StAR) via Western blot

296

7. SOD expression via immunohistochemistry
8. Histopathological examination using Johnsen's scoring system
9. Urinary cotinine levels [3].

Results demonstrated protection across multiple pathways. Hookah smoke exposure significantly decreased plasma testosterone, estradiol, and luteinizing hormone levels while increasing inhibin B and decreasing androgen-binding protein. Gum Acacia co-administration significantly mitigated these hormonal disruptions, bringing levels closer to air-exposed controls [3].

Plasma biochemical markers showed smoke-induced damage. Alkaline phosphatase, lipopolysaccharide-binding protein, lactate dehydrogenase, and uric acid all increased significantly with hookah smoke exposure. Gum Acacia treatment significantly reduced alkaline phosphatase, lactate dehydrogenase, and uric acid (though not lipopolysaccharide-binding protein), indicating partial metabolic protection [3].

Inflammatory cytokines in testicular homogenate increased dramatically. IL-1β, IL-6, TNF-α, and TGF-β1 all rose significantly in smoke-exposed animals. Gum Acacia co-administration significantly reduced all four inflammatory markers, demonstrating anti-inflammatory efficacy. Oxidative stress markers revealed severe damage. Malondialdehyde (lipid peroxidation), 8-oxo-2'-deoxyguanosine (DNA oxidative damage), and cytochrome C all increased significantly with smoke exposure, while glutathione reductase activity decreased. Gum Acacia co-administration significantly reversed all these changes, preserving antioxidant defenses and reducing oxidative damage [3].

Nitrosative stress showed complex patterns. Hookah smoke significantly decreased nitrite and total nitric oxide levels (though nitrate and nitrate/nitrite ratios remained unchanged). Gum Acacia co-administration

297

significantly increased nitrite and total nitric oxide levels, suggesting restoration of nitric oxide signaling which is important for vascular and reproductive function [3].

Transcription factor analysis revealed mechanistic insights. NF-κB p65 (inflammatory signaling) and Nrf2 (antioxidant response) both increased significantly in smoke-exposed testicular tissue. Gum Acacia co-administration significantly reduced both, indicating modulation of inflammatory and antioxidant pathways at the transcriptional level. Steroidogenic function showed impairment whereby StAR protein expression (measured by Western blot) decreased significantly with hookah smoke exposure, indicating disrupted testosterone synthesis machinery at the cellular level. Gum Acacia treatment significantly reversed this decrease, preserving steroidogenic capacity restoring StAR protein expression [3].

Histopathology using Johnsen's scoring revealed subtle damage. The air-exposed control group showed mean testicular biopsy score of 8.979, with 51% of seminiferous tubules showing complete spermatogenesis. The hookah smoke group scored 8.418, with only 39% showing complete spermatogenesis and 23% showing no spermatozoa (versus 12% in controls). Block differentiation at spermatocyte and spermatid levels increased from 2% and 10% (controls) to 15% and 8% respectively. The Gum Acacia plus hookah smoke group scored 8.94, with 59% showing complete spermatogenesis and only 12% showing no spermatozoa which is significantly better preservation than smoke alone [3].

SOD immunohistochemistry visually confirmed oxidative stress. Germ cells within seminiferous tubules of hookah smoke-exposed mice showed lower SOD expression compared to controls. Gum Acacia co-administration restored almost normal SOD expression, corroborating the biochemical antioxidant findings. Urinary cotinine (major nicotine metabolite) increased 156% in hookah smoke-exposed animals versus air-exposed controls, confirming significant nicotine absorption. Gum Acacia co-administration reduced cotinine levels by 57% compared to smoke-only groups, suggesting either reduced absorption or enhanced elimination. Body weights showed nonsignificant trends as hookah smoke caused slight nonsignificant reductions in both parameters. Gum Acacia treatment showed slight nonsignificant improvements when given with smoke exposure [3].

Why does this study matters for environmental reproductive toxicology? The study demonstrated that Gum Acacia protects against everyday environmental toxins affecting billions globally and not just pharmaceutical exposures requiring specialized medical settings. Air pollution, smoking, hookah use, and secondhand smoke represent ubiquitous reproductive hazards in urban centers and agricultural regions worldwide. An affordable, accessible intervention requiring no medical supervision addresses public health-level impact.

The mechanism validated across diverse stressors showing Acacia gum's protection extends beyond pharmaceutical toxins (like cisplatin in other studies) to environmental oxidants. The mechanisms (antioxidant support through Nrf2 modulation, anti-inflammatory effects via NF-κB suppression, preservation of steroidogenic machinery, and protection of germ cells) work across diverse insults, suggesting broad therapeutic utility.

The steroidogenic preservation matters beyond fertility. By maintaining StAR expression and testosterone levels, Acacia gum protects not just sperm development but also libido, erectile function, energy, mood, and bone density. The quality-of-life factors extend beyond conception outcomes. Testosterone represents both a fertility hormone and a wellness hormone.

299

The researchers concluded that daily hookah smoke exposure caused adverse effects on reproductive hormone levels and testicular oxidative/nitrosative stress and inflammation markers, which Gum Acacia significantly alleviated through mechanisms involving Nrf2 and NF-κB pathway changes, and StAR preservation. They recommended further studies on functional reproductive consequences and stated that, pending additional research, Gum acacia supplementation may prove useful for mitigating tobacco-related reproductive damage [3].

IV. 2020 - When Metabolism Fails: The Diabetes-Fertility Intersection

Abha, Saudi Arabia, 2020. Chemotherapy and environmental toxins represent acute or intermittent stressors while diabetes represents chronic metabolic dysfunction affecting every organ system, including reproductive tissues. Before presenting the King Khalid University study, we need to frame diabetic reproductive toxicity (how hyperglycemia and its downstream consequences specifically damage testicular function).

An important concept is *Endocrine Diabetotoxicity* and it explains how chronic hyperglycemia derails reproduction. Diabetes doesn't just elevate blood glucose; it triggers a cascade of pathological processes that converge on reproductive tissues. Diabetic men experience subfertility at rates substantially higher than the general population. Resulting in lower sperm counts, reduced motility, increased sperm DNA fragmentation, erectile dysfunction from vascular and neural damage, and reduced libido from hypogonadism. Managing diabetic fertility requires addressing the underlying metabolic dysfunction, not just symptomatic treatment.

A. A. Al-Doaiss and M. A. Al-Shehri at King Khalid University investigated whether Gum arabic alone or combined with insulin could protect testicular tissue from diabetes-induced histological damage in rats. The study used alloxan-induced diabetic rats (a model where alloxan destroys pancreatic beta cells at 150 mg/kg intraperitoneally, creating type 1 diabetes). Wistar rats were divided into groups (n=10 each). 1-Non-diabetic controls receiving normal saline, 2-diabetic rats (alloxan-induced), 3-diabetic rats plus Gum arabic (15 mg/kg/day by gavage in drinking water), 4-diabetic rats plus insulin (4 IU/day subcutaneously), 5-diabetic rats plus both insulin and Gum arabic, and 6-non-diabetic rats receiving Gum arabic alone. Treatment lasted 30 consecutive days, after which animals were sacrificed for histopathological examination. Measured outcomes included only testicular histopathology [4].

Results demonstrated varying degrees of histological protection. Non-diabetic control rats showed normal testicular architecture with hexagonal or rounded seminiferous tubules separated by thin intertubular connective tissue. Germinal epithelia contained normal spermatogenic layers including spermatogonia, primary and secondary spermatocytes, spermatids, and spermatozoa.

Diabetic rats showed severe testicular pathology (testicular atrophy, degenerative changes in spermatogenic cells, incomplete spermatogenesis, shrunken seminiferous tubules greatly depleted of germ cells, wider and vacuolated interstitial tissue, heterogeneity of spermatogenesis with some tubules showing complete absence of spermatogenesis, spermatid giant cells, edema and widening of interstitial tissue, sloughing germinal epithelium, irregular basement membranes, and germinal cell atrophy) [4].

Diabetic rats treated with Gum arabic alone showed substantial improvement with apparent normal seminiferous tubules and interstitial tissue occupied by Leydig cells. Most seminiferous tubules close together with regular outlines and narrow interstitium. Gum arabic treatment also showed restoration of spermatogenic cells in most tubules (though some showed absent spermatozoa), and mild interstitial hemorrhage with edema.

Diabetic rats treated with insulin alone showed moderate improvement with normal structure of most seminiferous tubules, restoration of spermatogenic cells in most tubules. However, some tubules showed absent or few spermatozoa with detached spermatogenic cells from basement membranes. Insulin treatment alone also showed mild interstitial hemorrhage with widened interstitial tissue [4].

Diabetic rats treated with both insulin and Gum arabic showed the best preservation with histological appearance approaching non-diabetic controls more closely than either treatment alone. Non-diabetic rats receiving Gum arabic alone showed minimal changes: essentially normal architecture with slight abnormalities in spermatogenesis, minimal interstitial edema, and rare degenerative changes; demonstrating Gum arabic's safety profile [4].

The study demonstrated that insulin therapy alone, while improving testicular histology compared to untreated diabetes, does not fully restore normal testicular architecture. Gum arabic provided additive histological protection when combined with insulin, suggesting mechanisms beyond glycemic control alone [4].

The researchers concluded that oral administration of Gum arabic alone or combined with insulin for four weeks successfully ameliorated diabetes-induced testicular histological alterations, with improvements in seminiferous tubule structure, spermatogenic cell preservation, and reduced degenerative changes. They attributed these effects to antioxidant, anti-inflammatory, and histological protective properties, recommending further investigation with functional fertility outcomes and biochemical markers [4].

The combination therapy approach validated a practical clinical strategy. Rather than competing with standard diabetes care, Gum arabic augments it, addressing tissue-level damage that glycemic control alone cannot fully prevent. This positions Gum arabic within integrative medicine frameworks that enhance rather than replace evidence-based treatments [4].

V. 2023 - Depth, and Dose: The Menoufia Confirmation

Menoufia, Egypt, 2023. Amany E. Nofal, Yosry A. Okdah, Mohamed I. Rady, and Hamada Z. Hassaan at Menoufia University and Al-Azhar University investigated whether Gum arabic (Hashab gum from Acacia Senegal) could mitigate cisplatin-induced testicular damage in rats, extending previous observations with additional mechanistic assessments [5].

The experimental design used forty adult male albino rats divided into four groups: control, Hashab gum only, cisplatin only, and co-treatment group receiving both cisplatin and Hashab gum concurrently. The study aimed to investigate cytological abnormalities causing spermatogenesis dysfunction through comprehensive biochemical, histometric, immunohistochemical, and ultrastructural analyses [5].

Measured outcomes included sperm parameters (count, motility, morphological abnormalities), oxidative stress markers (malondialdehyde for lipid peroxidation, catalase, superoxide dismutase, glutathione activities), reproductive hormones (testosterone and luteinizing hormone via blood sera), histometric measurements (seminiferous tubule diameter, germinal epithelial height, Johnsen's testicular biopsy score for spermatogenesis assessment, 4-level Cosentino's histological grading scale), immunohistochemical markers (proliferating cell nuclear antigen/PCNA for proliferation, Caspase-3 for apoptosis), and transmission electron microscopy examination for ultrastructural assessment of germinal epithelial cells, spermatozoa, and interstitial tissue [5].

Results demonstrated comprehensive protection across multiple parameters. Cisplatin caused significant increases in oxidative stress (elevated MDA) and significant decreases in antioxidant activities (CAT, SOD, GSH), disturbing testicular machinery. This produced significant histological and ultrastructural damage including atrophied seminiferous tubules with severely reduced germinal epithelium [5]. Reproductive hormones declined significantly. Testosterone and luteinizing hormone levels decreased in cisplatin-treated rats compared to controls and gum arabic-only groups. Cellular proliferation and apoptosis markers showed cisplatin toxicity. PCNA immunoexpression (measuring nucleic proliferation) declined significantly, while cytoplasmic Caspase-3 protein expression (apoptotic marker) increased significantly in testicular tissue. Sperm parameters deteriorated markedly as cisplatin treatment impaired spermatogenesis, decreased sperm number and motility, and increased morphological abnormalities [5].

Hashab gum co-administration provided significant protection (P<0.01) with reduced oxidative stress (MDA decreased significantly) and increased antioxidant activities (CAT, SOD, GSH activities rose significantly). Additionally, testosterone and luteinizing hormone levels elevated in blood sera, histometric measurements improved substantially (seminiferous tubule diameter increased, epithelial height restored, Johnsen's score of spermatogenesis improved, Cosentino's histological grading scale scores improved), immunohistochemical expression showed enhanced nuclear PCNA (indicating better proliferation) and reduced cytoplasmic Caspase-3 (indicating decreased apoptosis) [5].

Transmission electron microscopy examination confirmed ultrastructural protection. Hashab gum co-treatment restored germinal epithelial cell ultrastructure, showed elongated and transverse sections of spermatozoa in tubular lumens (indicating successful spermatogenesis), and demonstrated healthier interstitial tissue compared to cisplatin-only animals. Overall sperm quality improved significantly in co-treated animals compared to cisplatin-only group, with significant declines in morphological abnormalities of sperm. Rats receiving Hashab gum alone showed minimal changes compared to controls, demonstrating the supplement's safety profile when administered without concurrent chemotherapy [5].

Why this study advances cisplatin-fertility research? The study extended the 2020 Cairo findings (Azouz et al.) by adding mechanistic depth through proliferation markers (PCNA), ultrastructural examination via transmission electron microscopy, and detailed histometric scoring systems (Johnsen's score, Cosentino's grading). These additional assessments captured finer-grained pathological changes and recovery patterns beyond standard histopathology [5].

The researchers concluded that Hashab gum is a valuable agent for ameliorating chemotherapy-related infertility. This supports Hashab as a promising adjunct to preserve reproductive function [5].

Before we continue to Brain Health
The same bacterial metabolites that reach reproductive tissues reach neurological tissues. The same short-chain fatty acids that preserve testicular function in diabetic rats and protect against cisplatin damage cross the blood-brain barrier and modulate brain chemistry. The same prebiotic fermentation also shifts gut microbiome composition into producing molecules that affect memory, mood, neuroinflammation, and neurodegeneration.

The fertility story and the brain health story aren't separate. They're the same story told in different organs. When Hashab gum ferments in your distal gut, the metabolites don't choose whether to help your reproductive system or your nervous system; they help both, through the same mechanisms, traveling the same highways.

The question shifts from "Can Hashab gum help fertility?" to "What happens when those same bacterial metabolites reach the aging brain, the inflamed brain, and the metabolically challenged brain?" The answer, as you'll see, builds directly on everything you've just learned about the microbiota-gut-brain axis. The anatomy is the same. The metabolites are the same. Only the target tissues change.

References:

1. Azouz, R. A., and E. I. Hassanen. "Modulating Effect of Gum Arabic on Cisplatin-Induced Testicular Damage in Albino Wistar Rats." Revista Brasileira de Farmacognosia (Brazilian Journal of Pharmacognosy), 30(1): 90–98 (2020). DOI: 10.1007/s43450-020-00015-7

2. Nasir, Omaima, et al. "Comparative Efficacy of Gum Arabic (Acacia senegal) and Tribulus terrestris on Male Fertility." Saudi Pharmaceutical Journal 28 (2020): 1791–1796.

3. Ali, Badreldin H., et al. "Ameliorative Effect of Gum Acacia on Hookah Smoke-Induced Testicular Impairment in Mice." Biomolecules, vol. 10, no. 5, 2020, p. 762.

4. Al-Doaiss, Amin Abdullah, and Mohammed Ali Al-Shehri. "Protective Effect of Gum Arabic/Insulin Against Histological Changes in Testes of Diabetic Rats." International Journal of Morphology 38.2 (2020): 340–347

5. Nofal, Amany E., et al. "Gum Acacia Attenuates Cisplatin Toxic Effect Spermatogenesis Dysfunction and Infertility in Rats." International Journal of Biological Macromolecules, vol. 240, 2023, p. 124292.

CHAPTER 19

NEUROLOGICAL HEALTH

The Research that Revealed the Brain's Quiet Ally

When Membrane Protection Travels North

The brain might seem distant from the gut, liver and kidneys. However, neurological health is exquisitely dependent on signals originating far from the skull. From gut microbiota communicating with the brain through vagal pathways and metabolite signaling. Systemic inflammation reaches the brain through cytokines crossing the blood-brain barrier and activating microglia, while metabolic dysfunction in liver and kidneys generates uremic toxins and oxidative stress that impair neural function. Additionally, the vasculature feeding the brain with oxygen and nutrients responds to the same endothelial dysfunction, lipid peroxidation, and inflammatory damage that affects vessels throughout the body. The brain is not isolated; it's the most metabolically demanding, most oxidatively vulnerable, most inflammation-sensitive organ we have; making it both fragile and responsive to systemic interventions that create favorable conditions for neural health.

I. Feeding the Hippocampal Engine: When Diabetes Starves Memory Circuits

We enter the hippocampus (the brain region essential for forming new memories, for spatial navigation, for converting immediate experience into lasting recall) and ask whether metabolic dysfunction damages these circuits in ways that Gum arabic can prevent or reverse.

Concept: Neuronal Mitochondrial Bioenergetics

Neurons are metabolic race cars. While representing only 2% of body mass, the brain consumes 20% of resting oxygen. This is an extraordinary energy demand driven by the constant work of maintaining ion gradients (the electrical potentials across neuronal membranes that allow signaling), synthesizing neurotransmitters, trafficking proteins along axons and dendrites, and supporting synaptic transmission. This is especially true in regions like the hippocampus responsible for encoding new information through synaptic plasticity.

That energy comes from the mitochondria which is the cellular powerhouse that burns glucose and oxygen through the electron transport chain to generate ATP. Neurons are packed with mitochondria, particularly at synapses where energy demand is highest. The mitochondrial electron transport chain consists of five enzyme complexes (Complex I through V) embedded in the inner mitochondrial membrane, passing electrons from NADH and $FADH_2$ through a series of redox reactions that pump protons across the membrane, creating an electrochemical gradient that Complex V (ATP synthase) uses to generate ATP from ADP and phosphate. This is cellular respiration which is the fundamental energy-generating process that keeps neurons firing.

In diabetes, mitochondrial function becomes compromised through multiple mechanisms. Chronic hyperglycemia generates reactive oxygen species that damage mitochondrial DNA, proteins, and lipids (mitochondria are particularly vulnerable to oxidative damage because they generate ROS as byproducts of respiration and lack the robust DNA repair mechanisms that nuclear DNA enjoys). AGE formation in mitochondria impairs enzyme function. Altered substrate supply (fluctuating glucose, lipotoxicity from elevated free fatty acids) disrupts metabolic flexibility and inflammatory signaling activates pathways that suppress mitochondrial biogenesis (the process of making new mitochondria). The result is an energy crisis where neurons can't generate sufficient ATP to maintain their high-demand operations, synaptic function falters, neuroplasticity is impaired, and cognitive deficits emerge.

When we talk about mitochondrial dysfunction in the brain, we're not being abstract. We can measure it by assaying the enzyme complex activities (Complex I, II, III, IV, V activities measured in tissue homogenates or isolated mitochondria), by measuring ATP production capacity, and by measuring markers of mitochondrial biogenesis like PGC-1α (peroxisome proliferator-activated receptor gamma coactivator 1-alpha). When PGC-1α expression increases, it signals that cells are building more mitochondria and enhancing mitochondrial function which results in adaptive responses to energy demand or metabolic stress. When PGC-1α and mitochondrial enzyme activities are suppressed (as happens in diabetes), it indicates metabolic insufficiency.

Additionally, mitochondria are fueled not just by glucose but by alternative substrates including short-chain fatty acids (specifically acetate and propionate) which can enter the TCA cycle (Krebs cycle) after conversion to acetyl-CoA and succinyl-CoA respectively. This creates a direct connection between gut microbial fermentation (which produces SCFAs from prebiotics) and neuronal energy metabolism. The acetate and propionate generated in colon can enter bloodstream, cross the blood-brain barrier, and serve as fuel for neurons. This is particularly important when glucose metabolism is impaired (as in diabetes). SCFAs provide an alternative energy substrate that can partially bypass the defects in glucose oxidation.

With that foundation, we can appreciate what Ebrahim Rajab and colleagues tested in their 2021 collaborative study. They tested whether Gum arabic supplementation could preserve hippocampal structure and function in diabetic rats.

II. Act I - Preserving Hippocampal Memory Machinery in Metabolic Crisis

Bahrain and Ireland, 2021. This collaboration brought together diabetes researchers, neuroscientists, and mitochondrial biologists to ask whether Gum arabic's effect on systemic metabolism would translate into brain protection. Specifically, protection of the hippocampal circuits that encode memory and that are particularly vulnerable to metabolic dysfunction.

The study used a genetic type 2 diabetes model with Gum arabic supplementation (10% w/v in drinking water) over 16 weeks. Type 2 diabetic rats and controls were assigned to four groups: Control + Water, Control + GA, Diabetes + Water, Diabetes + GA. The comprehensive assessment included behavioral testing. Specifically, the Morris water maze, a standard test of hippocampal-dependent spatial learning and memory where rats learn a hidden platform's location using spatial cues. Memory is assessed by how quickly they find the platform (learning) and whether they search correctly when the platform is removed (memory retention). Hippocampal damage impairs water-maze performance predictably. Hippocampal tissue analysis examined neuronal architecture, and immunofluorescence for mitochondrial markers (PGC-1α and ATP synthase β-subunit/ATPB) [1].

The results demonstrated that Gum arabic preserves hippocampal function through mitochondrial support. Behavioral performance in the Morris water maze improved significantly whereby latency to find the platform was shorter for Diabetes + GA compared to Diabetes + Water ($P < 0.05$).

While not completely restored to non-diabetic levels, the improvement was substantial. Probe trial performance also improved (greater % time in target zone) in Diabetes+GA vs Diabetes+Water. This is the outcome that matters most; actual cognitive function, measured by behavior requiring intact hippocampal circuits [1].

PGC-1α expression density per cell was significantly higher in Diabetes + GA compared to Diabetes + Water (P < 0.05), indicating enhanced mitochondrial biogenesis meaning cells were building more mitochondria and enhancing their energy-generating capacity in response to metabolic stress. A similar trend was observed for ATP synthase β-subunit expression while Gum arabic increased PGC-1α expression density per cell [1].

The study identified specific cellular machinery being supported including the mitochondria and the energy generators. That organelle-level precision matters because it makes the mechanism testable, manipulable, and translatable. If mitochondrial dysfunction drives cognitive impairment in diabetes (and substantial evidence supports this), then interventions supporting mitochondrial function should protect cognition which is exactly what this study demonstrated [1].

We can deduce a relationship from the study connecting Gum arabic's fermentation in the gut (producing SCFAs) to neuronal energy metabolism in the hippocampus. Those SCFAs can serve as alternative fuel substrates for mitochondria, bypassing impaired glucose metabolism and supporting ATP generation. Additionally, SCFAs signal through receptors, and function as histone deacetylase inhibitors, potentially modulating gene expression programs (including PGC-1α) that regulate mitochondrial biogenesis. The gut-to-brain metabolic connection is mechanistically credible.

312

The water-maze improvement demonstrates functional outcomes; not just biochemical markers looking better but actual cognitive performance improving. For translation to human use, behavioral outcomes are what matter. If diabetic patients experience memory problems, and an intervention can measurably improve memory performance while supporting underlying mitochondrial mechanisms, that's the complete package for clinical translation [1].

This is systems medicine demonstrating that by improving metabolic health globally (through gut fermentation, SCFA signaling, inflammatory modulation, oxidative stress reduction), you create conditions where all tissues (including brain) can function optimally. The hippocampal benefit isn't separate; it's part of the integrated metabolic rescue that Gum arabic provides.

Contrast with pharmaceutical approaches: Current diabetes treatments focus on glucose control (insulin, metformin, GLP-1 agonists) and cardiovascular risk reduction. They don't directly target mitochondrial function or specifically aim to prevent cognitive decline, though some drugs may have indirect neuroprotective effects. Gum arabic's mitochondrial support creates a complementary approach. It does not replace diabetes medications but adds metabolic and mitochondrial support that those medications don't directly provide.

The 2021 hippocampal study positioned Gum arabic as a metabolic neuroprotector; protecting brain not through neurotransmitter manipulation or targeted receptor activation but through supporting the fundamental energy metabolism that neurons require to function. That distinction proves important for neurological challenges because mitochondrial dysfunction and energy crisis are common pathways in many neurological diseases beyond diabetes. Neurodegenerative diseases, ischemic injury, epilepsy, and aging-related cognitive decline all involve mitochondrial impairment.

313

If Gum arabic supports mitochondrial function broadly, its neuroprotective potential extends across multiple conditions.

III - Protecting the Spinal Cord from Reperfusion Chaos

We move now from hippocampus rejuvenation to acute injury. The kind of catastrophic oxidative burst that occurs when blood flow is interrupted then restored, creating an ischemia-reperfusion injury that devastates neural tissue within hours.

Concept: Ischemia-Reperfusion Injury in the Spinal Cord

Imagine a garden hose running water to plants. If you clamp the hose (ischemia), water flow stops, and plants begin to suffer from lack of water and nutrients. This is the ischemic phase where tissue is deprived of oxygen and glucose, ATP production falters, cells begin losing ion gradients, and damage accumulates. The paradox is that when you suddenly release the clamp (reperfusion), the rush of returning water doesn't simply rescue the plants as it arrives as a high-pressure surge that can damage delicate roots and dislodge soil. In biology's case, reperfusion triggers a massive burst of reactive oxygen species, inflammatory activation, edema, and cellular death that sometimes exceeds the damage from ischemia alone.

In clinical medicine, ischemia-reperfusion injury occurs in multiple scenarios: stroke (when a clot blocks brain blood flow then dissolves or is removed), heart attack (when coronary artery is blocked then reopened), organ transplantation (when organs are removed, cooled, then reperfused after transplant), and importantly, spinal cord injury (when trauma or surgical interventions disrupt then restore blood flow). The pathophysiology follows a predictable cascade.

During *ischemia*: Lack of oxygen halts mitochondrial ATP production, energy-dependent pumps fail, neurons depolarize, calcium floods into cells, excitotoxic neurotransmitters (particularly glutamate) accumulate, and cells shift to anaerobic metabolism generating lactate and lowering pH. This metabolic crisis damages cells but isn't immediately fatal for all of them as there's a window where reperfusion could rescue tissue.

During *reperfusion*: When blood flow returns, oxygen suddenly floods back into metabolically disrupted tissue where mitochondria are damaged and where reactive metabolites have accumulated. This triggers explosive ROS generation as damaged mitochondria can't properly use the oxygen and instead generate superoxide. Xanthine oxidase (an enzyme activated during ischemia) converts the restored oxygen to more superoxide, and inflammatory signaling is activated (NF-κB turns on, cytokines are produced, neutrophils are recruited through restored circulation). Additionally, the restored blood flow delivers inflammatory mediators from the systemic circulation, edema develops as damaged blood vessels become leaky, and the combination creates a "reperfusion injury" that kills cells that might have survived if reperfusion had been managed more carefully.

In the spinal cord specifically, ischemia-reperfusion can occur during surgical repair of aortic aneurysms (where spinal arteries are temporarily compromised), after traumatic injury with vascular disruption, or in experimental models where researchers temporarily clamp the spinal artery then release it to study protective interventions. The clinical consequences are devastating including paralysis, loss of sensation, and autonomic dysfunction affecting bladder and bowel control. Current treatments are limited (supportive care, early surgical decompression if trauma caused mechanical compression, blood pressure management to maximize perfusion) but nothing directly addresses the oxidative and inflammatory cascade driving reperfusion injury.

315

If Hashab gum can suppress the ROS burst and NF-κB activation that define reperfusion injury, it could provide neuroprotection in this acute-injury scenario.

IV. Act II - Preconditioning the Spinal Cord for Ischemic Challenge

Iran, 2024. Hesam Yahak, Gholam Hossein Farjah, Bagher Pourheydar, and Mojtaba Karimipour designed a spinal cord ischemia-reperfusion study to test whether Gum arabic (Hashab gum from Acacia Senegal) pretreatment could protect neural tissue from acute oxidative injury. Rats received oral gavage Hashab for 21 days before surgery undergoing temporary abdominal aortic clamping to induce spinal cord ischemia (60 min) followed by reperfusion [2]. After allowing time for acute injury to develop, researchers measured:

- *Functional outcomes* - Neurologic function was assessed with the Motor Deficit Index (MDI, 0–6) at 24/48/72 h and hind-limb sensation with Withdrawal Reflex Latency (WRL; 56 °C hot-plate).
- *Histopathology* - examining spinal cord sections for neuronal loss, tissue disorganization, inflammatory cell infiltration, and vascular damage.
- *Oxidative/antioxidant indices in plasma* - (SOD, CAT, TAC, MDA). No NF-κB or cytokines were measured.

The results demonstrated that Hashab gum pretreatment provides significant neuroprotection against ischemia-reperfusion injury. Motor function recovery was substantially better in animals that had received Hashab gum before ischemia-reperfusion compared to those that underwent the injury without pretreatment. While not completely preventing injury (the ischemia-reperfusion challenge is severe), Hashab gum significantly improved functional outcomes where animals showed better hind-limb movement, faster recovery, and less severe paralysis [2].

Histopathology showed substantial tissue protection. Neuronal loss was reduced (more neurons surviving the ischemia-reperfusion challenge), tissue architecture was better preserved, inflammatory cell infiltration was lower, white-matter damage (cavitation) scores were lower and motor-neuron counts higher. The tissue looked less catastrophically damaged. Oxidative stress markers showed the familiar protective pattern with reduced lipid peroxidation, and preserved antioxidant defenses [2].

Why the 2024 spinal ischemia-reperfusion study matters for acute neuroprotection? Most Hashab gum neurological studies examined chronic conditions. These include diabetic neuropathy developing over months, cognitive decline in chronic metabolic disease, and progressive gut inflammation. The ischemia-reperfusion study showed that Hashab gum protective mechanisms work in acute injury where the oxidative and inflammatory cascade develops over hours. This expands the applicability demonstrating that Hashab gum isn't just for slowly progressive conditions but can protect against acute neural insults [2].

The study used pretreatment (giving Hashab gum before the injury occurred) which is how ischemic preconditioning works. For clinical translation, this suggests value in perioperative use. Patients undergoing surgeries with risk of spinal ischemia (thoracoabdominal aortic aneurysm repair particularly) could supplement with Hashab gum before surgery, potentially reducing the devastating complication of post-operative paralysis.

The CCl_4 study showed that Hashab gum suppresses NF-κB in systemic toxicity. The spinal I/R study confirmed it works in acute neural injury.

The mechanism is robust and not confined to one injury type but operating across diverse challenges. That robustness is what clinical translation requires as you can't develop a therapeutic intervention if it only works in one experimental model. The consistency across chronic metabolic stress, systemic toxicity, and acute ischemia-reperfusion injury builds confidence that the mechanism will translate to human disease.

The spinal cord study also bridges to the next domain (seizures and network stability) because both ischemia-reperfusion and seizures involve excessive neuronal activation (glutamate excitotoxicity, calcium overload, mitochondrial stress) that Hashab gum's oxidative and inflammatory modulation can address. The transition from protecting individual neurons and axons (peripheral neuropathy, spinal injury) to protecting network-level function (preventing pathological synchronization that defines seizures) is the natural next step in understanding Hashab gum's neuroprotective range.

V. When Neural Networks Tip into Runaway Firing

We've seen Hashab gum protect neural structure (hippocampal neurons, spinal cord architecture). Now we ask whether it can stabilize neural function at the network level, prevent the pathological synchronization that defines epileptic seizures and modulate the gene programs that regulate learning plasticity and circadian timing.

Concept: Epileptic Kindling, EGR-1, and Rev-erbα
Epileptic kindling is a laboratory model and a clinical phenomenon where repeated, initially subthreshold electrical or chemical stimulation gradually lowers the seizure threshold until stimuli that initially didn't cause seizures begin triggering full convulsions. It's a form of pathological learning where the brain becomes progressively better at seizing. The most common

chemical kindling model uses pentylenetetrazole (PTZ), a GABA_A receptor antagonist that reduces inhibitory tone in brain, creating brief seizures when given at moderate doses but requiring repeated administration over days to weeks to produce the kindling effect where the brain becomes progressively more seizure-prone.

Kindling matters clinically because it models epileptogenesis; the process by which a normal brain becomes epileptic, often following initial insults like head trauma, stroke, prolonged febrile seizures in childhood, or status epilepticus. Understanding kindling mechanisms is critical for developing interventions that could prevent epilepsy development in at-risk individuals rather than just suppressing seizures after epilepsy is established. The mechanisms of kindling involve oxidative stress (repeated seizures generate massive ROS that damage neurons and alter their excitability), inflammatory activation (microglia become chronically activated, cytokines are elevated, creating pro-excitatory environment), altered gene expression (repeated seizures activate transcriptional programs that change the expression of ion channels, neurotransmitter receptors, and synaptic proteins in ways that make networks more excitable), and structural remodeling (sprouting of new connections, particularly in hippocampus, that create aberrant circuits prone to synchronization).

Two genes are specifically relevant to kindling and measured in the study we're about to examine. *1-EGR-1 (Early Growth Response 1)* is an immediate-early gene. A transcription factor rapidly induced by neuronal activity that regulates expression of genes involved in synaptic plasticity, learning, and memory. In normal physiology, EGR-1 is the "learning switch". When neurons fire during memory encoding, EGR-1 is activated and helps consolidate those memories by driving expression of structural proteins that strengthen synapses. However, in kindling, excessive EGR-1 activation can drive pathological plasticity thereby strengthening connections that shouldn't be strengthened and creating hyperexcitable

319

circuits. Measuring EGR-1 provides a window into whether pathological plasticity mechanisms are engaged. *2-Rev-erbα* is a nuclear receptor that functions as a transcriptional repressor and is a core component of the molecular circadian clock. This is the cellular timekeeping mechanism that generates 24-hour rhythms in gene expression, metabolism, and physiology. Rev-erbα is the "clock dimmer" as it suppresses expression of clock genes and metabolic genes in a rhythmic pattern, creating the oscillations that define circadian time.

Circadian disruption is increasingly recognized as relevant to seizure disorders. Many epilepsy patients have seizures that occur preferentially at specific times of day, sleep-wake disruption lowers seizure threshold, and metabolic rhythms controlled by clock genes influence neural excitability through effects on energy metabolism, oxidative stress, and inflammatory tone. Measuring Rev-erbα provides insight into whether circadian and metabolic timing are being affected.

If Gum arabic can reduce oxidative stress and inflammation in kindling (making networks less excitable), modulate EGR-1 expression (preventing pathological plasticity), and influence Rev-erbα (stabilizing circadian-metabolic timing), it could act at multiple levels to prevent or reduce seizure susceptibility.

VI. Act III - Stabilizing Neural Networks: PTZ Kindling, Oxidative Stress, and Clock Genes

Turkey, 2024. Funda Yakmaz, Ahmet Sarper Bozkurt, and Şenay Görücü Yılmaz at Gaziantep University investigated whether Gum arabic supplementation after kindling by oral gavage (2 mg/kg/day) for 10 days could alter the molecular programs underlying network hyperexcitability. Rats were subjected to PTZ i.p. 35 mg/kg/day for 11 days, then a 75 mg/kg

dose 48 h later; behaviors recorded with the LABORAS system.
After establishing full kindling, researchers measured:

1. Seizure parameters using standardized severity scales
2. Oxidative stress status via antioxidant capacity assays (total antioxidant status/TAS and total oxidant status/TOS) measuring the overall ability of hippocampal tissue to neutralize reactive species, gene expression; specifically, EGR-1 and Rev-erbα mRNA levels in hippocampus measured by quantitative PCR
3. Automated behavior metrics (locomotor activity, immobilization, rearing, grooming, eating, drinking) via LABORAS; the authors infer possible anxiolytic effects. [3]

The results demonstrated that Gum arabic modulates multiple levels of seizure biology. Gum arabic significantly increased TAS levels and decreased TOS levels, thus exhibiting antioxidant properties by reducing oxidative stress burden. This indicates that the oxidative stress generated by repeated seizures was being better managed, preventing the oxidative damage that contributes to progressive hyperexcitability [3].

Gene expression changes were particularly striking. EGR-1, which was upregulated in the seizure group (reflecting pathological plasticity and neuronal activation), was significantly downregulated with Gum arabic treatment. This indicates that Gum arabic normalized the excessive immediate-early gene expression associated with kindling-induced network remodeling. Rev-erbα, which was downregulated in the seizure group, was significantly upregulated after Gum arabic treatment, suggesting restoration of normal circadian-metabolic timing mechanisms. The gene-level changes indicate that Gum arabic isn't just neutralizing ROS after they form but is modulating the cellular programs determining network excitability and metabolic state [3].

Behavioral measures demonstrated anxiolytic effects, consistent with reducing stress responses. This is relevant because stress lowers seizure

321

threshold and anxiety is comorbid with epilepsy. The abstract concludes that Gum arabic may be an antiepileptic and anxiolytic therapeutic in improving epileptic seizures by reducing oxidative stress burden through EGR1 and Rev-erbα pathways [3].

The kindling study demonstrated that Gum arabic's neuroprotective effects aren't confined to specific brain regions or injury types. The mechanism is sufficiently general (oxidative stress reduction, inflammatory modulation, metabolic support, gene expression normalization) that it provides resilience across diverse challenges to neural system stability.

VII. Closing Reflection for Readers

The science is still young; human neurological trials are a necessary next step before clinical recommendations become standard. However, as we have demonstrated, the preclinical foundation is remarkably strong. Consistent mechanisms across diverse models, clear dose-response relationships, validated molecular targets, functional outcomes that matter to patients, and a safety profile that permits long-term use.

The neurological story also reinforces the book's central theme. Health is integrated, not compartmentalized. You can't separate brain health from gut health, metabolic health, inflammatory status, and oxidative balance. Interventions that repair terrain (creating favorable conditions where systems can self-regulate and function optimally) have value across every organ and every condition. Hashab gum is that kind of intervention, and its effects in neural systems validate the approach while opening doors to applications not yet explored.

Atherosclerosis, hypertension, endothelial dysfunction, vascular stiffness, diabetic neuropathy, ischemia-reperfusion injury, and neurodegenerative disease are all manifestations of systematic problems. The root cause usually being dysbiosis, oxidative stress, chronic inflammation, mitochondrial dysfunction, and metabolic dysregulation expressing themselves in different anatomical locations. Vascular health is neural health (without perfusion, neurons die within minutes) and neural health is vascular health as dysregulated autonomic tone from brain dysfunction damages vessels. The separation is artificial; the biology is integrated; and Hashab gum's effects span the circuit because the mechanisms are universal.

References:

1. Rajab, Ebrahim, et al. "Gum Arabic Supplementation Prevents Loss of Learning and Memory Through Stimulation of Mitochondrial Function in the Hippocampus of Type 2 Diabetic Rats." Journal of Functional Foods, vol. 87, Dec. 2021, article 104757
2. Yahak, Hesam, et al. "Protective Effect of Gum Arabic on Spinal Cord Ischemia-Reperfusion Injury in Rats." Caspian Journal of Neurological Sciences, vol. 10, no. 1, 2024, pp. 47-56
3. Yakmaz, Funda, et al. "PTZ-Kindled Rat Model; Evaluation of Seizure, Hippocampal EGR-1 and Rev-erbα Gene Regulation, Behavioral Analysis and Antioxidant Capacity of Gum Arabic." Molecular Biology Reports, Volume 51, article number 279 (2024)

CHAPTER 20

The Research Demonstrating the Ultimate "Healthifier"

From Solo Performance to Orchestra

The last chapter ended with a quiet revelation about the brain. It demonstrated that when the gut is calmed, mitochondria is fueled, and inflammatory volume knobs are turned down. This results in neural circuits that remember who they are as they encode memories more reliably, resist tipping into seizures, and preserve cognitive function under stress. That same pattern (terrain first, targets second) explains why Hashab gum does more than act alone. It also acts with things, with living probiotics that hate heat and acid, with omega-3 oils that oxidize and separate, with fragile antioxidants that break before they help, and with oral rehydration solutions that depend on elegant intestinal physics.

This chapter tells that story as a journey through time and application. From hospital yogurt cups handed to patients with irritable bowel syndrome, through factory benchtops where curcumin particles are engineered for stability, to pediatric emergency wards in Sudan where oral rehydration solutions amplified by Hashab gum save children from dehydration. Besides its intrinsic prowess as a multi-faceted healer, Hashab gum also boosts other healing ingredients and compounds; it's the ultimate platform. It's not just an active ingredient doing one thing well, but a multifunctional polymer that is simultaneously film-forming (wrapping fragile partners in protective layers), mucoadhesive (helping compounds stick where they need to act), prebiotic (feeding beneficial organisms while creating favorable terrain), and interfacial (organizing the oil-water boundaries that determine whether lipids can be digested and absorbed).

The through-line connecting these diverse applications is mechanistic rather than coincidental. Hashab gum's arabinogalactan-protein structure creates favorable microenvironments at multiple scales including the molecular (protecting sensitive compounds from oxygen and water), colloidal (stabilizing emulsion droplets at oil-water interfaces), microbial (providing slow-fermenting substrate that selected strains thrive on), and physiological (modulating intestinal transport through multiple pathways beyond the classic sodium-glucose cotransporter). When you pair Hashab gum with interventions that fail because of delivery problems (probiotics die in storage or stomach acid, omega-3s oxidize before absorption, polyphenols precipitate uselessly, rehydration solutions leak back out through secretory channels), it addresses exactly those failure modes through mechanisms we've been documenting since the inflammation chapter, but now deployed in service of making partners work rather than acting solo.

What emerges from the studies we'll examine is a design principle that transforms supplement formulation from shotgun approaches (throw everything together and hope) into rational engineering. The studies will demonstrate Hashab gum as the carrier matrix that organizes, protects, delivers, and enhances other actives while contributing its own terrain-repair effects. These include anti-inflammatory tone, antioxidant support, microbiome modulation, and metabolic benefits documented across this book. When formulated correctly, one plus one equals considerably more than two, not through mystical synergy but through addressing complementary failure modes simultaneously. The probiotic arrives alive because Hashab gum protected it, engrafts successfully because Hashab gum created favorable gut terrain, and produces its beneficial effects in an environment where inflammation isn't overwhelming the signals. That's multiplicative benefit through mechanistic stacking.

This chapter walks through the evidence chronologically, showing how industries and clinics discovered Hashab gum's platform potential across different applications, and synthesized the lessons into practical guidance for formulators, clinicians, and ultimately patients who deserve products that actually work as labeled rather than failing in the bottle or the gut.

I. New Concepts You'll Need: A Traveler's Glossary for the Synergy Landscape

Before we step into the studies, let's establish a few technical concepts you haven't met in earlier chapters.

Synbiotics and the Logic of Designed Pairs

A *synbiotic* is an intentionally designed combination. It's a combination of a probiotic (the living microorganism—usually Lactobacillus, Bifidobacterium, or other beneficial bacteria) plus a prebiotic (the fermentable substrate that feeds it) packaged or administered together. The design logic is beautiful in its simplicity. Probiotics face hostile environments during manufacturing (heat, oxygen, mechanical shear), storage (residual moisture, oxidative stress over months), transit through stomach (gastric acid at pH 1-2, pepsin digestion), and arrival in intestine (bile salts that dissolve membranes, competition from resident bacteria). Most probiotics die before doing useful work.

Pairing these probiotics with a powerful prebiotic raises the probability that organisms survive the gauntlet, engraft successfully, and produce the metabolic and immunomodulatory effects that justify taking the product. Success is tracked through *encapsulation efficiency* (what percentage of the probiotic strain got successfully incorporated into protective particles

327

during manufacturing), *viable counts* (how many organisms remain alive, measured as colony-forming units or CFU per gram, after storage under defined conditions), and *survival through simulated digestion* (how many cells remain viable after exposure to synthetic gastric fluid at low pH followed by bile salts at intestinal pH). These aren't arbitrary metrics; they predict whether swallowing a capsule or eating yogurt will actually deliver living organisms to your colon where they can colonize, function and delivery results.

Encapsulation: Building Walls That Dissolve on Cue

Encapsulation is the art and science of wrapping sensitive materials (living cells, oils, vitamins, polyphenols) inside protective walls so they tolerate hostile environments during processing and storage, then release their contents exactly where and when needed. Think of it as building a time-release safe where the walls must be strong enough to protect the contents from premature degradation (oxygen exposure, moisture, pH extremes, temperature fluctuations) but designed to open predictably when triggered by the right stimulus (usually moisture, pH change, or enzymatic digestion in the target location).

For probiotics specifically, encapsulation means surrounding bacterial cells with polymer matrices (Hashab gum, alginate, chitosan, maltodextrin, proteins) that form protective films. The challenge is multifold. Walls too thick and impermeable, and cells suffocate or fail to release. Walls too thin or porous, and protection fails. The engineering sweet spot is often a multi-layer system with an inner layer for moisture control, an outer oxygen barrier layer with controlled porosity that allows some gas exchange (cells need to breathe minimally even in dormancy) while limiting water activity enough to prevent microbial growth of contaminants.

Lipid Delivery: The Dance at Oil-Water Boundaries

When we talk about delivering omega-3 fatty acids, fat-soluble vitamins, or lipophilic polyphenols like curcumin, we're dealing with a different fundamental challenge. These molecules don't dissolve in the aqueous environment of the gut lumen. Digestion and absorption require converting large oil droplets into microscopic structures called *mixed micelles* (aggregates of bile salts, phospholipids, digested lipids, and the lipid-soluble nutrients we're trying to absorb) that are small enough (~5-10 nanometers) to diffuse through the unstirred water layer coating the intestinal epithelium and deliver their cargo to the brush border membrane where uptake occurs.

The key to successful lipid delivery is *interfacial chemistry*; what happens at the boundary between oil and water. Large oil droplets are thermodynamically unstable in water because they want to coalesce and separate into a distinct oil phase (picture salad dressing that separates if you don't shake it). *Emulsifiers* are molecules that adsorb at oil-water interfaces, with hydrophobic regions orienting toward the oil and hydrophilic regions toward the water, creating a stabilizing film that prevents droplet coalescence. Hashab gum is an excellent natural emulsifier because its arabinogalactan-protein structure contains both hydrophobic regions (from the protein component and some sugar residues) and highly hydrophilic regions (from the charged and hydroxyl groups on the polysaccharide chains).

However, stability in the bottle isn't enough because the emulsion must also perform well during digestion. Pancreatic lipase accesses oil droplets at the interface, cleaving triglycerides into fatty acids and monoglycerides. If the interfacial film is too rigid or impermeable, lipase can't reach the substrate and digestion stalls. If it's too labile, droplets coalesce before digestion completes.

Hashab gum's interfacial film hits a sweet spot. It's stable enough for storage, but digestible enough to allow lipase access, yielding well-formed mixed micelles. The technical term you'll encounter is *bioaccessibility* (the fraction of a nutrient that's released from the food matrix and incorporated into micelles and thus potentially absorbable), measured by analyzing the micellar phase after in vitro digestion. This predicts but doesn't guarantee *bioavailability* (the fraction that actually reaches systemic circulation), which requires animal or human studies.

Oral Rehydration: More Than Sodium-Glucose Cotransport
The elegant physiological principle underlying oral rehydration therapy (ORT) for diarrheal diseases is the *sodium-glucose cotransporter* (SGLT1) in the intestinal brush border. This protein simultaneously transports one glucose molecule and two sodium ions from the lumen (the hollow space inside the intestine where food passes through, is digested, and nutrients are absorbed) into the epithelial cell, using the energy from the sodium gradient (maintained by the sodium-potassium ATPase on the basolateral membrane) to drive glucose uptake against its concentration gradient. Water follows the solutes osmotically through water channels (aquaporins) and paracellular pathways (between cells). By providing glucose and sodium in appropriate ratios (typically aiming for osmolality of 200-310 mOsm/L to avoid osmotic penalties), standard ORS enhances fluid absorption even when secretory diarrhea (driven by enterotoxins activating chloride secretion) is ongoing.

However, the intestine has additional transport pathways beyond SGLT1 including sodium-independent glucose transporters (GLUT2, GLUT5), amino acid cotransporters, organic solute transporters, and water channels that respond to osmotic gradients. Acacia gum's effects on oral rehydration appear to work through multiple mechanisms such as stimulating these alternative uptake pathways (increasing total absorptive capacity), providing fermentable substrate that produces short-chain fatty acids which enhance colonocyte absorption and barrier function, and potentially reducing secretory flux by modulating chloride channel activity (CFTR,

330

the cystic fibrosis transmembrane conductance regulator). Additionally, Acacia gum can serve as a *micronutrient chaperone* facilitating absorption of minerals like zinc that are critical for mucosal repair and immune function during recovery from diarrheal illness. Zinc normally interacts with multiple intestinal transporters and can compete with other metals for absorption. Acacia gum appears to enhance zinc uptake through mechanisms that aren't fully characterized but may involve creating favorable microenvironments at the brush border or forming soluble complexes that are more readily transported.

With these concepts established, we're ready to follow how different research communities (clinical gastroenterology, food engineering, pharmaceutical sciences, and emergency medicine) discovered Acacia gum's synergy potential in their respective domains, creating convergent evidence that this polymer is genuinely special as a platform technology.

II. Act I - A Yogurt Cup Proves the Point

Seoul, South Korea, 2012. Sungkyunkwan University School of Medicine is where we begin to explore what survives beyond theory when treating patients with irritable bowel syndrome. IBS is the quintessential "terrain disease" as there's rarely a single identifiable pathogen or anatomical lesion, just a constellation of symptoms (abdominal pain, bloating, altered bowel habits) driven by visceral hypersensitivity, altered gut-brain signaling, low-grade inflammation, and dysbiosis. Current treatments are frustratingly limited as dietary modification helps some patients. Antispasmodics and antidepressants provide symptomatic relief for others, but many patients cycle through interventions without sustained benefit.

The probiotic approach to IBS has face validity because if dysbiosis contributes to symptoms, restoring balanced microbiota should help.

However, probiotic trials in IBS show variable results, likely because strain selection matters, delivering sufficient viable organisms to the colon is challenging, and because a chaotic gut environment may not provide favorable conditions for engraftment. The synbiotic concept addresses both issues by pairing a strain with demonstrated IBS benefits with a prebiotic that feeds that strain preferentially while creating generally favorable gut terrain.

Yang Won Min and colleagues ran a randomized, double-blind, controlled 8-week trial in IBS outpatients, testing a composite yogurt that combined Acacia dietary fiber with high-dose Bifidobacterium animalis subsp. lactis Bb-12 (plus starter cultures) against a control yogurt that contained B. lactis but no Acacia fiber or enhancer. Outcomes were assessed with a structured questionnaire using visual-analog scales (VAS), the Bristol stool scale, and an overall IBS-symptom VAS. A total of 130 patients were randomized and 117 completed the study.

The key findings demonstrated that compared with control, the composite yogurt produced significantly greater improvement in overall IBS-symptom VAS (64.2 ± 17.0 vs 50.4 ± 20.5; $P < 0.001$) and bowel-habit satisfaction (Δ 27.16 vs 15.51; $P = 0.010$). In prespecified subtypes, IBS-C showed a larger gain in overall symptom improvement with the composite yogurt, while IBS-D showed a greater increase in bowel-habit satisfaction. Other symptom domains (e.g., pain/discomfort and bloating) improved within groups but did not show significant between-group differences in the overall cohort. No significant adverse events were reported.

This well-designed clinical trial supports an additive benefit of pairing Acacia fiber with B. lactis in IBS, with the strongest signals in overall symptom relief, bowel-habit satisfaction, and differential benefits by IBS subtype (overall symptoms in IBS-C; satisfaction in IBS-D).

This was among the first to demonstrate clinical benefits of Acacia gum–probiotic pairing in a disease state rather than just showing microbiological endpoints (survival, colonization) in healthy volunteers. By targeting IBS (a common, costly, quality-of-life-impairing condition with limited effective treatments) the study positioned Acacia gum synbiotics in medical gastroenterology rather than just wellness markets. It foreshadowed the design principle that would emerge from subsequent work whereby Acacia gum isn't just delivering organisms; it's creating the terrain where those organisms can thrive and produce beneficial effects.

III. Act II - Omega-3s: Fragile Oils Safely to the Wall

Bordeaux, France, 2022. The omega-3 fatty acid story has been one of modern nutrition's most frustrating sagas. It has enormous potential (cardiovascular protection, anti-inflammatory effects, neural development and cognitive support) documented through mechanistic studies and some clinical trials. On the other side it has inconsistent benefits in real-world supplementation, possibly because much of what people consume either oxidizes before absorption or is never absorbed at all. DHA (docosahexaenoic acid, a long-chain omega-3 from marine sources including microalgae) is polyunsaturated to an extreme degree (DHA has six double bonds) making it exquisitely vulnerable to lipid peroxidation. One free radical hitting one double bond initiates a chain reaction where each oxidized lipid generates another radical attacking a neighboring lipid, ripping through membranes like falling dominoes.

Worse, bulk omega-3 oil sitting in capsules or bottles has enormous surface area exposed to oxygen, light, and trace metals (from processing equipment) that catalyze oxidation. By the time consumers buy supplements, oxidation may be extensive. Then comes the absorption challenge when omega-3s arrive in the stomach as oil droplets. Without emulsification creating small, stable droplets that can be efficiently digested by pancreatic lipase in the small intestine, much of the oil passes unabsorbed. Even if digestion occurs, the mixed micelles that should form to carry fatty acids and monoglycerides to the brush border can be unstable, coalescing before absorption completes. The net result is that label claims and actual bioavailability can diverge dramatically.

A French research team led by Leslie Couëdelo and Carole Vaysse at ITERG, working with the company Nexira, wanted to see whether adding Acacia gum to omega-3 oil could help the body absorb these healthy fats more effectively. To test this, they used a controlled experiment in rats that had been fitted with a small tube in their intestinal lymph duct. This setup allowed the researchers to collect lymph fluid (the liquid that carries absorbed fats from the intestines) at regular intervals after the rats swallowed a single dose of oil. One group received plain microalgae oil (a source of DHA and EPA), while the other received the same oil mixed into an emulsion stabilized with Acacia gum, where the oil droplets were coated with a thin film of the gum [2].

The results were striking. Rats that received the Acacia gum emulsion absorbed much more omega-3 into their intestinal lymph fluid (about three to four times more than those given plain oil) and the peak absorption happened earlier, after roughly four hours instead of six. The study measured how much DHA and EPA appeared in the lymph during the first six hours, showing that Acacia gum made the oil easier for the digestive system to process and transfer into the body's fat-transport pathways [2].

Mechanistically, Acacia gum acted like a natural emulsifier. It helped the oil form tiny, stable droplets that enzymes could easily break down, while also preventing the oil from clumping or oxidizing. By stabilizing the droplets and protecting them during digestion, Acacia gum improved how well the fatty acids entered the intestinal lymph for absorption [2].

334

IV. Act III - Antioxidants: Packaging the Delicate

A 2023 Egyptian experiment in Helwan University tested whether Gum arabic (Hashab gum from Acacia Senegal) and turmeric (TUR) could lessen glycerol-induced acute kidney injury in rats, a standard model that mimics rhabdomyolysis-related kidney damage. Sixty-six male rats were fed diets containing Hashab(GA) alone, Turmeric(TUR) alone, or GA+TUR at 1%, 2%, or 4% (w/w) for 28 days. They were then given a single glycerol injection to trigger kidney injury (50% glycerol in saline, 5 ml/kg) and kept on the same diets for 3 more days before testing. Outcomes included blood kidney function markers (urea, creatinine, uric acid), kidney antioxidant status (GSH, GPx, and MDA as a lipid-peroxidation index), and microscopic kidney histology [3].

Compared with injured controls, the combination diets generally performed best, especially the 4% GA + 4% TUR group. In that group, urea, creatinine, and uric acid were markedly lower, kidney GSH and GPx were higher, and MDA was reduced, indicating less oxidative stress. On histology, several sections from the 2%+2% and 4%+4% combination groups appeared close to normal, although some sections still showed vacuolization [3].

The evidence proves Hashab gum is valuable for polyphenol and botanical delivery. The benefits extend from pure encapsulation science to genuine biological synergy where Hashab gum contributes therapeutic effects beyond just delivery.

V. Act IV - ORS That Absorbs Faster and Leaks Less

Manhasset, 2001. Researchers Michael Wingertzahn and Richard Wapnir from the New York University School of Medicine made a surprising discovery about Gum arabic's effect on the intestines. They wanted to know whether this natural fiber could change how the gut absorbs water and electrolytes; a question inspired by traditional uses of Gum arabic for digestive health and hydration in desert regions [4].

To test this, they perfused segments of rat small intestine with a standard oral rehydration solution containing glucose and electrolytes, with or without added Gum arabic. In some experiments, they chemically blocked the normal sodium-glucose cotransporter (the mechanism that most rehydration drinks rely on) to see if Gum arabic could still promote absorption. They also measured how water, sodium, glucose, and marker molecules moved across the intestinal wall [4].

The results showed that Gum arabic enhanced absorption of water, sodium, and glucose even when sodium transport was blocked. This means it can stimulate alternative absorption routes that don't depend on the usual sodium-glucose transport system. The study also found increased uptake of a large inert molecule (PEG 4000), suggesting that Gum arabic slightly increased the permeability of the intestinal lining, possibly allowing more passive or paracellular transport [4].

In plain terms, Gum arabic helped the intestine draw in more water and nutrients through backup pathways; something standard oral rehydration theory hadn't recognized. The researchers concluded that Gum arabic acts as a "pro-absorptive adjuvant", meaning it can help the gut recover fluid and electrolytes even when normal transport systems are impaired, such as during diarrhea or intestinal injury.

Zinc escort services: In 2004, a follow-up study by researchers Mahmoud Ibrahim, Nina Kohn, and Raul Wapnir from Schneider Children's Hospital at North Shore investigated whether Gum arabic could improve the absorption of zinc; a nutrient essential for intestinal repair and immunity, and a key supplement in diarrhea treatment. Earlier work from the same research group had shown that GA enhances water and electrolyte uptake in the gut. This study asked if that benefit might extend to micronutrients such as zinc [5].

The team gave lightly anesthetized rats oral doses of isotonic solutions containing glucose, sodium, and glutamate, either with GA (25 g/L) or without GA. They also tested hypertonic solutions with varying GA levels. Blood samples were collected for three hours and analyzed for zinc, sodium, glucose, glutamate, and tritiated water.

In the isotonic solutions, rats that received Gum arabic showed significantly higher blood zinc concentrations within 15 minutes (about 20 percent greater than controls) and maintained that difference throughout the 180-minute test. The total zinc absorbed, expressed as the area under the curve, was roughly 30 percent higher with Gum arabic. Levels of the other measured solutes did not change, showing that GA's effect was specific to zinc uptake under these conditions. In hypertonic mixtures, however, zinc absorption declined overall, likely because high osmotic pressure counteracted absorption.

Closing the back door: reducing secretory flux: Cholera causes life-threatening diarrhea by switching on a chloride-secretion pump (CFTR) in the small intestine through very high cAMP levels. In a rat model using cholera toxin, Turvill, Wapnir and colleagues from The Royal London School of Medicine & Dentistry asked whether adding Gum arabic to the perfused solution could counter that secretion. After the jejunum was exposed to cholera toxin for two hours, the researchers perfused the segments in vivo with electrolyte solutions containing 0, 2.5, or 5.0 g/L GA and tracked water and sodium (^{24}Na) movement [6].

Gum arabic reduced cholera-toxin-induced secretion and promoted net movement of water and sodium from the lumen back into the blood. They also noted wider intercellular spaces in villi (but not crypts), consistent with altered junctional pathways that favor absorption. In short, even with cholera toxin driving secretion, GA shifted the balance back toward absorption. The study supports GA as a practical additive to make oral rehydration solutions work better under strong secretory conditions.

Gum arabic could be framed as a double-action ORS enhancer as it unlocks extra absorptive doors (increasing flux through non-sodium-dependent pathways and facilitating zinc uptake) while simultaneously reducing the secretory burden. This is precisely the kind of synergy that transforms incremental improvements into meaningful benefits. A 20% increase in absorption might shorten treatment by hours and a 30% reduction in secretion might prevent progression to hypovolemic shock. Combining both effects could be life-saving in settings where IV access is limited and every hour of inadequate oral intake brings mortality risk closer.

Real-world validation in Sudan: The laboratory findings would mean little if they didn't translate to actual pediatric care. In a randomized hospital trial at Omdurman Paediatric Emergency Hospital (Sudan) during March–August 2011, SSA Salih and colleagues conducted a real-world scenario study. 180 children aged 6–60 months with acute non-bloody diarrhea received either standard WHO oral rehydration solution (ORS) alone or the same ORS with added Gum arabic (Sweetfibre; a mix of Acacia Seyal and Acacia Senegal). The study tracked practical, bedside outcomes: 1-whether diarrhea stopped within 24 hours, 2-whether electrolyte imbalance developed, 3-whether cases progressed to severe dehydration or shock, 4-how many were discharged within one day, 5-weight change by discharge, and 6-recurrence at 6-week follow-up [7].

Children who received Gum-arabic–supplemented ORS did better on several counts. 90% had diarrhea stop within 24 hours (vs 38.9% in controls), only 3% developed electrolyte imbalance (vs 23.3%), no cases progressed to severe dehydration or shock (vs three in controls), and 80% were discharged after one day (vs 30%). The trial summary did not report notable adverse effects. These results are consistent with the laboratory evidence that Gum arabic can promote intestinal absorption and improve ORS performance during diarrheal illness [7].

Why does the Sudanese pediatric study matter for global health? Diarrheal diseases kill hundreds of thousands of children annually, predominantly in resource-limited settings where IV access is limited, medical supervision is intermittent, and the margin between successful oral rehydration and death from hypovolemia is narrow. Anything that makes ORS more effective (faster rehydration, better electrolyte stability, reduced secretory losses) without requiring new equipment, training, or cold chain will save lives at scale. Gum arabic ticks every box. It's locally produced in Sudan and other African countries (eliminating import costs and supply-chain vulnerability), it's food-grade safe (no regulatory barriers to inclusion in ORS), it dissolves instantly in water (no preparation complexity), and it's shelf-stable (no refrigeration needed). The cost per life saved could be measured in cents.

The complete ORS synergy story: Taken together, the four ORS studies (non-sodium-dependent absorption enhancement, zinc bioavailability improvement, secretion reduction in cholera toxin model, and clinical validation in pediatric diarrhea) establish Acacia gum as a genuine ORS enhancer operating through multiple complementary mechanisms. This isn't a single trick or a marginal improvement; it's a systems-level upgrade to oral rehydration therapy that addresses fundamental limitations of current formulations while maintaining complete compatibility with established protocols. For public health programs in regions where diarrheal disease remains a major mortality driver, incorporating Acacia gum into ORS represents one of the most cost-effective interventions imaginable.

VI. Act V - SUPERIOR BIOLOGICAL STRESS RELIEF

Egypt, 2023. Some studies resist categorization because they operate across multiple organ systems simultaneously, demonstrating that synergy is a systems property rather than an organ-specific phenomenon. This study from Benha University is perfect to drive the point of this chapter. It demonstrates the inherent beneficial properties of Hashab gum beyond the synergistic discussion.

This 2023 study by Tharwat A. Imbabi and colleagues followed 40 male rabbits through a hot summer period to see whether three low-cost supplements 1-Acacia gum (Hashab Gum from Acacia Senegal - 100 mg/kg), 2-vitamin C (30 mg/kg), or 3-lycopene (50 mg/kg)) could blunt the wide-ranging damage caused by heat stress. Animals were split into four groups (control, Hashab, vitamin C, lycopene) and dosed orally every day for 90 days [8].

The team measured semen quality (motility, live/dead cells, normal/abnormal forms), brain neurotransmitters (serotonin, dopamine, glutamate, aspartate), and semen-plasma antioxidant/energy markers (GSH, SOD, CAT, TAC, MDA, NO, L-carnitine, Na^+/K^+-ATPase, ATP, total calcium). They also performed chemical analyses of Hashab gum phospholipids by HPLC and antioxidant enzymes. All three supplements helped under heat stress, but Hashab gum frequently gave the strongest responses.

Versus controls, all treatments improved semen traits (more motile/live sperm, fewer abnormalities) and strengthened antioxidant status (higher GSH/SOD/CAT/TAC; lower MDA and NO). For the neurotransmitters, serotonin and dopamine rose, while glutamate and aspartate fell which is consistent with easing stress effects. In many readouts the Hashab group was best (often $p<0.001$), though some differences (e.g., GSH, CAT) were not significantly higher than vitamin C.

The authors also detected phosphatidylcholine and phosphatidylserine in Hashab gum by HPLC and argued these membrane lipids could contribute to antioxidant protection. Overall, the data indicates that Hashab gum is a practical additive that can bolster reproduction-related measures, brain chemistry markers, and antioxidant defenses during heat stress; often more than vitamin C or lycopene at the tested doses.

The heat-stress rabbit study crystallizes an important point we are trying to make. Food formulators often view Hashab gum from the perspective of making formulations better and that is true. However, this book is about demonstrating that Hashab gum can stand alone and outcompete others beyond synergistic prowess. Its highest and best value is what it does alone while its ability to make others better is only secondary.

That said, it's time we started talking about some of the limitations we discovered on our research journey. This is important because as we address all the amazing features of Hashab gum, we need to also establish the edges of the benefits so that our readers don't leave thinking Hashab gum is a miracle. Even the best of things have limitations.

References:

1. Min, Yang Won, et al. "Effect of Composite Yogurt Enriched with Acacia Fiber and Bifidobacterium lactis." World Journal of Gastroenterology, vol. 18, no. 33, 7 Sept. 2012, pp. 4563-69
2. Couëdelo, Leslie, et al. "Effect of Gum Acacia on the Intestinal Bioavailability of n-3 Polyunsaturated Fatty Acids in Rats." Nutrients, vol. 14, no. 13, 2022, p. 2694
3. Abd El-Aziz, Ashraf, Rasha Ismail, and Sherihan Mousa. "Effect of Turmeric and Gum Arabic Supplementation on the Kidney Alteration Caused by Glycerol Toxicity in Rats." Egyptian Journal of Nutrition, vol. 38, no. 2, 2023, pp. 96-126
4. Wingertzahn, Michael A., et al. "Stimulation of Non-Sodium-Dependent Water, Electrolyte, and Glucose Transport in Rat Small Intestine by Gum Arabic." Journal of Nutritional Biochemistry, vol. 12, no. 5, 2001, pp. 266-69
5. Ibrahim, Mahmoud A., Nina Kohn, and Raul A. Wapnir. "Proabsorptive Effect of Gum Arabic in Isotonic Solutions Orally Administered to Rats: Effect on Zinc and Other Solutes." Journal of Nutritional Biochemistry, vol. 15, no. 3, Mar. 2004, pp. 185-89
6. Turvill, J. L., Wapnir, R. A., Wingertzahn, M. A., Teichberg, S., and Farthing, M. J. G. "Cholera Toxin-Induced Secretion in Rats Is Reduced by a Soluble Fiber, Gum Arabic." Digestive Diseases and Sciences 45 (2000): 946–951
7. Salah, S. S. A., et al. "Gum Arabic - A Superb Anti-Diarrhoeal Agent." Sudan Journal of Medical Sciences, vol. 7, no. 3, 2012, pp. 155-66
8. Imbabi, Tharwat A., et al. "Enhancing semen quality, brain neurotransmitters, and antioxidant status of rabbits under heat stress by acacia gum, vitamin C, and lycopene as dietary supplements: an in vitro and in silico study." Italian Journal of Animal Science 22, no. 1 (2023): 321–336.

CHAPTER 21

THE CONTRARIAN STUDIES

1% of Published Studies Show the limits of Hashab Gum

The Value of Honest Boundaries

The previous chapter demonstrated that Hashab gum acted like a quiet systems engineer by stabilizing probiotics, ferrying omega-3 fatty acids and polyphenols across treacherous terrain and even upgrading oral rehydration solutions by unlocking absorption pathways that standard formulations never access. Its intrinsic prebiotic, anti-inflammatory, antioxidant, and antimicrobial properties were demonstrated across 19 chapters.

Now we turn to face some (less than 1% of the reviewed 540 studies) of the published studies where Hashab gum didn't sing the same song. Not to undercut the case we've built across nearly 350 pages, but to understand the limits. Good science doesn't move forward by ignoring inconvenient data or dismissing results that don't fit the narrative. Science advances by finding the edges of a big idea while understanding exactly where a principle applies and where it doesn't.

Before we open each story, recall the core signatures of Hashab gum that emerged so far:

- Selectively slow fermentation across days with excellent tolerability even at high doses (15-30 grams daily)
- Creating short-chain fatty acid production without the explosive

gas generation that plagues inulin and fructo-oligosaccharides

- Antioxidant and anti-inflammatory control through NF-κB suppression and Nrf2 activation, operating at the transcriptional level to shift cellular programs
- Membrane protection through arabinogalactan-protein film formation that reduces permeability and shields sensitive structures
- Microbiome signaling that favors beneficial organisms while creating generally hostile conditions for pathogens
- Low viscosity in the gut lumen at effective intake levels, which is both advantage and limitation depending on what outcome you're chasing.

Those same signatures explain both Hashab gum's extraordinary wins and its occasional misses when investigators ask it to perform jobs that require opposite properties. A violinist is a poor choice for a weightlifting competition, not because violinists lack skill but because the contest demands different capabilities. Similarly, Hashab gum underperforms in specific applications not because its mechanisms fail but because those mechanisms are mismatched to endpoints that require rapid proximal action, high viscosity, or mineral donation rather than polymer film formation. Understanding these mismatches doesn't weaken the clinical case for Hashab gum but instead refines the prescription. It tells us when to deploy it as sole intervention, when to pair it strategically with complementary agents, and when to select a different tool entirely.

I. Fecal Incontinence Responds to Viscosity, Not Finesse

Minnesota, **United States, 2014.** We begin with a rigorously conducted randomized clinical trial that tested whether dietary fiber supplementation could improve fecal incontinence in adults; a deeply distressing condition affecting quality of life, social participation, and psychological well-being.

344

Fecal incontinence, the involuntary loss of liquid or solid stool, results from various etiologies including sphincter damage from childbirth or surgery, neurological conditions affecting bowel control, severe diarrhea overwhelming continence mechanisms, or chronic constipation with overflow incontinence. Current management includes behavioral interventions (scheduled toileting, pelvic floor exercises), medications to alter stool consistency, and in severe cases, surgical repair of damaged anatomy. The hypothesis that fiber supplementation might improve incontinence by normalizing stool consistency is mechanistically plausible. If watery stools are the problem, bulking and gelling those stools should help continence mechanisms work more effectively [1].

Donna Z. Bliss (featured in Kidney chapter study from 1996 proving Hashab's Kidney effects) and colleagues at the University of Minnesota School of Nursing conducted this test in a well-designed trial comparing different fiber types head-to-head in adults with fecal incontinence. The trial randomized participants to receive psyllium (a classic gel-forming fiber from Plantago seed husks), Gum Arabic (unlike 1996 Hashab study she did not specify which type of Gum arabic), carboxymethylcellulose (CMC), or placebo. They carefully monitored incontinence episodes, stool consistency, and quality-of-life outcomes over the intervention period. This wasn't a preliminary exploration; it was a single-blind, randomized, placebo-controlled clinical trial with head-to-head fiber arms using validated instruments to measure outcomes that matter to patients including fewer incontinence episodes, better stool form, and improved bowel control [1].

Before we examine the results, we need to understand the physics of fecal continence and why fiber type matters. Fecal continence depends on a sophisticated system: internal and external anal sphincters provide muscular closure, rectal compliance allows temporary stool storage, sensory nerves signal the need to defecate, and critically, *stool consistency*

345

determines whether the sphincter system can maintain closure under challenge. Think of continence as a dam holding back water versus holding back mud versus holding back pebbles. The material properties of what's being held determine how much engineering the dam requires. Liquid stool challenges continence mechanisms maximally because fluids flow through any small opening, exert hydrostatic pressure that overcomes weak sphincters, and cannot be compressed or shaped by voluntary muscle contraction. Formed stool is far easier to control as it doesn't flow under gravity, it can be held by moderate sphincter pressure, and voluntary contraction can delay passage until appropriate time and place.

This is where fiber physics becomes critical. Dietary fibers differ enormously in their effects on stool consistency, and those differences predict success in fecal incontinence better than almost any other fiber property. The key physical parameters are *water-holding capacity* (how much water a given mass of fiber can bind), *gel strength* (essentially how thick and cohesive the resulting stool is), and *yield stress* (the force required to make the material flow, which directly translates to whether stool will leak through a moderately competent sphincter or remain contained).

Psyllium is the champion of stool bulking and gelling. Its seed husks contain mucilage which is a mixture of hemicelluloses that swell enormously when hydrated, forming highly viscous gels with substantial yield stress. When psyllium transits through the colon, it absorbs water that would otherwise remain as free liquid in stool, binding that water into a gel matrix. The resulting stool is larger in volume (which helps by stimulating more normal defecation reflexes rather than allowing small, unpredictable leakage), substantially more formed and cohesive, and has physical properties that continence mechanisms can manage. The gel doesn't flow through small openings, it responds to voluntary contraction by compressing rather than leaking, and it provides sensory feedback that allows individuals to sense and respond to impending bowel movements rather than experiencing unpredictable accidents. Psyllium's stool-thickening effects are so reliable that it's used clinically in both diarrhea (to bulk and gel watery stool) and constipation (to soften hard stool and provide bulk that stimulates peristalsis). It's the rare fiber that normalizes in both directions.

Gum arabic occupies the opposite end of the viscosity spectrum. Its molecular structure (branched arabinogalactan chains with protein cores) creates excellent water solubility but minimal gel formation at concentrations that humans normally consume. Even at high doses, Gum arabic is still lower in viscosity compared to Psyllium husk. That low viscosity is precisely why Gum arabic has such excellent tolerability. It doesn't create the sense of fullness, bloating, or cramping that high-viscosity fibers cause. It doesn't slow gastric emptying or nutrient absorption in ways that would be problematic. It ferments slowly enough and selectively enough that gas production remains manageable rather than becoming socially embarrassing or physically painful. For individuals with irritable bowel syndrome, inflammatory bowel disease, or other conditions where gut hypersensitivity makes high-viscosity fibers intolerable, Gum arabic's low viscosity is its greatest asset, enabling delivery of prebiotic and metabolic benefits without triggering symptoms.

However, in fecal incontinence, that same low viscosity becomes a liability. If the problem is liquid stool leaking through compromised continence mechanisms, providing a fiber that remains low-viscosity and doesn't substantially change stool mechanical properties is asking the wrong tool to do a job outside its capabilities. It would be like asking a thin paint to fill cracks that require thick spackle; the paint is excellent for its intended purpose (smooth coverage over intact surfaces), but it can't solve a problem that demands filling and thickening properties the paint doesn't possess.

347

The trial results confirmed exactly what stool physics predicts: At 16 grams each for each fiber daily; Psyllium supplementation significantly improved fecal incontinence outcomes by reducing the number of incontinence episodes from 5.5 per week (placebo) to 2.5 per week and forming gel in feces that improved stool consistency. The effect sizes were clinically meaningful, whereby patients experienced real improvements in their ability to control bowel movements. Gum arabic supplementation did not match those benefits. Incontinence episode frequency was 4.3 per week (compared to placebo at 5.5 per week), and no gel formation occurred. Surprisingly, CMC (Cellulose derived fiber) actually worsened incontinence to 6.2 episodes per week. Quality of life scores did not differ significantly among any groups.

Why Gum arabic underperformed in this specific application and what that teaches:
Mechanism-to-endpoint mismatch: Fecal incontinence is fundamentally a stool-consistency problem requiring gel-formation solutions. Gum arabic's mechanisms (microbiome modulation, antioxidant, barrier enhancement, anti-inflammatory terrain repair) operate at the cellular and metabolic level, creating benefits that manifest over weeks in systemic endpoints like glucose control, inflammatory markers, kidney function, and cognitive performance. Those mechanisms simply don't change stool rheology in ways that help continence. Expecting Gum arabic to perform like psyllium in fecal incontinence is mechanistically equivalent to expecting an anti-inflammatory drug to work as an antibiotic; wrong tool, different mechanism required.

In theory, if you pushed Gum arabic doses high enough, you might begin achieving some stool-thickening effects through sheer mass. Additionally, adherence would collapse as nobody maintains fifty-gram-per-day fiber intake unless needed in sever situations. Psyllium achieves therapeutic stool changes at sixteen grams per day (the dose used in this study) precisely because its gel-forming capacity is so high per gram consumed. The dose required for Gum arabic to match that effect would exceed what any normal person would take under normal conditions.

II. The Iron Window: A Sprint GOS/FOS Can Win That Gum Arabic Shouldn't Try

Zurich, Switzerland, 2022. We move from stool mechanics to absorption kinetics with a carefully designed study from ETH Zurich investigating whether prebiotic supplementation could enhance iron absorption in iron-depleted women. Iron deficiency and iron deficiency anemia affect billions of people globally, particularly women of reproductive age who face monthly iron losses through menstruation. Current iron supplementation strategies have frustrating limitations. High-dose iron causes significant gastrointestinal side effects (nausea, constipation, metallic taste) that destroy adherence. Absorption efficiency is often poor (typically ten to twenty percent of an oral dose), and there's increasing concern that poorly absorbed iron remaining in the colon may promote growth of pathogenic bacteria while generating oxidative stress. If prebiotics could increase the proportion of supplemental iron that's absorbed, it would allow lower doses with better tolerability, fewer colonic side effects, and improved outcomes.

Ambra Giorgetti and colleagues ran a randomized, single-blind, crossover study in 30 iron-depleted young women to test whether adding common prebiotic fibers to an iron pill changes how much iron the body absorbs. They used the gold-standard stable-isotope method whereby each woman swallowed 100 mg of iron as ferrous fumarate labeled with a harmless iron isotope, taken with either 15 g GOS, 15 g FOS, 15 g Acacia gum (Fibregum™ - Species not specified), or a sugar control on different study days. Fourteen days later, the team measured how much of the labeled iron had been built into new red blood cells. This gives a precise fractional iron absorption (FIA) for each condition [2].

Before examining why the results differ between prebiotics, we need to understand the temporal and spatial constraints on iron absorption. Iron absorption from the gut occurs almost exclusively in the duodenum and proximal jejunum which is roughly the first thirty to fifty centimeters of small intestine beyond the stomach. This geographic restriction reflects the localization of the key iron transporters. Divalent metal transporter 1 (DMT1) on the apical (lumen-facing) membrane of enterocytes, which brings iron into the cell, and ferroportin on the basolateral (blood-facing) membrane, which exports iron into circulation. These transporters are most highly expressed in the duodenum and decline sharply in the more distal intestine. Additionally, iron absorption is pH-sensitive and form-dependent whereby ferrous iron (Fe^{2+}) is more absorbable than ferric iron (Fe^{3+}), and acidic pH helps maintain iron in the ferrous form and in solution rather than precipitating as insoluble hydroxides. Once intestinal pH rises above about 6 (which occurs rapidly past the duodenum as bicarbonate secretions neutralize gastric acid), iron increasingly precipitates and becomes unavailable for absorption.

The stable-isotope methodology used in this study captures a very specific absorption window. The iron from a single test meal transiting through the duodenum over approximately one to three hours after consumption. If a prebiotic intervention is going to enhance absorption measured by this method, it must create favorable conditions within that narrow temporal and spatial window. This is where fermentation kinetics become decisive.

GOS and FOS are rapidly fermentable oligosaccharides. When they reach the proximal colon (or even terminal ileum in some individuals), colonic bacteria ferment them quickly. That fermentation generates short-chain fatty acids within hours, creating a localized pH drop and increased SCFA concentrations that can extend proximally through retrograde mixing and through systemic effects if enough SCFA is absorbed.

In studies where GOS/FOS and iron are co-administered, there's a plausible mechanistic window where the rapid fermentation in the proximal colon creates conditions that improve iron availability during the critical duodenal absorption phase as the pH drop helps maintain iron in ferrous form, the SCFAs themselves may enhance enterocyte function or transporter expression, and there may be improved mucus properties or reduced inflammation that facilitates absorption. The timeline is tight as fermentation must begin within hours of consumption and create effects that extend proximally enough to influence the duodenum. It's mechanistically feasible with fast-fermenting substrates.

Acacia Gum, in contrast, is a slow-fermenting fiber with activity peaking in the distal colon over 6+ hours to days rather than a few hours. The selectivity of its fermentation (favoring specific bacterial populations that can break down the complex arabinogalactan structure) combined with its resistance to rapid degradation means that acute, single-meal administration won't create the proximal pH drop or SCFA spike needed to influence iron absorption measured in a stable-isotope study. Gum arabic's effects on gut barrier integrity, inflammatory tone, mucus production, and microbiome composition develop gradually and manifest most strongly in the distal colon where fermentation is most active.

Those effects absolutely can improve overall iron status over weeks or months of supplementation; by reducing intestinal inflammation that impairs absorption, by improving mucosal integrity, by modulating hepcidin (the iron-regulatory hormone) through anti-inflammatory effects, and by creating favorable microbiome conditions that reduce pathogen overgrowth and oxidative stress. However, those chronic benefits won't appear in a stable-isotope measure capturing single-meal absorption in the

351

duodenum.

The trial results: When iron was taken with GOS or FOS, iron absorption increased by about 45% and 51%, respectively, compared with iron alone (P < 0.001 for both). When iron was taken with Acacia gum (15 g), absorption did not change versus control (P = 0.688) [2].

Translating the result through fermentation kinetics and spatial mismatching. The difference between GOS/FOS and Gum arabic in this application isn't about one being "better" but about matching fermentation profile to measurement window. GOS/FOS can plausibly create proximal effects quickly enough to influence duodenal absorption within hours of consumption. Gum arabic creates distal effects gradually over longer time periods which is perfect for sustained metabolic and barrier benefits but mismatched to acute proximal absorption endpoints. This is like comparing sprinters and marathon runners in a hundred-meter dash. The sprinter wins the sprint, but that tells you nothing about who would win a marathon or who has better overall cardiovascular health [2].

The iron-absorption study teaches us an important lesson. Temporal and spatial mismatches between when and where an intervention acts versus when and where outcomes are measured can create apparent ineffectiveness that dissolves when the time-scale and geography are appropriate. Gum arabic's benefits are real but they unfold gradually over days to weeks and operate most powerfully in the distal colon therefore asking it to bend an acute duodenal absorption curve is asking it to violate its kinetic profile.

III. Conflicting Iron Study: Proving Gum arabic helps with Iron Absorption

352

China, 2024. This study investigated how a specific part of Gum arabic helps the body absorb non-heme iron (the kind found in plants and most supplements). Gum arabic isn't just fiber; about 3% of it is a collagen-like protein rich in the amino acid hydroxyproline. When this protein is digested, it releases tiny peptide fragments such as Hyp-Hyp, Pro-Hyp, and Ser-Hyp.

The researchers from Ocean University of China used human intestinal cell models (Caco-2 monolayers) and rats. They found that the protein fraction, not the polysaccharide (fiber) fraction, increased iron reduction, uptake, and transport across the intestinal barrier. Mechanistically, these Gum-arabic-derived peptides inhibit an enzyme called prolyl hydroxylase (PHD). When PHD is blocked, a sensor protein called HIF-2α becomes more stable. Stabilized HIF-2α then switches on genes that code for the main iron-handling proteins in the duodenum: duodenal cytochrome b (Dcytb), divalent metal transporter 1 (DMT1), ferroportin, and hephaestin [3].

In simple terms, Gum arabic–derived peptides tell intestinal cells to "upgrade" their iron-absorption machinery, so more non-heme iron can move from the gut into the blood. This positions Gum arabic not just as a gentle prebiotic fiber, but also as a potential adjunct strategy to improve iron absorption and support anemia management.

So how did 2 studies exploring Gum arabic's influence on Iron absorption come up with opposite findings? Firstly, the second study abstract did not state when results were recorded unlike the first study which recorded results after 3 hours. Secondly, neither study specified the type of Gum arabic and we don't know whether they used Hashab gum (Acacia Senegal) or Talha gum (Acacia Seyal) and the difference is critical based on the findings of this second iron absorption study. Since the 2nd

353

study attributes the iron absorption to the protein content; Hashab gum has multiples times more protein content compared to Talha and therefore knowing the Acacia gum type is critical.

If Gum arabic's iron effect comes from hydroxyproline-rich peptides, then Hashab gums's (Acacia Senegal) higher protein/AGP fraction is not a minor detail; it's the dose. Per gram of powder, Hashab gum should release more Hyp-Hyp, Pro-Hyp, and Ser-Hyp, giving stronger inhibition of PHD, more HIF-2α stabilization, and bigger upregulation of Dcytb, DMT1, ferroportin, and hephaestin. Talha gum may match Hashab gum on fiber and SCFA, but it likely underperforms on this peptide signal. For an iron-focused formula, that extra protein in Hashab gum could translate into a clinically meaningful difference. In borderline deficiency or low-dose fortification, that leverage could be decisive.

This is another example of the catastrophic naming conventions (simply calling it Gum arabic or Acacia gum) associated with this ingredient. A clearer and finalized naming convention must be enacted to end these discrepancies and second guessing.

IV. Infants on Iron: The Opening Sprint Versus the Long Game

Switzerland and France, 2024. The third edge case brings us to the delicate and rapidly shifting ecology of infant intestinal microbiota under iron supplementation stress. Iron supplementation in infants, while sometimes medically necessary to prevent or treat anemia, creates a microbiological dilemma that pediatricians and microbiome researchers have been documenting with increasing concern. Supplemental iron, particularly in the high doses often prescribed, can suppress beneficial bifidobacteria (the dominant organisms in healthy breastfed infant guts, producing lactate and acetate that acidify the intestine and inhibit pathogens) while favoring enterobacteria and other potentially pathogenic taxa that thrive when iron becomes available. The problem is that many pathogens are iron-limited in the gut (the host intentionally sequesters iron through various mechanisms to starve pathogens) so flooding the intestinal lumen with poorly absorbed supplemental iron can inadvertently feed exactly the organisms you don't want to promote.

Paula Momo Cabrera and colleagues, in a collaboration between ETH Zurich and French research institutions (Danone), used an elegant in-vitro continuous fermentation system (the African infant PolyFermS gut model) inoculated with fecal samples from Kenyan infants. They modeled this iron-supplementation stress to test whether different prebiotics could maintain bifidobacterial populations and overall microbiome stability under iron challenge. The model simulated infant colonic conditions (pH 5.8, temperature, retention time of 8 hours, nutrient availability mimicking Kenyan infant diet) and introduced iron at concentrations mimicking supplementation (12.5 mg/day), then compared how short-chain GOS with long-chain FOS (9:1 ratio), native inulin, and Acacia gum influenced microbiome composition over the timeframe of the simulation. This wasn't a human trial measuring clinical outcomes but a sophisticated mechanistic study examining ecological competition under controlled conditions [4].

Before examining why the prebiotics performed differently, we need to understand the unique challenges of infant microbiome ecology under metabolic stress. The infant intestinal microbiome during the first year of life is not a miniature version of the adult microbiome. It's a distinct ecosystem with different dominant organisms, different metabolic priorities, and critically, different ecological rules. Healthy breastfed infant microbiomes are typically dominated by bifidobacteria, which have specialized genetic capabilities for metabolizing human milk oligosaccharides (complex sugars in breast milk that the infant cannot

355

digest but that selectively feed beneficial bacteria). These bifidobacteria create an acidic, lactate-rich environment that's hostile to many pathogens, stimulate immune system development in ways that establish appropriate inflammatory tone for life, and provide metabolic products that support intestinal barrier maturation.

When iron supplementation is introduced, this carefully balanced system faces acute disruption. Iron availability in the gut lumen shifts within hours to days as doses accumulate. Enterobacteriaceae (a family that includes *E. coli*, *Klebsiella*, *Enterobacter*, and various pathogens) are particularly adept at scavenging iron through siderophores (iron-binding molecules they secrete) and high-affinity iron transporters. Given access to iron, these organisms can outcompete slower-growing bifidobacteria for other resources like colonization sites on the mucosa, utilization of available carbohydrates, and dominance of the intestinal niche. Once enterobacteria gain a foothold, they can be difficult to displace because they generate a more inflammatory environment (through lipopolysaccharide and other pathogen-associated molecular patterns) that further impairs bifidobacterial growth while creating conditions that favor their own persistence.

To rescue the microbiome under this acute challenge, you need interventions that act quickly (within the first days of iron exposure) to give bifidobacteria a competitive advantage that allows them to maintain dominance despite iron making the environment more favorable to pathogens. This is the ecological equivalent of a land rush. If beneficial organisms can claim territory and resources quickly, they can often hold that territory even when conditions shift in favor of competitors. However, if the competitors get established first, dislodging them requires sustained effort and may never fully restore the original balance.

This ecological timing explains why "fast" prebiotics have advantages in acutely stressed systems. GOS and FOS are oligosaccharides with low

356

degrees of polymerization; they're short chains of sugars (typically three to ten units) that bifidobacteria can metabolize rapidly using enzymes that many other bacteria lack. When GOS/FOS reach an infant colon that's under iron stress, bifidobacteria that have the right enzymatic machinery can immediately begin fermenting these substrates, generating lactate and acetate quickly, reproducing faster because energy is available, and outcompeting enterobacteria for space and resources. The rapidity of this response (measured within hours) is crucial when the threat (iron-driven pathogen expansion) is also rapid. Inulin, while slightly slower than GOS/FOS, still provides relatively fast fermentation by specialized bifidobacterial strains.

Acacia gum, in contrast, is a complex, high-molecular-weight polysaccharide requiring sophisticated enzymatic systems to degrade. This is excellent for creating sustained, gradual fermentation that doesn't cause gas explosions and that maintains stable microbiome composition, but it's slow off the starting line. In an infant microbiome facing acute iron-driven disruption, Acacia gum is like bringing a comprehensive urban-planning document to a land rush; valuable for long-term development, less useful for winning the immediate scramble for territory.

The study results in the Kenyan infant microbiota model: Under iron supplementation conditions, scGOS/lcFOS and inulin were more effective than Acacia gum at maintaining bifidobacterial populations and limiting pathogen expansion. The fast-fermenting oligosaccharides allowed bifidobacteria to maintain dominance despite iron stress, with increased production of acetate (up to 40 mM increases), propionate, and butyrate, while Acacia gum showed no effect on any of the four microbiota tested. Acacia supplementation (5 g/day dose mimicked) did not significantly alter bifidobacterial concentrations, SCFA production, or overall microbiota composition. Iron supplementation alone did not induce major microbiota shifts except promoting Clostridioides difficile in one donor microbiota,

357

which was prevented when prebiotics were co-supplemented [4].

The authors explained these results by stating that Acacia gum is a more complex molecule and needs a specific set of bacterial enzymes to be broken down. Those enzymes are made by particular "acacia-eating" bacteria (some *Bacteroides* and *Bifidobacterium* strains). In these partially breastfed Kenyan infants, those specialist bacteria (and the genes for the full enzyme set) were rare or missing. As a result, Acacia gum mostly passed through without being fermented. In adults, where those specialist microbes are more common, Acacia gum can work as a prebiotic. However, in this specific infant population at weaning age, their microbiomes just weren't equipped to use it, so it looked weak compared with the other fibers [4].

V. Teeth Need Minerals; A Polymer Cannot Pretend to Be Fluoride

Cairo, Egypt, 2023. The fifth edge case takes us to dental health, specifically to the clinical challenge of remineralizing early enamel lesions. These are the white-spot lesions or incipient caries that represent the earliest detectable stage of tooth decay, where minerals have been lost from enamel but the surface hasn't yet cavitated into an actual hole. These early lesions are theoretically reversible if you can deliver calcium, phosphate, and fluoride to the demineralized enamel under conditions that favor crystal growth rather than further dissolution. This way you can rebuild the hydroxyapatite crystalline structure and arrest or reverse the decay process.

Current remineralization strategies include fluoride varnishes (which deliver high concentrations of fluoride that incorporates into enamel as fluorapatite, a more acid-resistant form of the mineral), casein phosphopeptide-amorphous calcium phosphate (CPP-ACP, a milk-derived protein that stabilizes calcium and phosphate in a bioavailable form for delivery to enamel), and combinations of these approaches.

Ahmed H. Samaha, Rawda H. Abd ElAziz, and Rasha R. Hassan at Cairo University conducted a randomized controlled trial comparing Gum arabic (Hashab gum from Acacia Senegal) varnish to fluoride varnish and CPP-ACP-fluoride varnish for remineralizing initial carious lesions over six months. The researchers tracked outcomes at baseline, 1, 3, and 6 months using two accepted measures: 1-DIAGNOdent (a laser-fluorescence reading that reflects mineral loss/gain) and the 2-Nyvad criteria (a clinical scoring system that classifies whether a lesion is active or arrested) [5].

The trial results where exactly what chemistry predicts: Fluoride and CPP-ACPF groups both showed significant mineral gain by DIAGNOdent at 3 and 6 months, and by Nyvad they arrested essentially all active lesions by 3–6 months. The Gum arabic group did not show significant DIAGNOdent improvement over time (so, no effective remineralization at 6 months). However, by Nyvad, GA arrested about 85% of active lesions possibly by forming a protective surface coating, but without restoring minerals like the fluoride-containing products did within the study period [5].

This study runs counter to the studies (see oral health chapter 16) documenting Gum arabic's genuine benefits showing remineralization and antibacterial potential. The mechanistic explanations have yet to be finalized, and more research is needed in this regard.

VI. The Pill-Timing Footnote: A Pharmacokinetic Caution, Not an Indictment

Khartoum, Sudan, 2004. The Sixth and final edge case is brief, specific, and easily addressed. It's a pharmacokinetic study examining whether Gum arabic affects absorption of amoxicillin, a commonly prescribed antibiotic. I. B. Eltayeb, A. I. Awad, and colleagues from the University of Khartoum gave healthy Sudanese volunteers a single oral dose of amoxicillin (500 mg, typical therapeutic dose) under four different conditions: alone (control), concurrently with Gum arabic, 2 hours after Gum arabic, or 4 hours after Gum arabic. Blood samples were collected at multiple timepoints over six hours, and amoxicillin concentrations were measured. The study wasn't designed to assess clinical outcomes (whether infections were cured, whether side effects occurred). It was pure pharmacokinetics asking *does Gum arabic change how quickly and completely amoxicillin enters the bloodstream* [6]?

Before interpreting the results, we need to understand what pharmacokinetic parameters tell us. Pharmacokinetics describes what the body does to a drug including how it's absorbed from the gut, distributed to tissues, metabolized, and eliminated. For antibiotics like amoxicillin, pharmacokinetics matter clinically because achieving adequate concentrations at the infection site is essential for efficacy. If absorption is delayed or reduced, you might not achieve bactericidal concentrations when you need them, potentially allowing bacteria to develop resistance or infection to progress. For some drugs, timing is less critical (chronic medications where you're establishing steady-state levels over days), but for antibiotics, getting the drug in quickly and completely is usually desirable.

Many dietary fibers, not just Gum arabic, can modestly affect drug absorption through several mechanisms:
- Increased viscosity in the gut lumen can slow diffusion of drugs to the absorptive epithelium (imagine wading through syrup versus water, the drug molecules move slower)
- Physical binding or trapping of drugs in gel matrices can sequester

360

them away from absorptive surfaces

- Altered gastric emptying or intestinal transit time can change how long drugs spend in regions of maximal absorption
- In some cases, fibers can compete with drugs for transporters or alter the activity of drug-metabolizing enzymes.

These are well-known fiber-drug interactions, not unique to Gum arabic, and they're managed through simple timing strategies.

The study results: Amoxicillin absorption was significantly reduced when co-administered with Gum arabic or given 2 hours after Gum arabic; Cmax decreased from 7.31 mg/L (control) to 2.00 mg/L (concurrent) and 3.19 mg/L (2h post-gum arabic), and AUC decreased proportionally. However, when amoxicillin was administered 4 hours after Gum arabic, absorption parameters were not significantly different from control, indicating complete resolution of the interaction [6].

Given the nature of fibers in general. We can deduce that this is not unexpected and it's not unique to Gum arabic as other fibers will likely also have similar effects with varying time windows. Every intervention (fiber, food, other medications, even time of day) affects drug absorption to some degree. The solution is rational scheduling, not abandoning either the medication or the fiber

---

VI. The Honest Shape of a Great Tool

These six papers (fecal incontinence, iron absorption, infant microbiota rescue, dental remineralization, antibiotic pharmacokinetics) don't debunk Hashab gum's therapeutic value across metabolic, renal, cardiovascular, neurological, reproductive, and synergistic applications documented in hundreds of other studies. Instead, they write Hashab gum's job description with precision. This is the systems fiber you deploy for the problems modern life actually presents in epidemic proportions. These include but are not limited to chronic inflammatory tone that's too high, oxidative stress creating cumulative damage, intestinal barriers that are too leaky, microbiota communities that are dysbiotic, and adherence that's too low because other interventions cause intolerable side effects. For stool-gel problems requiring viscosity, mineral repair requiring ion donation, or acute challenges requiring immediate proximal action, select tools optimized for those specific physics or chemistry. Pair Hashab gum intelligently with those specialized tools so the system as a whole wins rather than asking any single ingredient to be all things.

The one-percent check reveals that Hashab gum's limitations are predictable from first principles, and manageable through rational formulation and timing. These limitations can be resolvable through combination approaches where Hashab gum contributes its unique strengths (tolerability, systemic terrain repair, sustained action, delivery enhancement) while partners contribute capabilities Hashab gum lacks (rapid fermentation, mineral donation, high viscosity, acute proximal effects). Understanding these boundaries doesn't undermine confidence; it refines precision and allows us to capture the extraordinary benefits documented across nineteen chapters while avoiding predictable pitfalls.

The ninety-nine percent of research showing benefits across kidney disease, diabetes, metabolic syndrome, cardiovascular dysfunction, liver injury, reproductive challenges, neurological stress, and synergistic applications remains valid and compelling. The one percent shows real boundaries in fecal incontinence, iron absorption, infant dysbiosis rescue, dental remineralization, and drug timing. It teaches us where and how to use Hashab gum.

References:

1. Bliss, Donna Z., et al. "Dietary Fiber Supplementation for Fecal Incontinence: A Randomized Clinical Trial." Nursing Research, vol. 63, no. 6, Nov.-Dec. 2014, pp. 434-48

2. Giorgetti, Ambra, Frederike M. D. Husmann, Christophe Zeder, Isabelle Herter-Aeberli, and Michael B. Zimmermann. "Prebiotic Galacto-Oligosaccharides and Fructo-Oligosaccharides, but Not Acacia Gum, Increase Iron Absorption from a Single High-Dose Ferrous Fumarate Supplement in Iron-Depleted Women." The Journal of Nutrition 152 (2022): 1015–1021

3. Li, Shiyang, et al. "Gum Arabic-Derived Hydroxyproline-Rich Peptides Stimulate Intestinal Nonheme Iron Absorption via HIF2α-Dependent Upregulation of Iron Transport Proteins." *Journal of Agricultural and Food Chemistry*, vol. 72, no. 7, 2024, pp. 3622–3632

4. Cabrera, Paula Momo, et al. "Comparative Prebiotic Potential of Galacto- and Fructo-Oligosaccharides, Native Inulin, and Acacia Gum in Kenyan Infant Gut Microbiota during Iron Supplementation." ISME Communications, vol. 4, no. 1, 2024, article ycae033

5. Samaha, Ahmed Hesham, Rawda Hesham Abd ElAziz, and Rasha Raafat Hassan. "Remineralization Efficacy of Gum Arabic Varnish Vs Fluoride Varnish and CPP-ACPF Varnish in Initial Carious Lesions Over 6 Months Follow Up: A Randomized Controlled Clinical Trial." Advanced Dental Journal, vol. 5, no. 4, 2023, pp. 919-33

6. Eltayeb, I. B., et al. "Effect of Gum Arabic on the Absorption of a Single Oral Dose of Amoxicillin in Healthy Sudanese Volunteers." Journal of Antimicrobial Chemotherapy, vol. 54, no. 2, Aug. 2004, pp. 577-78

CHAPTER 22

The Research that Blew the Cover on the Fiber Trend

EARNING THE RIGHT TO COMPARE FIBERS

The last chapter was an honest engagement with Hashab gum's boundaries and areas requiring additional studies and accurate species identification. It also acknowledged where mechanism-to-endpoint mismatches limit effectiveness while showing how rational combinations capture benefits across complementary timescales and mechanisms. It gave us a clear, credible lens for examining the competing fibers that crowd supplement shelves and fill "health food" aisles with promises of digestive wellness, metabolic improvement, and microbiome optimization. Many of those popular fibers, have problems that aren't occasional edge cases requiring mechanistic explanation and strategic pairing. Their problems are built into their fundamental properties. This chapter will seek to explore the many troubling studies regarding these fibers. The aim is to add another layer to your understanding before finalizing the book.

We dissected Hashab gum layer by layer so we can get a comprehensive picture of the ingredient. Now it's time to do a Macro analysis of the entire genre because not all "fibers" are made equal. The notion of "just add fiber" needs to be challenged because the term is too broad and needs to account for the actual micro effects and long-term physiological consequences.

In making this argument, the destination isn't fear or rejection of all fibers except Hashab gum. The destination is a sophisticated choice and recognition that "fiber" is not a single entity but a diverse family of molecules with profoundly different effects on fermentation kinetics, immune tone, hepatic metabolism, intestinal mechanics, and adherence potential.

By chapter's end, you'll understand why professional gastroenterology societies now explicitly warn that soluble fibers are not interchangeable and why certain fermentable fibers worsen symptoms in irritable bowel syndrome despite being theoretically beneficial for microbiome health. You will understand why liver researchers watch bile-acid perturbations with concern when fast-fermenting fibers are used in metabolically vulnerable populations, and why the mechanistic elegance demonstrated in short-term trials so often fails to translate into sustained real-world use when tolerability destroys adherence before benefits can accrue. Let this chapter be an additional disclaimer for all so called "fibers".

I. When Fermentation Outruns Physiology: The Liver Lesion Nobody Expected

Multiple institutions, 2018. The fiber community faced an uncomfortable moment when Vishal Singh and colleagues published findings in *Cell* that seemed to indict a category of interventions generally considered safe and beneficial. In mouse models with an abnormal gut microbiome and innate-immune defects (such as TLR5-knockout mice), a purified, compositionally defined diet containing 7.5% inulin led (over months) to blocked bile flow (cholestasis), liver injury, and eventually liver cancer.

The same pattern (early bilirubin elevation and high circulating bile acids

365

progressing to tumors) did not occur with a cellulose-only control diet. Wild-type mice on a high-fat diet with added inulin also showed a lower-penetrance version of the problem.

The lesson wasn't that "fiber is bad". However, in certain microbiome contexts, rapid and sustained fermentation can alter the handling of bile acids in ways that stress the liver. Bile acids act as signals that help set liver metabolism. In these mice, the bile-acid pool and transport pathways shifted, total bile acids in blood spiked early, and the liver showed injury, inflammation, and scarring before tumors formed. It was the fermentation-dependent interaction between inulin and a susceptible microbiome that mattered; blocking fermentation or removing soluble fiber prevented disease.

The right ingredient, fermented at the wrong tempo in the wrong microbial community in the wrong genetic background, can crash a physiological performance. The study wasn't attacking fiber broadly or suggesting inulin should be banned, but it exposed a reality the field had been slow to acknowledge. That is fermentation speed, microbial ecology, and host genetics interact in ways that can transform benefit into harm, and fast-fermenting fibers carry risks in certain contexts that slow-fermenting alternatives don't.

When bile-acid pools shift composition or concentration rapidly due to microbial metabolism (bacteria can deconjugate, dehydroxylate, and otherwise modify bile acids), the liver must adapt its synthetic pathways, its export mechanisms, and its metabolic programming. In healthy, metabolically flexible hosts, this adaptation occurs smoothly. In genetically vulnerable hosts (the mice in this study carried specific susceptibility alleles) with pre-existing metabolic disease, or in contexts where other stressors are present, the adaptation can fail, leading to bile-acid accumulation, cholestasis, inflammatory activation in hepatic tissue, and eventually progression toward cancer.

Why this 2018 finding changed clinical practice and fiber recommendations? Before Singh's publication, "fiber is beneficial" was treated as a universal truth requiring no qualification. The study forced recognition that fiber is not a monolithic category and that molecular structure determines fermentation kinetics. Kinetics determine metabolic and microbial effects, and that those effects can be harmful rather than beneficial in certain host contexts. People who had been indiscriminately recommending "add fiber" began asking: which fiber, at what fermentation speed, in what dose?

II. The Liver Levers: When Temperature Control Didn't Save the Story

Germany, 2020. A fair scientific response to the 2018 alarm bells was skepticism about confounding variables. Maybe the liver effects weren't about inulin's fermentation kinetics at all. Perhaps they reflected peculiarities of rodent housing conditions that don't translate to humans. Mouse researchers know that housing temperature profoundly affects metabolism. Mice housed below their thermoneutral zone (around 30°C) experience cold stress at standard temperatures, causing them to burn more energy for thermogenesis, which can alter hepatic lipid metabolism, bile-acid synthesis, and inflammatory tone. Maybe, critics suggested, the 2018 findings were artifacts of housing conditions rather than genuine fiber effects.

In a 2020 mouse study, M. J. Pauly and colleagues designed a careful study to test exactly that alternative explanation. They asked whether inulin's effects on the liver depend on room temperature. They fed a 30% inulin diet to healthy male C57BL/6J mice for 12 days. All mice stayed at about

367

22 °C for the first 5 days, then were moved for the last 7 days to either 30 °C (thermoneutral) or 6 °C (cold) [2].

The industry expectation was that thermoneutral housing would validate inulin's safety. Instead, the study delivered a sobering answer demonstrating that even over this short period, inulin changed cholesterol and bile-acid handling. Plasma cholesterol, fecal cholesterol, and bile acid excretion also fell simultaneously while cholesterol accumulated in the liver. Bile acids in the blood (especially unconjugated forms) rose markedly, and ileal Fgf15 (a bile-acid feedback hormone) was almost undetectable. These changes signal cholestasis (impaired bile-acid flow/clearance). Cold exposure made several of these effects worse, boosting hepatic Cyp7a1 (the main bile-acid synthesis enzyme) and further increasing circulating bile acids. Histology and fibrosis markers showed only mild liver injury at 12 days. Inulin also raised SCFAs in the gut and portal blood, indicating robust fermentation [2].

Understanding why bile-acid disruption concerns hepatologists and metabolic researchers requires recognizing that bile acids are not passive digestive molecules but active metabolic regulators. Think of bile acids as dimmer switches controlling multiple metabolic rooms simultaneously. One switch affects lipid absorption and synthesis (determining whether dietary fats are absorbed or pass unabsorbed, whether the liver synthesizes cholesterol de novo, whether cholesterol is exported into bile for elimination). Another switch affects glucose homeostasis (modulating insulin sensitivity, gluconeogenesis, and glycogen storage). A third affects inflammatory tone and energy expenditure through TGR5 signaling in multiple tissues. When bile-acid composition, concentration, or signaling is altered; multiple metabolic rooms flicker simultaneously (some brightening (increased activity), others dimming (reduced activity)) and the whole-body metabolic pattern shifts.

The 2020 temperature-controlled study mattered because it removed alternative explanations. Yes, inulin's effects on bile acids and hepatic lipid metabolism are real, not artifacts. Yes, they occur even at thermoneutral conditions. All deduced explanations point to the very fast fermentation that also causes the bloating and stomach upset from Inulin.

III. Real Humans, Real Adherence: When Elegant Mechanisms Meet Daily Life

Stanford University, 2021. Now we leave the carefully controlled mouse facilities and temperature chambers to walk into Stanford where real humans with real lives tried to implement dietary interventions and researchers tracked what actually happened. Tracking not just microbes and molecules but also adherence, tolerability, and the lived experience determining whether interventions translate from protocol to practice.

Hannah C. Wastyk, Christopher D. Gardner, and colleagues conducted an ambitious randomized trial comparing two dietary approaches: one group received high-fiber diets (Not prebiotics and instead categorized into fruits, vegetables, legumes, grains, nuts, seeds etc. aiming for substantial increases in total fiber intake through whole foods and, when necessary, supplements), while another received fermented-food diets (yogurt, kefir, kimchi, sauerkraut, kombucha, and other traditionally fermented foods). The study tracked participants deeply across seventeen weeks using comprehensive multi-omic profiling (analyzing microbiome composition, immune markers, metabolomic profiles) while also carefully documenting adherence and tolerability through food diaries, symptom surveys, and the million small data points that reveal whether people can actually sustain these interventions [3].

The results taught lessons about biological heterogeneity that laboratory

369

studies often miss. The high-fiber arm reliably boosted microbial carbohydrate-active enzymes; the bacterial machinery for breaking down complex carbohydrates increased when feeding fiber to microbiomes. Microbiome diversity increased in some individuals but not cohort-wide. The critical finding was that immune responses to fiber wasn't uniform. People with higher baseline microbial diversity tended to show decreases in steady-state immune-cell signaling (a calmer immune tone), while a lower-diversity subgroup showed increases in these signaling markers. The trial's primary outcome (a composite cytokine response score) did not change significantly in either arm. On tolerability, fiber eaters reported softer stools during ramp and maintenance [3].

By contrast, the fermented-foods arm showed something remarkable. Inflammatory markers consistently decreased across participants. C-reactive protein, IL-6, and other inflammatory cytokines dropped. Immune profiles shifted in favorable directions. Microbiome diversity increased steadily across the intervention, reaching peak diversity during the choice phase when consumption remained elevated but lower than maximum which suggests ecosystem remodeling rather than transient effects. Fermented-food participants experienced temporary bloating during the initial ramp phase that was resolved by maintenance [3].

In summary, fiber changed function (more carbohydrate-processing capacity) and provoked person-specific immune shifts tied to starting diversity, while fermented foods raised diversity and lowered multiple inflammation markers cohort-wide. Both strategies were achievable with guidance; fiber tended to soften stools, and fermented foods caused transient bloating early on. The Stanford study revealed that whole food fiber interventions produce heterogeneous responses depending on baseline microbiome composition. Meaning benefit isn't universal but contingent on starting conditions.

IV. Precision Prebiotics Arrive: When One Size Fails Everyone

Stanford University, 2022. A team led by Samuel M. Lancaster asked whether different purified fibers produce distinct/personal effects and whether dose matters. Eighteen adults completed three 3-week cycles of escalating fiber doses (10 g/day in week 1, 20 g/day in week 2, 30 g/day in week 3). One cycle with arabinoxylan (AX), one with long-chain inulin (LCI from chicory), and one with a mixed-fiber blend (equal parts inulin, arabinoxylan, glucomannan, resistant starch, and acacia). The researchers collected stool and blood repeatedly and profiled everything from microbiome genes to lipids, bile acids, cytokines, and standard clinical metrics [4].

The central finding revealed both fiber-specific effects and concerning safety signals. AX showed clear dose-responsive biology with LDL and total cholesterol falling with rising doses, and bile-acid measurements shifting alongside microbial pathways that break down xylans. This is evidence that AX changes lipid handling while ramping up xylan-fermenting microbes.

Inulin increased beneficial Bifidobacterium at highest dose(30g). However critically, at 30g daily, inulin caused adverse effects in multiple participants with three experiencing elevated liver enzymes (alanine aminotransferase/ALT), and others showing inflammatory cytokine spikes including IL-6, TGF-β, and VEGF-A. The study confirmed previous mouse findings proving high-dose inulin can cause inflammation and liver stress markers in humans, not just rodents. Participants with ALT rises were taken off inulin promptly [4].

The mixed-fiber cycle produced smaller, intermediate shifts with muted lipid changes and fewer inflammatory signals than pure inulin. Suggesting that diversity of fibers can temper strong single-fiber effects at high doses [4]. This wasn't experimental error or poor study design; it was biology revealing dose-dependent toxicity. Proving that "more fiber" isn't universally better and that fermentation kinetics determine whether effects benefit or harm.

V. When Gels Go Wrong: The Psyllium Cautionary Tales

United States, Canada, United Arab Emirates, 2018-2025. Now we shift from fermentation biology to mechanical physics, examining how even beneficial fibers create genuine safety hazards when their physical properties interact with human anatomy and physiology in problematic ways. Psyllium is not a villain; it's a profoundly useful fiber that helps millions of people manage constipation, improve stool form, reduce cholesterol modestly, and support glycemic control. However, psyllium's superpower (its ability to absorb water and swell dramatically, forming highly viscous gels) is also a hazard when misused. Its risks include choking, esophageal impaction, and intestinal obstructions that have resulted in emergency department visits, intensive care admissions, surgical interventions, and at least one documented fatal outcome [5-7]. Let's examine three cases that teach different dimensions of mechanical fiber safety.

Case one: Pneumatosis intestinalis during bowel preparation (2025). Tampa, Florida, 2025. Parker Penny and Steven Lorch report a 53-year-old man who developed small-bowel obstruction (SBO) with pneumatosis intestinalis after a medication error during colonoscopy prep. The patient was prescribed polyethylene glycol (PEG) but mistakenly took psyllium instead (he confused the products because their brand names were similar) ingesting roughly 14 tablespoons (~47.6 g) over ~6 hours. On CT, clinicians saw SBO with a transition point and pneumatosis (gas within the bowel wall). Pneumatosis can indicate advanced ischemia, but it can be reversed with prompt care.

He was treated conservatively with IV fluids, medications for symptoms, and nasogastric decompression (about 1.4 liters of gelatinous output initially). The next day, PEG solution was given through the NG tube, his distention improved, the tube was removed by hospital day 3, and he was discharged on day 4. The authors emphasize that psyllium is generally safe, but in large, rapidly ingested amounts (especially without enough water) it can form a nondigestible hydrogel/bezoar that mechanically obstructs the intestine. The case underscores the need for clear patient education and labeling to prevent look-alike/sound-alike mix-ups during bowel-prep instructions [5].

Case two: Fatal choking (2025). The Institute for Safe Medication Practices Canada documented a fatal choking in a long-term-care resident with dysphagia after inappropriate use of psyllium. When psyllium is not mixed with enough liquid (or when given to someone with swallowing difficulty) it can swell into a cohesive gel that lodges in the esophagus and compresses the airway, making it hard or impossible to clear by coughing. Unlike thin liquids (which usually pass or can be suctioned) or foods that break apart, a gelled bolus can create a rapid, complete blockage and cause asphyxiation [6].

Case three: Intestinal obstruction (2018). A. F. Hefny and colleagues reported a case of intestinal obstruction caused by psyllium and reviewed similar cases from medical literature. The pattern across reports is clear showing when psyllium is taken without enough water, its powerful ability to absorb fluid and expand turns from helpful to harmful. In people with gut narrowing from previous surgery, inflammation, or slow bowel movement due to illness or medications, the gel-like mass can enlarge until it blocks the intestine. The 21-year-old man in their case had taken

373

psyllium husks for constipation while fasting, which prevented him from drinking fluids. The swollen fiber accumulated, distending his colon and causing incomplete obstruction. He recovered after hospitalization and repeated enemas, avoiding surgery. The review highlighted that similar obstructions (sometimes in the esophagus, sometimes in the bowel) occur when psyllium is swallowed dry, with little water, or by patients with motility problems [7].

This doesn't mean abandoning psyllium; it means recognizing that psyllium occupies a different risk-benefit category. When stool-form correction is the primary goal and you can ensure appropriate use (adequate hydration, careful dosing, monitoring for side effects, avoiding in at-risk individuals), psyllium remains valuable. When the goal is daily prebiotic and metabolic support over weeks to years in diverse users with variable adherence and understanding, Hashab gum's forgiving profile reduces the risk of serious adverse events essentially to zero while delivering the systemic benefits that long-term use of tolerable interventions creates.

VI. What the Guidelines Quietly Say: When Conservative Panels Acknowledge Fiber Isn't Universal

United Kingdom and United States, 2021. Professional gastroenterology societies have begun explicitly acknowledging through clinical guidelines that fiber types differ in their effects on irritable bowel syndrome. It's being recognized that soluble fibers improve symptoms while insoluble fibers may worsen them, and that dietary recommendations must distinguish fiber types rather than treating "fiber" as undifferentiated. The British Society of Gastroenterology recommends soluble fiber (ispaghula/psyllium) to improve overall IBS symptoms and abdominal pain, and advises against insoluble fiber (e.g., wheat bran) because it can worsen symptoms. Start low (3–4 g/day) and increase gradually to minimize bloating. For diet beyond fiber, the guideline supports a low-FODMAP diet as second-line therapy for patients who do not respond to first-line measures and it should be implemented with a trained dietitian and followed by structured re-introduction of FODMAPs according to tolerance (weak recommendation; very low-quality evidence) [8].

The American College of Gastroenterology makes the same key distinctions. Use soluble, not insoluble fiber for global IBS symptoms (strong recommendation; moderate-quality evidence). The ACG also recommends a limited trial of a low-FODMAP diet to improve global symptoms (conditional recommendation; very low-quality evidence). These recommendations classify fiber by solubility and mechanistic explanations [9].

These guidelines provide clinicians permission to be selective by recommending specific fiber types (soluble like ispaghula) while avoiding others (insoluble like bran) and offering low FODMAP diet for patients requiring additional symptom management. For patients, the guidelines validate that different fibers create different outcomes and legitimize stopping fibers that consistently worsen symptoms rather than assuming "adaptation will occur eventually" [8,9].

References:

1. Singh, Vishal, et al. "Dysregulated Microbial Fermentation of Soluble Fiber Induces Cholestatic Liver Cancer." Cell, vol. 175, no. 3, 18 Oct. 2018, pp. 679-694.e22,

2. Pauly, Mira J., et al. "Inulin Supplementation Disturbs Hepatic Cholesterol and Bile Acid Metabolism Independent from Housing Temperature." Nutrients, vol. 12, no. 10, 20 Oct. 2020, p. 3200

3. Wastyk, Hannah C., et al. "Gut-Microbiota-Targeted Diets Modulate Human Immune Status." Cell, vol. 184, no. 16, 5 Aug. 2021, pp. 4137-4153.e14

4. Lancaster, Samuel M., et al. "Global, Distinctive, and Personal Changes in Molecular and Microbial Profiles by Specific Fibers in Humans." Cell Host & Microbe, vol. 30, no. 6, 8 June 2022, pp. 848-862

5. Penny, Parker, and Steven Lorch. "Psyllium Overdose During Bowel Preparation Leading to Pneumatosis Intestinalis: A Case Report." ACG Case Reports Journal, vol. 12, no. 9, Sept. 2025, article e01820

6. Institute for Safe Medication Practices Canada. "Fatal Choking Incident Associated with Inappropriate Use of Psyllium." ISMP Canada Safety Bulletin, vol. 25, no. 6, 24 June 2025. PDF, ismpcanada.ca/wp-content/uploads/ISMPCSB2025-i6-Choking-Hazards.pdf.

7. Hefny, Ashraf F., et al. "Intestinal Obstruction Caused by a Laxative Drug (Psyllium): Case Report and Review of the Literature." Journal of Surgical Case Reports, vol. 2018, no. 10, Oct. 2018, article rjy270

8. Vasant, Dipesh H., et al. "British Society of Gastroenterology Guidelines on the Management of Irritable Bowel Syndrome." Gut, vol. 70, no. 7, 2021, pp. 1214-1240

9. Lacy, Brian E., et al. "ACG Clinical Guideline: Management of Irritable Bowel Syndrome." American Journal of Gastroenterology, vol. 116, no. 1, 2021, pp. 17-44

CHAPTER 23

Another Layer that Buried Hashab Gum Until it Was Buried No More!

When the Quiet Hero Lost Its Badge (Then Got It Back)

The previous chapter taught us a deceptively simple reality that keeps saving people from supplement-aisle disappointment and gastrointestinal distress. How a fiber behaves inside the body matters infinitely more than what the marketing label promises or what the ingredient name suggests.

Viscous gel-formers like psyllium can choke or obstruct when misused by individuals with swallowing difficulties or when consumed without adequate hydration; creating genuine medical emergencies documented in case reports and safety bulletins across multiple countries. Sprint-speed fermenters like inulin can light up bloating and cramping that destroys adherence within days. Critically, in narrow but concerning contexts revealed by careful animal models and human metabolic studies, Inulin can wobble bile-acid choreography and stress hepatic function in ways that raise legitimate safety questions for vulnerable populations. Perhaps most importantly for translating elegant mechanisms into real-world health improvements is tolerability. Tolerability determines adherence, adherence determines sustained use, and sustained use determines whether the biological benefits demonstrated in two-week trials ever manifest as measurable improvements in health.

Against this evidence backdrop, Hashab gum looks like what might be called a boring hero. It dissolves invisibly into beverages without creating texture challenges that limit consumption. It disappears into daily routines rather than demanding precise timing, hydration protocols, or medical supervision. Importantly, it keeps doing small, steady, cumulatively good things day after day. Gradually shifting microbiome composition toward beneficial profiles by slowly producing short-chain fatty acids without explosive gas generation. Hashab quietly strengthens intestinal barriers through mucin stimulation and anti-inflammatory signaling while gently modulating glucose and lipid metabolism through mechanisms documented across preceding chapters. Hashab gum reliably supports kidney function, cardiovascular health, neurological resilience, and reproductive outcomes in populations ranging from healthy adults to patients with advanced chronic disease.

Now here's the riddle that should make you lean forward with curiosity or perhaps frustration. If Hashab gum is genuinely useful across organ systems and is superior to alternatives on the criteria that determine real-world success; then why did it spend the better part of a decade in regulatory limbo? Why was it counted as dietary fiber under one set of rules, then suddenly not counted, then finally counted again after years of petitions, denials, new studies, and bureaucratic processes? Why was another layer of confusion added to its naming quagmire mystifying industry observers and leaving consumers even more confused about whether this ancient, widely used ingredient was legitimate or suspect?

Was this regulatory caution reflecting appropriate scientific skepticism and evidence standards protecting public health? Was it geopolitical tensions affecting ingredient supply chains or was it industry lobbying by competitors with different economic interests? Were regulatory agencies responding to pressures invisible to outside observers? Or was it simply the mundane but consequential reality of doing science in public through administrative processes designed for thoroughness rather than speed? Is this ingredient doomed to undergo another round of conspiracy to hide it from the public that desperately needs it?

The answer, from 22 chapters teaching you to look past simple narratives and toward mechanistic complexity and contextual nuance, is "all of the above and none of the above". It's a perfect storm of legitimate regulatory requirements, genuine scientific challenges posed by material heterogeneity, misaligned commercial incentives, unfortunate timing, and Hashab's own subtle virtues that made it harder to prove in short-term trials than fibers producing immediate dramatic effects.

This chapter tells that regulatory story not to fuel conspiracy theories or assign villains, but to help you understand how evidence becomes policy. It will educate you as to why categories and definitions shape what becomes visible and accessible to consumers. Finally, you will understand why the 2021 resolution (when the U.S. Food and Drug Administration finally granted petitions and announced its intent to add Acacia gum arabic to the official list of dietary fibers based on human evidence of beneficial physiological effects) represents not just bureaucratic housekeeping but validation of everything this book has been teaching across hundreds of pages.

By chapter's end, you'll understand the timeline from early acceptance through redefinition, denial, and eventual recognition. You'll grasp why the scientific challenge was real; how mixing two Acacia species under one ingredient name muddied research signals and made regulatory dossiers look noisier than they should have. You'll see how incentives shaped the pace. Why some industry players had incentives to keep Hashab gum hidden while others invested years and substantial resources proving what traditional use and growing research already suggested. You'll appreciate why the delay, frustrating as it was for advocates and confusing as it was

379

for consumers, ultimately strengthens rather than weakens the case for Acacia gum. When regulatory agencies that demand rigorous proof finally grant recognition, that recognition means something more than marketing permission; it means the evidence survived scrutiny designed to protect public health against exaggerated claims and unproven ingredients.

The destination isn't vindication through revelation of wrongdoing or conspiracy. The destination is understanding how regulatory science works, why it sometimes moves slowly even when evidence accumulates, and how that very slowness, when it eventually yields to proof, creates confidence that the recognition is deserved and durable.

I. Before the Storm: Acacia the Anonymous Workhorse

Long before "prebiotics" became a supermarket buzzword and "gut health" emerged as a wellness category driving billions in supplement sales, Acacia (gum arabic) was everywhere in the American food supply while being essentially invisible to consumers. Walk into any convenience store in 1990, 2000, or 2010, and Acacia gum was there. It was emulsifying the citrus oils that give your soda its bright flavor without letting them separate into unappetizing oil slicks floating on top. It kept candy shells glossy and smooth through the humidity changes of cross-country shipping. It stabilized the flavors in chewing gum so they release consistently rather than dumping all at once or fading within seconds. It performed a dozen other functional tasks that food technologists understood intimately but that consumers neither knew nor needed to know because the ingredient did its job invisibly and safely.

Acacia gum was used in the most miniscule doses required to fulfil the elementary functional jobs of stabilizing, emulsifying and encapsulating. For example, a rumor has it that a globally renowned drink that sells more than 1 billion drinks daily uses approximately .2 grams of Acacia gum which is enough to do the functional emulsification job while providing zero health benefits to consumers. Same rumor has it that this same drink company is responsible for consuming 70-80% of all Acacia gum production over the past 100 years. Do you see where the incentives would lie for such an organization? Let's not delve into these rumors and instead continue following the evidence trail we started since the beginning of this book.

The regulatory status supporting this ubiquitous-but-anonymous use was straightforward and uncontroversial. The United States Food and Drug Administration had affirmed Acacia (Gum arabic) as Generally Recognized as Safe (GRAS) direct food substance, codified in the Code of Federal Regulations at 21 CFR section 184.1330. This GRAS affirmation represents the agency's determination that qualified expert consensus approved this substance as safe under conditions of intended use. This meant that food manufacturers could incorporate Acacia gum into products without requiring pre-market approval as long as it meets regulatory conditions. This is the regulatory equivalent of a green light for an ingredient with such a long history of safe use [1].

The GRAS designation covered Acacia's functional properties (its work as emulsifier, stabilizer, thickener, and film-former) but during this pre-2016 era, it also implicitly supported something else. The pre-2016 era implicitly acknowledged that Acacia gum was a dietary fiber because it is an analytically measurable, non-digestible arabinogalactan polysaccharide. It is roughly 85–90% non-digestible carbohydrate by weight, which fits the analytical concept of dietary fiber [1].

Under the regulatory framework existing before 2016, companies could legitimately count that analytically measured fiber when calculating the dietary fiber values printed on Nutrition Facts labels. This created a quiet, functional equilibrium. Acacia did its technical jobs (emulsifying, stabilizing) while also contributing to the fiber number on labels. Manufacturers were content because they had versatile ingredients with clean labeling and established supply chains. No drama, no controversy, no particular incentive for anyone to draw attention to Acacia's existence. It was the quintessential commodity ingredient; valuable precisely because it was reliable, boring, and invisible.

Then, in 2013, this quiet equilibrium shifted slightly when FDA finalized a response to a 2011 petition requesting expanded permitted uses for Acacia gum in foods. The agency's action, documented in federal dockets and reported in trade publications serving the food-ingredient industry, issued a final rule expanding the permitted food uses for Acacia (Gum arabic). In that rule, FDA also made explicit what lab methods had long shown: "We concur that Acacia supplies dietary fiber". This action (published in the Federal Register on December 6, 2013) confirmed expanded use categories and acknowledged Acacia's fiber contribution under the labeling framework then in force. Trade publications in early 2014 picked up the story, and interest grew as formulators who had used Acacia gum mainly for texture and stability began highlighting its fiber contribution. This positioned Acacia as a gentler fiber source for products aiming to raise fiber intake without the digestive side effects common to some high-fiber supplements [2].

This was Acacia's moment of transition from purely functional ingredient toward something that might be actively promoted for health benefits; a transition that seemed straightforward and unremarkable at the time. The 2013 FDA action appeared to be administrative housekeeping, clarifying and expanding uses for a long-accepted ingredient while confirming what food scientists already knew about its fiber content. There was no hint that within three years, the entire regulatory ground would shift beneath Acacia, creating years of uncertainty and requiring a level of scientific proof that this ancient ingredient had never needed to muster before. However, that shift was coming, driven not by any concern about Acacia specifically but by FDA's comprehensive overhaul of how dietary fiber would be defined, measured, and proven for labeling purposes.

II. The 2016 Reset: FDA Draws a New Line in the Sand

In May 2016, the Food and Drug Administration published its final rules comprehensively revising the Nutrition Facts label that appears on packaged foods. The nutritional facts label is the familiar black-and-white box that Americans have relied on since 1994 to understand serving sizes, calories, nutrients, and daily value percentages. The revision was the most significant label update in two decades, reflecting evolving nutritional science, changing dietary patterns, and public health priorities that had shifted substantially since the original label's introduction. The changes included updating serving sizes to reflect realistic consumption rather than aspirational portions. Adding a line for added sugars to distinguish naturally occurring sugars in fruit and milk from sugars added during manufacturing. Updating the vitamins and minerals required on labels to emphasize nutrients Americans under-consume rather than nutrients where deficiency has become rare. Importantly, it made the calorie count visually prominent to help consumers make more informed choices about energy intake [3].

Buried in this comprehensive revision was a change that would prove consequential far beyond its technical-sounding description. FDA redrew the definition of dietary fiber to emphasize physiological function rather than just chemical structure and analytical methods. The new definition drew a bright regulatory line. Going forward, isolated or synthetic non-digestible carbohydrates would count as dietary fiber on Nutrition Facts labels only if manufacturers could demonstrate through adequate scientific evidence that these ingredients produce beneficial physiological effects in humans. Specifically, Dietary fibers needed one or more of the effects FDA recognized as clinically relevant based on authoritative health organization recommendations and consistent evidence. The recognized effects included lowering blood glucose and insulin responses (glycemic attenuation), reducing blood cholesterol levels (cardiovascular benefit), improving laxation (bowel health), reducing blood pressure, or increasing mineral absorption such as calcium [3].

FDA's reasoning was sound and reflected appropriate regulatory caution in an era where "functional fibers" had proliferated in the supplement and food-additive marketplace. Food manufacturers and supplement companies had developed numerous isolated, purified, and synthetic non-digestible carbohydrates that met the narrow analytical definition of fiber (resisting digestion by human enzymes, measured by approved laboratory methods) but that might or might not actually provide the health benefits. The agency wanted to ensure that when consumers saw "dietary fiber" on a label, that number represented ingredients with demonstrated physiological value rather than just analytical convenience. This was done to prevent manufacturers from bulking up fiber claims with materials that looked like fiber in the laboratory but didn't act like fiber in the human body [3].

This was not, fundamentally, an attack on any specific ingredient or industry segment. It was a raise-the-bar move aimed at truthful labeling and public health protection. It forced manufacturers to prove that isolated fibers do more than pad a number on a Nutrition Facts panel. It ensured that the term "dietary fiber" retained meaning and value rather than becoming diluted to meaninglessness by inclusion of every non-digestible carbohydrate regardless of physiological effect. FDA provided an initial list of seven isolated or synthetic fibers that the agency had already determined met the new standard based on existing published literature: beta-glucan, psyllium, cellulose, guar gum, pectin, locust bean gum, and hydroxypropylmethylcellulose. For other fibers (including many that had been counted under the previous analytical definition) the agency opened a petition pathway allowing manufacturers or trade associations to submit evidence demonstrating beneficial physiological effects, with FDA reviewing submissions and adding qualified fibers to the official list through subsequent regulatory actions [3].

The 2016 redefinition created an overnight regulatory discontinuity for numerous ingredients. Materials that had been legitimately counted as dietary fiber for years under the analytical approach (including Acacia gum arabic) suddenly found themselves in limbo. They weren't rejected or declared non-fibers in some absolute sense. They simply weren't on the initial approved list, meaning they couldn't be counted as dietary fiber on labels unless and until manufacturers submitted evidence through the petition process and the FDA granted approval. The analytical chemistry hadn't changed (Acacia was still roughly ninety percent non-digestible prebiotic according to labs and older studies) but the regulatory framework had shifted from "fiber is what resists digestion and measures as fiber" to "fiber is what resists digestion, measures as fiber, and demonstrably provides beneficial physiological effects in humans". That additional requirement (proof of human benefit) would prove to be the challenging hurdle that extended Acacia's limbo period for five years [3].

For readers encountering this regulatory history from the outside, it's important to appreciate that FDA's action was both reasonable in principle and disruptive in practice. The agency was responding to legitimate concerns about truth in labeling and was establishing standards that should, in theory, benefit consumers by ensuring the fiber values on labels represent functional ingredients rather than analytical artifacts. At the same time, the abrupt shift imposed substantial costs and delays on ingredients like Acacia that had extensive histories of food use, substantial existing research suggesting benefits, but that hadn't yet been tested specifically on the endpoints FDA now required, using the study designs and evidence standards that regulatory approval would demand. An ingredient could be perfectly safe, genuinely beneficial in ways supported by decades of traditional use and growing mechanistic research yet still find itself excluded from fiber labeling until manufacturers invested the considerable time, resources, and scientific expertise required to generate FDA-acceptable human evidence addressing FDA-recognized endpoints. This challenging process could take years even under the best circumstances [3].

What made the 2016 shift particularly consequential for Acacia was that the fiber's subtlety (its gentle, slow fermentation and gradual, sustained effects rather than dramatic acute changes) meant that the most obvious benefits might not appear in the short-term studies that are most practical and affordable to conduct. Acacia's advantages emerge over weeks and months of daily use. The sustained improvements in microbiome composition, gradual anti-inflammatory effects, kidney function preservation across years, and metabolic improvements all accrue through adherence-enabled sustained exposure. These are exactly the outcomes that matter for real-world health but that are challenging to demonstrate in the randomized controlled trials that represent the sweet spot of feasibility for ingredient manufacturers submitting regulatory petitions.

The stage was set for a frustrating period where Acacia's genuine value would be difficult to prove on the timeline and with the endpoints that regulatory requirements demanded, despite substantial biological plausibility and growing research interest that would eventually generate the needed evidence. These years of regulatory uncertainty created confusion among consumers, hesitancy among formulators, and frustration among advocates who could see the disconnect between Acacia's real-world utility and its bureaucratic invisibility.

III. Evidence, Re-Evidence, Then Finally Yes

The period from 2016 through 2021 represented what might be called Acacia's regulatory exile. A frustrating limbo where the ingredient remained perfectly legal to use in foods and supplements (the GRAS affirmation for safety never changed), where existing research continued accumulating evidence of benefits, yet where the specific regulatory recognition allowing fiber-content labeling remained elusive because the evidence submitted through petition processes didn't yet meet FDA's standards for the kinds of human studies and clinical endpoints the new framework required.

Acacia's suppliers and trade organizations did exactly what the 2016 rule changes demanded. They assembled comprehensive dossiers pulling together existing published research. They coordinated with academic researchers to design and conduct new human trials targeting FDA-recognized physiological endpoints. They met with agency officials to understand evidence expectations and study-design requirements, and they submitted formal petitions through the established administrative pathways providing the mechanism for manufacturers to present evidence and request regulatory determinations. This was the boring, necessary, expensive work of translating scientific knowledge into regulatory language and meeting evidentiary standards that, while demanding, serve legitimate public health protection purposes by requiring proof rather than accepting plausibility [4].

The early submissions encountered obstacles. The existing published research on Acacia, while substantial and growing, wasn't necessarily designed around the specific endpoints FDA had designated as evidence of beneficial physiological effects. Studies might have examined stool frequency, gastrointestinal symptoms, tolerance, microbiome composition changes, or longer-term metabolic markers like hemoglobin A1c or lipid profiles. All of these are valuable scientifically but not necessarily matching the acute meal-challenge studies with glucose and insulin measurements that regulatory authorities prefer for demonstrating glycemic attenuation, or the specific cholesterol-measurement protocols required for cardiovascular benefit claims, or the precise laxation metrics needed for bowel-function claims [4].

Additionally, much existing research didn't distinguish between Acacia senegal and Acacia seyal sources (a material heterogeneity issue we'll examine in detail shortly), possibly creating additional analytical noise that made effects look less consistent than they might have been if source material had been better controlled and characterized [4].

In January 2020, FDA issued a denial letter responding to one petition, writing that "the strength of the evidence is insufficient" to support adding Acacia gum to the list of dietary fibers meeting the beneficial physiological effect requirement. The denial was neither a declaration that Acacia doesn't provide benefits nor a rejection of Acacia as inherently unworthy of fiber status. However, it was the agency's way of saying "the human data you've submitted so far don't meet our evidentiary standards; please bring better studies addressing the endpoints we recognize, with appropriate sample sizes, controls, and statistical analyses". This kind of denial isn't unusual in regulatory science. It's often a waypoint rather than a final destination, a signal about what additional work is needed rather than a permanent rejection [5].

The denial focused minds and resources. It became clear that meeting FDA's standard would require commissioning new human clinical trials specifically designed around post-prandial (after-meal) glucose and insulin responses. This is one of the most straightforward and well-accepted endpoints for demonstrating beneficial physiological effects because blood sugar control is fundamental to metabolic health, and measurement techniques are standardized and widely accepted. Additionally, this focus was superior because the FDA and other regulatory agencies have long recognized glycemic attenuation as clinically relevant given the global epidemic of insulin resistance, prediabetes, and type 2 diabetes. Industry groups and academic researchers collaborated on designing exactly these studies. They conducted randomized, controlled human trials where participants consumed standardized carbohydrate-containing meals with or without Acacia gum, followed by serial blood glucose and insulin measurements across several hours to capture the full postprandial response curve.

These studies took time to design properly, secure ethics approvals for human research, recruit appropriate participants, conduct with sufficient rigor to meet good clinical practice standards, analyze statistically, and publish in peer-reviewed journals. Peer review and acceptance is the gold standard that regulatory agencies like FDA rely on because peer review provides independent expert validation that study designs, analyses, and conclusions are sound. By late 2020 and into 2021, the evidence FDA had requested began appearing in accessible form. All this effort manifested in well-designed human trials showing that consuming Acacia gum (roughly 13–40 g) with carb-containing meals showed lower peak glucose (often about 5–16% vs. control, depending on design) and significant reductions in post-prandial insulin while some studies also reported reduced glucose or insulin AUC. These are the kinds of improvements that, sustained over months and years through daily use, would translate into better glycemic control and reduced diabetes risk in at-risk populations.

On December 17, 2021, FDA publicly granted the citizen petition and announced its intent to add "Acacia (Gum Arabic)" to the regulatory list of dietary fibers, citing the evidence demonstrating reduced post-prandial blood glucose and insulin responses when Acacia is consumed with carbohydrate-containing meals. Simultaneously, the agency announced that it would exercise enforcement discretion; meaning FDA would not object to manufacturers immediately counting Acacia as dietary fiber on "Nutrition Facts" labels even before the formal rulemaking was complete. This was recognition that the evidence threshold had been met and that requiring manufacturers to wait for final administrative completion of rulemaking would serve no public health purpose [6].

The 2021 decision represented vindication, validation, and regulatory closure of a five-year process that had been frustrating for everyone involved. From FDA's perspective, the system had worked as designed. The agency had established evidence standards, manufacturers had submitted evidence that didn't initially meet those standards, the agency had communicated what additional evidence was needed, manufacturers had generated that evidence through appropriate human studies, resulting in the agency granting recognition once proof was adequate.

From the industry's perspective, years of effort and substantial investment in clinical research had finally produced the regulatory outcome that traditional use and growing scientific literature had established. From the consumers' perspective (though few consumers tracked the regulatory minutiae as Acacia has always been a hidden ingredient), Acacia could once again be labeled with its fiber content. This made it easier for formulators to incorporate it into supplements and functional foods, easier for nutritionists and clinicians to recommend, and easier for consumers to identify it as a source of dietary fiber when scanning supplement labels or researching prebiotic options [6].

What changed between the 2020 denial and the 2021 approval was simple but consequential. The human evidence on an FDA-recognized endpoint (postprandial glycemic and insulinemic control) reached the threshold of quality, quantity, and consistency that regulatory standards required. The biological mechanisms hadn't changed. Acacia had always worked through

390

slow fermentation, SCFA production, microbiome modulation, and the various pathways documented across this book's preceding chapters. However, mechanism, no matter how well understood, doesn't satisfy regulatory requirements for labeling claims. Proof of beneficial physiological effects in humans does, and once that proof arrived in acceptable form, FDA granted recognition appropriately and promptly.

IV. Why Did It Take That Long? Unpacking Delay Without Invoking Conspiracy

Looking back at the five-year journey from the 2016 redefinition through the 2021 approval, it's tempting to search for villains, conspiracies, or deliberate obstruction explaining why Acacia spent years in regulatory limbo while other fibers sailed through with initial approval or faced shorter petition timelines. The reality, as is so often the case in complex regulatory and commercial systems, is that the delay emerged from the intersection of multiple legitimate factors. These include scientific challenges, material heterogeneity, misaligned incentives, timing, and Acacia's own virtues creating paradoxical difficulties for proof. None of these individually constituted wrongdoing, but together they created a perfect storm that buried a genuinely valuable ingredient under bureaucratic process for half a decade.

The possible suspect is the species-mixing problem: Acacia is two trees in a regulatory trench coat. Perhaps the single most important scientific complication slowing clear evidence accumulation and regulatory recognition is one that most consumers and even many researchers don't fully appreciate: "acacia gum" or "gum arabic" as defined in food regulations and international standards includes exudates from two distinct Acacia species, Acacia senegal and Acacia seyal, which are close botanical cousins but not completely identical in their molecular composition, functional properties, or physiological effects. In commercial trade, particularly in Sudan and other major producing regions, Acacia senegal gum is often referred to as "Hashab" and is generally considered the premium grade with superior emulsifying properties and higher arabinogalactan-protein content, while Acacia seyal is called "Talha" and typically commands lower prices with somewhat different functional characteristics.

The two species produce gums that are similar enough that regulatory authorities and international standards bodies have treated them as a single substance for safety and functional purposes. Both are safe, both are effective (to different extents) emulsifiers and stabilizers, both are non-digestible complex carbohydrates that meet the analytical definition of prebiotic fiber. However, at the molecular level, they differ in ways that can affect fermentation kinetics, SCFA production patterns, interactions with gut bacteria, and potentially the magnitude and timing of physiological effects in human studies. Acacia senegal gum typically has higher protein content (particularly the arabinogalactan-protein fraction that gives Acacia many of its unique properties), may ferment somewhat faster and more completely than Acacia seyal gum, and may produce different ratios of acetate, propionate, and butyrate when bacteria metabolize it. These differences are subtle but could influence study outcomes.

The regulatory and research problems emerge because many published studies and many commercial products don't specify which species are used, don't report molecular characterization that would allow independent assessment of material quality, and don't control source material rigorously across batches used in long-term studies. When you're trying to demonstrate beneficial physiological effects for regulatory purposes, this heterogeneity creates noise that makes effects look less consistent than they might actually be. One study might use Hashab material, show robust glycemic attenuation, and publish positive findings. Another study might use primarily Talha material or a mixed batch, show more modest effects or higher variability, and publish neutral or equivocal findings. When regulatory reviewers look at the collective evidence, the inconsistency reduces confidence that the effect is reliable and reproducible. This is probably the biggest missed opportunity regarding this ordeal as the FDA could have forced a classifying distinction of both gums. Unfortunately, they didn't and this problem will continue to haunt us into the future.

Acacia is a victim of its own subtlety and virtues. The very properties that make Acacia superior for long-term daily use (slow fermentation, gentle effects, excellent tolerance, sustained benefits developing over days and weeks rather than dramatic acute changes) create challenges for demonstrating effects in short-term studies that are most practical for regulatory petitions. Inulin produces rapid, proximal fermentation with dramatic bifidogenic effects visible within hours and substantial gas production that's unpleasant but at least provides immediate feedback that something is happening biochemically. Psyllium produces obvious changes in stool form and transit time within one to three days that are easily measured and that participants and clinicians notice immediately. These rapid, obvious effects make it straightforward to design twelve-week studies showing clear differences between treatment and placebo groups.

Acacia's benefits are quieter and more gradual. Microbiome composition shifts that take time to establish, anti-inflammatory effects that emerge over sustained use as transcriptional programs respond to SCFA signaling, and metabolic improvements that accrue through adherence-enabled long-term exposure rather than acute dramatic changes. These are exactly the kinds of benefits that matter for managing chronic metabolic disease but they're harder to capture in the compressed timelines that make clinical trials affordable and practical. A study might show statistically significant but modest glucose reductions after four weeks that would become

393

clinically substantial after six months of sustained use, but FDA is evaluating the four-week data and may not find it compelling enough for regulatory recognition even though the long-term trajectory is what matters for health. Conducting trials for longer periods is also very expensive.

Ecosystem incentives weren't aligned toward fast resolution. The commercial dynamics surrounding Acacia created a situation where different industry players had very different interests regarding dietary fiber recognition, and those misaligned incentives contributed to pace. On one side, the major buyers (beverage companies, confectionery manufacturers, and other food producers using Acacia primarily for its functional properties as emulsifier and stabilizer) had limited incentive to push for dietary fiber recognition that might increase ingredient costs or create supply constraints. These companies valued Acacia for solving technical problems (keeping citrus oils dispersed in sodas, preventing ice crystal formation in frozen desserts) where its performance was excellent and where no alternative ingredient matched its combination of effectiveness, safety, clean label appeal, and established supply chains.

If Acacia suddenly became recognized and promoted as a valuable prebiotic fiber, demand would increase, prices might rise, and supply competition would intensify. None of which served the interests of buyers who were already satisfied with the ingredient's functional performance and who had no need for fiber labeling on their products.

On the other side, ingredient suppliers (the companies purchasing Acacia from producers in Sudan and other growing regions, processing it into purified grades suitable for food and pharmaceutical use, and selling it to manufacturers) had every economic incentive to achieve dietary fiber recognition because it would open new markets (dietary supplements, functional foods marketed for gut and metabolic health) and allow premium pricing for ingredient positioning beyond food additive status.

However, even with this group there could have been an incentive to not rush and stock up as much raw Acacia gum (at depressed prices due to dietary fiber fallout) and then profit greatly after the Dietary fiber classification was back. This is supposition but we are discussing incentives.

However, it was these suppliers who mustered the resources and funded the new clinical research required for FDA petitions, coordinated industry efforts through trade associations, and invested the resources and time required to navigate regulatory processes. The ingredient suppliers are typically small-to-medium companies without the market power of the major food manufacturers who are their customers. This meant that their ability to drive rapid change was constrained by their position in the commercial ecosystem. The players with the strongest incentive to achieve fiber recognition had limited resources to accelerate the process, while the players with the most resources had limited incentive to prioritize fiber recognition over the hidden status quo.

The system moved when the ingredient suppliers generated sufficient evidence and made a compelling enough case that regulatory processes yielded approval. However, this took years of sustained effort that might have been compressed if the entire commercial ecosystem had been aligned behind rapid resolution. The fact that recognition eventually came suggests the system worked as designed even if the timeline was longer and more frustrating than advocates hoped or than seems optimal in retrospect.

V. The Designation Puzzle: Why "Gum Arabic" Should Be Split for Science

Acacia (Gum arabic), as legally defined in food regulations across multiple jurisdictions (United States, European Union, Codex Alimentarius international standards), refers to exudates from two Acacia species: Acacia senegal and Acacia seyal. Both species are members of the Fabaceae (legume) family, both grow primarily in the Sahel region of Africa (particularly Sudan, which produces the majority of world supply), both produce dried gum nodules through natural exudation or tapping that are harvested, cleaned, and processed into powdered or granular forms, and both have long histories of food use extending back millennia. In regulatory terms, particularly for safety assessment, treating them together makes sense because both have been consumed by humans for thousands of years without significant toxicity signals.

The differences lie in color (or lack thereof), in protein composition, and in the proportions of other chemical components. These differences play a big role in the formulation capabilities as food scientists are well aware. More importantly, they also yield different outcomes for health purposes even if both are beneficial in different ways. The differences are way beyond the scope of this book but are important to highlight for the benefit of the reader.

The scientific and regulatory challenge emerges at the intersection of these two realities. Regulations treat Hashab and Talha as a single substance (Acacia gum) while chemistry recognize they're similar-but-distinct materials whose differences might matter for physiological effects even if they don't matter for safety. When research studies investigate Acacia's prebiotic effects, metabolic benefits, or kidney protective properties, most studies use carefully sourced Hashab-grade Acacia senegal material. Some studies use Talha (Acacia seyal) especially when exploring the differences. The problem is that the vast majority of research does not specify exactly which species they are testing even though we know the vast majority are using Acacia Senegal as its accepted internationally as the standard.

Keep in mind the inclusion of Acacia seyal to the regulatory definition of "Acacia Gum arabic" did not occur until much later in its history. Acacia seyal got formally "promoted" to full Gum arabic status in the late 1990s, anchored by JECFA in 1998 and Codex in 1999. Before Acacia seyal was formally written into the JECFA/Codex definition in 1998–1999, "Gum arabic" in international specs was essentially code for Acacia senegal. JECFA's 1997 specification (and earlier ones) defined Gum arabic as the dried exudate from Acacia senegal "or closely related species of Acacia," and then mentioned A. seyal only as an example of a closely related species whose gum is "sometimes referred to as gum talha". In the descriptive section they clearly treated Acacia senegal gum as the reference material and described gum from other species, including A. seyal, as different in appearance and properties. Older pharmacopoeias and standards (e.g., French Journal Officiel, Food Chemicals Codex, US Pharmacopeia) likewise defined "Gum arabic" as the exudate from Acacia senegal or "other related species," but the toxicology work that underpinned regulatory acceptance used authenticated A. senegal gum. So, practically, up to the late 1990s the internationally accepted Gum arabic of commerce was Acacia senegal (Hashab), with other African acacias (including Acacia seyal) sitting in a gray zone as "closely related" or "gum Talha" but not yet explicitly co-equal in the official definition.

This lack of specification wouldn't matter if Hashab and Talha were functionally identical, but they're not identical in many ways that could influence study outcomes. The AGP content difference is particularly relevant as the arabinogalactan-proteins are the fraction most responsible for Acacia's unique immune-modulating properties, barrier-protective effects, and some fermentation characteristics (as we discussed in the iron absorption study highlighting a different absorption pathway). Material with higher AGP might show stronger or faster effects in studies measuring inflammatory markers, microbiome shifts, or barrier permeability. Material with lower AGP might still be effective but with more modest effect sizes or slower onset. When you're trying to pool studies for meta-analysis or evaluate evidence for regulatory purposes, this uncontrolled variation makes collective evidence look weaker than evidence from any single well-controlled study using consistent source material.

The molecular weight distribution also matters. Lower-molecular-weight fractions may be more rapidly fermented by gut bacteria than higher-molecular-weight fractions, potentially affecting SCFA production kinetics and gas generation. Mineral content (Specifically calcium) is also significantly different between the 2 gums. These are relevant because they potentially affect microbial fermentation rates and some physiological effects as trace minerals in the Gum can influence host metabolism barrier functions. None of these variables is huge individually, but collectively they create enough variation that identical doses of nominally identical "Acacia gum" from different plant species might produce measurably different effects in careful human studies.

What should change going forward, to accelerate future research and provide consumer confidence in product consistency, is greater transparency and standardization around material characterization. For research purposes, grant-funded studies and industry-sponsored trials investigating health effects should as standard practice report the material characterization of the Acacia gum used in sufficient detail that others could replicate findings or assess whether differences in outcomes across studies might reflect source-material variation. When studies show differing results (one finding robust prebiotic effects while another finds modest effects, one showing significant glucose attenuation while another shows trends that don't reach significance) the research community should be able to assess whether they used comparable materials or whether material differences explain outcome differences.

Currently, that assessment is usually impossible because publications often provide minimal material characterization beyond "gum arabic, gum acacia, acacia gum, gum arabica, arabic gum, commercial grade acacia gum etc.". This is minimal information that precludes meaningful comparison.

Would adopting this recommendation require splitting regulatory definitions so that senegal and seyal are regulated separately? This would definitely be ideal and more beneficial to consumers. Industry experts have developed many heuristics over centuries regarding the gastrointestinal effects that both Hashab and Talha express in individuals. Given how this book discussed the many local ancient applications and how modern clinical studies proved them; it will be foolish to not take these differences seriously.

I purposely left out these differences from the content of this book as it requires its own concentrated studies. However, you probably noticed I referenced Acacia Seyal (Talha) only once in this book and it demonstrated its effects as an anti-diarrheal. Now you can imagine what taking an anti-diarrheal means to someone interested in relieving constipation in the long term. The anti-diarrheal properties of Talha (Acacia seyal) are known locally in producing regions and among industry experts. They are proof that the fermentation mechanics of both Acacia gums have different effects on consumers and regulatory agencies should take them into account.

VI. The Final Bridge : Gratitude, Recognition, and Forward Momentum

The regulatory journey from 2016 through 2021 wasn't just bureaucratic process grinding slowly forward through administrative procedures and evidentiary reviews. Behind every petition submission, every clinical trial, every published paper, every meeting with FDA officials, and every public comment supporting Acacia's recognition stood real people doing real work. Scientists designed studies and analyzed data. Clinicians enrolled participants and monitored safety. Engineers optimized extraction and purification to deliver consistent material for research. Producers in Sudan tended Acacia trees and harvested gum with techniques refined over generations. Industry advocates coordinated resources and navigated regulatory complexity. Animals sacrificed in labs to derisk future human studies. Consumer advocates amplifying voices of people whose health improved with Acacia supplementation and who wanted regulatory recognition to validate their experiences and enable broader access.

The next chapter is theirs; the researchers, clinicians, suppliers, producers, advocates, and traditional knowledge-keepers whose collective work pulled Hashab from commodity anonymity into scientifically validated and regulatorily recognized. They contributed to Acacia gum's increasingly accessible status as the most livable prebiotic fiber for everyday long-term support of metabolic, cardiovascular, inflammatory, and systemic health. Their dedication deserves recognition, their work deserves documentation, and their success deserves celebration.

References:

1. United States, Food and Drug Administration. "Acacia (Gum Arabic)." Code of Federal Regulations, title 21, sec. 184.1330.
2. United States, Food and Drug Administration. "Food Additives Permitted for Direct Addition to Food for Human Consumption; Acacia (Gum Arabic)." Federal Register, vol. 78, no. 235, 6 Dec. 2013, pp. 73434–73439
3. United States. Food and Drug Administration. "Food Labeling: Revision of the Nutrition and Supplement Facts Labels." Federal Register, vol. 81, no. 103, 27 May 2016, pp. 33742–33999.
4. United States, Food and Drug Administration. Guidance for Industry: Scientific Evaluation of the Evidence of Beneficial Physiological Effects of Isolated or Synthetic Non-Digestible Carbohydrates. 2 Mar. 2018; Nexira; Industry meetings with FDA, petition submissions, and regulatory correspondence, 2016-2020. Federal Register notices, FDA docket materials, and trade publication reporting.
5. Nexira; Alland & Robert; Importers Service Corp. "Citizen Petition (FDA-2020-P-2357)." 28 Dec. 2020; United States. Food and Drug Administration. "Final Response Letter to Keller and Heckman LLP Re: Citizen Petition FDA-2019-P-1911 (Acacia/Gum Arabic)." 31 Jan. 2020
6. United States. Food and Drug Administration. "FDA Grants Citizen Petition on Acacia (Gum Arabic) as a Dietary Fiber." Constituent Update, 17 Dec. 2021

CHAPTER 24

THE ACACIA HEROES

The Heroes, the Statistics, and the Future

A Thank You from Acacia

This chapter is the story of the researchers who spent careers investigating a tree exudate that kept producing surprising findings across seemingly unrelated domains. It's a thank you to the institutions that invested resources into studying this commodity ingredient. It's an appreciation of the countries that built research capacity around a natural resource central to their economies and cultures. It's a salute to the companies that recognized Acacia's potential decades before regulatory frameworks caught up. This is for everyone who invested the substantial time, money, and scientific expertise required to generate the evidence that modern medicine and policy demand. These are the Acacia heroes who did the hard work that will (I hope) bring Acacia gum to every household in need.

This chapter is not just a retrospective celebration of past achievement. It's also a forward-looking invitation to participate in the next phase of Acacia's journey. That journey requires more than passive readership; it requires active participation from people who understand Acacia's value and who want to help make this ancient, gentle, broadly beneficial ingredient accessible to the millions. This is an opportunity to brainstorm ways to benefit humanity and solve the global dysbiosis epidemic.

Before we look forward, though, we need to look back with appropriate gratitude and recognition to understand who built the foundation we're now standing on and appreciate the scope of work that accumulated over a century to reach this moment where scientific evidence and regulatory recognition finally aligned with millennia of traditional knowledge.

I. The Regulatory Victory and the Companies Who Made It Happen

Before celebrating researchers and institutions, we need to acknowledge the commercial actors whose investments, coordination, and persistence translated academic research into regulatory reality. Without the willingness to fund expensive human trials, navigate complex petition processes, and maintain commitment through years of uncertainty and setbacks; even the most compelling laboratory research would have been irrelevant to everyday people. The 2021 FDA recognition didn't emerge spontaneously from accumulating evidence; it emerged because specific companies decided Acacia gum was worth fighting for and invested accordingly.

Beginning around 2017 and 2018, as the implications of FDA's 2016 dietary fiber redefinition became clear and as initial petitions encountered evidence gaps that needed filling, major Acacia suppliers coordinated an unusual level of industry collaboration. Nexira, Ingredion (through its TIC Gums division), Importers Service Corporation (ISC Gums), Alland & Robert, and Kerry Group were the first to get involved. However, it was only a few of those companies who did the heavy lifting. They met with FDA officials, presented preliminary data, listened carefully to agency feedback and agreed to fund additional targeted human studies specifically addressing postprandial glucose, insulin responses, satiety effects, and bowel function outcomes. This coordination represented millions of dollars in research investment, years of commitment, and willingness to share findings even when proprietary advantage might have counseled secrecy.

The formal citizen petition that FDA ultimately granted came from three companies whose names deserve specific recognition. Those are Nexira, Alland & Robert, and Importers Service Corporation (ISC Gums). These petitioners assembled comprehensive dossiers, commissioned the pivotal human trials demonstrating glucose and insulin benefits. They coordinated with academic researchers to ensure study designs met regulatory standards and presented the evidence package. These were the companies that finally persuaded FDA that Acacia gum delivers real, beneficial physiological effects in humans warranting dietary fiber status.

Let's start with the companies who deserve recognition.

Nexira (France): For more than forty years, Nexira has invested in nutritional and gut-health research on Acacia, building dedicated ingredient platforms like Fibregum™ and Inavea™ Pure Acacia that frame the material explicitly as ninety-percent-plus soluble fiber. Nexira led regulatory engagement both in Europe and the United States, publicly championing Acacia's recognition and promoting it as carbon-neutral, FODMAP-friendly, and clinically prebiotic at doses as low as ten grams daily. They played a key role in positioning Acacia from invisible food additive towards a visible health ingredient that consumers specifically seek. Their willingness to fund human trials, publish findings openly, and share regulatory strategies represents industry leadership that benefits the entire field.

Alland & Robert (France) pursued complementary positioning emphasizing natural sourcing, sustainability, clean-label appeal, and digestive wellness. They conducted a substantial consumer study involving two hundred forty participants demonstrating that daily Acacia intake improved intestinal comfort, reduced abdominal pain and bloating, and enhanced quality of life, with over seventy percent of participants reporting better gut comfort within one month and over sixty-five percent experiencing less stomach pain. By emphasizing real-world consumer outcomes alongside mechanistic research, Alland & Robert helped establish that Acacia gum's benefits aren't just laboratory phenomena but translate into quality-of-life improvements that everyday users notice and value.

ISC (USA): Founded in 1941, this family-owned company in Edison, New Jersey became the original developer of gum acacia spray drying processes still used industry-wide today. They are known for their breakthroughs regarding Acacia seyal (Talha) gum. For centuries, Acacia seyal gum's dark color rendered it commercially useless. Then, in the 1990s, ISC developed decolorization methods that preserved the gum's natural properties while transforming it into a white powder. Suddenly, a wasted resource became viable. Before 1984, Talha gum was barely commercially available in the United States.

TIC Gums (United States): Founded in 1909 as the Tragacanth Importing Company and acquired by Ingredion in 2017. TIC Gums spent over a century mastering texture and stabilization. Their breakthrough came from Acacia innovation when in 2002, they patented TICAmulsion A-2010; gum acacia modified with OSA technology. This super-emulsifier could create high oil load emulsions up to 40%, dramatically increasing production efficiency. Independent research confirmed that their modified Acacia outperformed all modified starches for beverage stability.

Gum Arabic USA and their sourcing partnership with **Dar Savanna** (Sudan) represent a different but equally important strategy. They undertook a grassroots education and direct-to-consumer marketing project emphasizing Acacia's prebiotic and metabolic health benefits. Gum Arabic

USA's flagship product "Hashab Prebiotica®" is marketed as a pure natural prebiotic explicitly tied to gut flora and systematic health. Gum Arabic USA reaches consumers who read ingredient labels carefully, research supplement options thoroughly, and seek maximum-quality materials. They also spotlight the ethical dimensions of ingredient supply, framing Acacia as both a potent prebiotic and origin-linked wellness ingredient supporting rural livelihoods.

These commercial actors collectively created the market conditions and regulatory momentum that translated academic research into accessible products. Without Nexira, ISC and Alland & Robert funding the human trials that FDA required, regulatory recognition might have remained delayed indefinitely. Without Kerry group and Ingredion embedding Acacia into mainstream food formulation, reach would be limited to the small subset of consumers who actively purchase supplements. Without GumArabicUSA, Dar Savanna and similar grassroots companies educating consumers, the prebiotic fiber message would remain trapped in technical literature rather than reaching people who could immediately benefit from incorporating this potent yet gentle prebiotic into their daily routines.

This commercial ecosystem (companies pursuing different strategies but sharing commitment to Acacia's value) represents the practical infrastructure translating science into impact. The researchers generated the evidence; these companies generated the access, the awareness, and the regulatory permission enabling that evidence to matter in real life.

II. The Research Explosion: When Science Went Exponential

Understanding the current momentum and future trajectory of Acacia research requires grasping just how dramatically scientific attention has accelerated over the past hundred years. The five hundred forty peer-reviewed publications analyzed for this chapter (representing every study I could access through academic databases, institutional repositories, industry reports, and direct researcher outreach) reveal a field that evolved slowly for eight decades before exploding into exponential growth that shows no signs of slowing.

The early decades established chemical foundation with painstaking patience. From Alfred W. Thomas's pioneering 1928 physico-chemical study through the 1970s, research output averaged fewer than two studies annually. This means only twenty-two publications across more than fifty years, representing 4.1% of total historical research concentrated in a half-century span. These foundational studies, primarily from British and American institutions, focused on chemical structure, compositional analysis, and basic physical properties. The work was essential but unglamorous, establishing the vocabulary and analytical methods that later researchers would use to ask more sophisticated questions about function and effect.

The expansion phase spanning the 1990s through 2000s saw research accelerate to eighty-three studies (15.4% of total) as commercial food applications emerged and as analytical chemistry techniques improved enough to characterize complex natural polymers with precision previously impossible. Researchers discovered and documented Acacia's remarkable emulsification properties. These included its ability to stabilize oil-in-water emulsions at lower concentrations than synthetic alternatives, with better long-term stability and with sensory neutrality that preserved product flavor and appearance. These discoveries drove commercial interest from beverage, confectionery, and dairy industries. They created economic incentives for deeper investigation and established Acacia gum's value proposition for food technologists who needed reliable, natural, clean-label ingredients solving technical problems without downsides.

The acceleration phase beginning around 2010 marks the inflection point where research trajectory changed fundamentally. From 2010 through 2019, one hundred seventy studies appeared (31.5% of total); more in one decade than in the previous eight decades combined. Annual publication rates tripled from 10-15 studies per year in the 2000s to 30-45 studies per year through the 2010s. This acceleration reflected growing global concern about metabolic disease, obesity, and diabetes. These trends created an urgency around dietary interventions with emerging recognition of gut microbiome importance for systemic health which further accelerated prebiotic research.

Improved research capacity in Middle Eastern and African institutions allowed them to lead investigations. Interestingly, the data shows that MENA institutions were mostly researching health benefits while sub-Saharan African institutions were focused more on Agro-forestry. Developed nations were still more focused more on formulation studies.

The growth rate from 2015 to 2020 indicates not linear increases, but exponential acceleration where each year's output significantly exceeds the year before. The true explosion phase arrived with stunning force in 2020 and has sustained through 2025 at unprecedented intensity. These five years alone have produced 250+ studies (49% of all historical research concentrated in just 5 years) representing nearly half of everything ever published about Acacia gum. Annual output now routinely exceeds 40-50 studies.

What explains this explosive recent growth? Multiple reinforcing factors created positive feedback loops accelerating research across institutions and nations. FDA's 2016 dietary fiber redefinition created a regulatory incentive for generating human evidence, prompting industry funding that enabled larger and better-designed clinical trials than academic grants typically support. The global COVID-19 pandemic paradoxically accelerated health research by highlighting the critical importance of metabolic health, immune resilience, and gut-systemic connections for disease outcomes. Improved international collaboration enabled resource pooling, with researchers in Sudan partnering with French analytical chemists, Saudi biomedical scientists collaborating with British food technologists, and Egyptian clinical investigators sharing methods with American microbiome researchers. All these collaborations created efficiencies that solo-institution work couldn't match.

Perhaps most significantly, the research itself began revealing compelling findings that generated multiple follow-up investigations. When studies showed kidney protection in chronic disease models, nephrologists worldwide wanted to understand mechanisms, test different doses, examine various populations, and explore whether benefits extended to their specific patient groups. When fertility researchers documented reproductive improvements, that opened entire new research lines around hormonal pathways, oxidative stress in reproductive tissues, and sperm quality enhancement; questions that hadn't seemed relevant when Acacia was understood primarily as a food additive. When neurological studies suggested gut-brain axis benefits and cognitive protection, neuroscientists who'd never considered dietary fibers suddenly saw potential tools for addressing neuroinflammation, creating demand for mechanistic studies that previous decades hadn't imagined.

The explosion is real, sustained, and accelerating. Research output that took 150 years to reach its first one hundred studies took only 10 years to add the next one hundred, and only 3 years to add the one hundred after that. The trajectory suggests we'll surpass one thousand published studies within the next five to seven years as research capacity continues to expand in Asia, Africa, and South America while established research centers in Europe and North America maintain or increase their efforts. This is no longer a niche specialty pursued by a handful of dedicated researchers. It has evolved into a major multidisciplinary field spanning chemistry, food science, nutrition, medicine, pharmacology, materials engineering, nano technology and public health; attracting talent and resources commensurate with its potential to address pressing global health challenges.

III. The Geographic Heroes: Countries That Built Global Knowledge

The five hundred forty studies analyzed represent research conducted across 63 countries spanning every inhabited continent, but recent output concentrates heavily in certain regions where urgent health crises created strong incentives for investigating dietary and metabolic interventions. Understanding geographic patterns reveals not just who contributed but why different countries pursued different research questions and how international collaboration built comprehensive understanding that no single nation could have generated alone.

The United Kingdom occupies the historical foundation position, contributing the earliest systematic investigations and maintaining consistent research leadership across decades. British institutions were first to approach Acacia gum with rigorous analytical chemistry. They were the first to document emulsification mechanisms, and the first to establish quality standards and safety protocols that global trade required. The University of Edinburgh, University of Leeds, and the constellation of Welsh institutions (University of Wales, North East Wales Institute, Glyndŵr University) built the scientific vocabulary and methodological approaches that subsequent researchers worldwide adopted. British dominance in early decades reflects colonial-era scientific infrastructure, access to empire trade goods including Hashab from Sudan, and the robust university system supporting long-term curiosity-driven research without requiring immediate commercial returns. Institutional memory, established

410

collaboration networks, and recognized expertise mean British researchers continue influencing the field even as absolute research output shifts toward other nations.

Sudan represents the essential source-nation research perspective without which Acacia investigations would remain extractive rather than collaborative. As the country where approximately seventy percent of global Acacia gum supply originate; Sudan has cultural, economic, and scientific reasons to understand this resource thoroughly. The University of Khartoum emerges as the single most productive institution globally in Acacia research (more on institutional heroes shortly), driving investigations across agricultural optimization, sustainable harvesting, quality characterization, and increasingly, human health applications. Sudanese researchers didn't just study the material; they studied the people who've consumed it daily for generations. Sudan translated traditional knowledge into clinical trials to ascertain whether community anecdotal beliefs (Hashab supports kidney function) would hold under rigorous scientific scrutiny. That translation from tradition to evidence represents profound contribution validating indigenous knowledge through modern methodology while ensuring that source nations participate in value creation beyond raw material export. Sudan's research output has grown dramatically since the year 2000, reflecting investments in university infrastructure and research capacity that allowed local scientists to lead investigations rather than serving primarily as sample sources for research led elsewhere.

The United States provided mid-century food-science expertise that commercialized Acacia gum for modern industrial applications, then shifted toward nutritional and metabolic research as chronic disease epidemics created urgency around dietary interventions. American researchers pioneered large-scale food applications (understanding how Acacia stabilizes beverage emulsions, prevents ice crystallization, and enables reduced-fat formulations without texture penalties) generating knowledge that built the commercial market supporting later health investigations. More recently, U.S. institutions have led research on fiber benefits, cardiovascular outcomes, encapsulation technologies for drug delivery, and microbiome interactions. Recent research includes major medical centers and metabolism researchers investigating whether dietary fiber can meaningfully impact obesity, diabetes, and cardiovascular disease at population scale.

Saudi Arabia has emerged as a dominant force in biomedical research on Acacia's organ-protective effects, particularly for kidney, liver, and cardiovascular systems. With substantial research funding directed toward addressing the kingdom's growing metabolic disease burden (diabetes, chronic kidney disease, obesity have reached epidemic levels in Gulf nations), Saudi institutions have systematically investigated whether natural dietary interventions can complement or reduce dependence on pharmaceutical management. King Saud University leads this effort, producing dozens of studies documenting Acacia's nephroprotective, hepatoprotective, and cardioprotective effects while building scientific foundations for human trials.

France occupies a unique position as bridge between industrial food technology and cutting-edge nutritional biochemistry. French institutions (particularly INRA, University of Montpellier, and various research institutes) have excelled at deep structural analysis while also pioneering research on prebiotic effects, gut microbiota interactions, and the immunological consequences of fiber fermentation. France's research reflects its strong food culture (interest in how foods affect health through mechanisms beyond just nutrients), robust public research infrastructure, and geographic/historical ties to Francophone Africa including some Acacia-producing regions. French researchers often collaborate with both UK scientists (sharing analytical chemistry expertise) and Sudanese scientists (sharing access to diverse gum samples and traditional knowledge), serving as connectors in international research networks.

Egypt has rapidly scaled research output focusing on organ protection, diabetes management, and toxicology asking whether Acacia can mitigate harm from environmental pollutants, pharmaceutical side effects, and metabolic dysfunction. Egypt's population health challenges include high diabetes prevalence, chronic kidney disease, and heavy-metal environmental exposure in some regions. Egyptian researchers investigated whether accessible, affordable, culturally acceptable interventions like Acacia gum can reduce disease burden and improve outcomes in resource-limited settings where expensive pharmaceuticals and advanced medical care aren't universally available.

Oman, Iran Germany, India, China, Malaysia, and others each contribute specialized research niches reflecting their particular strengths and priorities. Oman through Sultan Qaboos University has become a powerhouse in chronic kidney disease research with exceptionally consistent output. Germany contributed critical early renal physiology and immunology studies establishing mechanistic understanding. India focuses on drug delivery and pharmaceutical applications, exploring how Acacia's properties enable controlled release, targeted delivery, and improved bioavailability. China leads nanotechnology and advanced materials applications, investigating how Acacia can be engineered into sophisticated delivery systems. Malaysia has built strength in food applications, shelf-life extension, and increasingly in prebiotic and metabolic research.

The geographic evolution tells a story of democratizing science and globalizing collaboration. Early research was dominated by former colonial powers with established scientific infrastructure. Modern research includes leadership from source nations, from countries facing urgent health crises, and from newly industrialized nations building research capacity around

413

materials and applications where they can contribute meaningfully. No single country could have generated current comprehensive understanding alone. This evolution required British analytical chemistry, Sudanese traditional knowledge, Saudi biomedical research, French structural biology, American clinical investigation, Egyptian toxicology combined with Chinese materials engineering. That international collaboration, with researchers across 63 nations contributing pieces to the puzzle, represents science working as it should. These are shared problems generating shared inquiry producing shared knowledge that benefits all of humanity.

IV. The Institutional Heroes: Universities That Built Research Legacies

While individual researchers deserve recognition (we'll honor them shortly), institutions create the stable infrastructure, long-term commitment, and collaborative environments enabling sustained research programs that span decades and survive individual career transitions. The institutional heroes are universities, research institutes, and medical centers that invested in Acacia research and maintained programs through periods when funding was scarce. These are the institutions that built expertise and networks making them go-to resources for anyone worldwide wanting to investigate Acacia's properties, applications, or effects.

The University of Khartoum (Sudan) stands unambiguously as the single most productive institution globally in Acacia research, with output spanning agricultural optimization, chemical characterization, food applications, and most impressively, clinical trials directly testing health benefits in human patients. The university's position in the heart of Acacia-producing regions provides advantages that foreign institutions cannot match. They have direct access to diverse germplasm for agricultural research, relationships with gum producers enabling supply-chain investigations, and patient populations with generations of Acacia consumption providing both traditional knowledge and baseline data for controlled studies. The university's institutional culture recognized this material as national heritage and an economic asset. Its researchers have led clinical trials in diabetes management, sickle cell anemia, rheumatoid arthritis, chronic kidney disease, cardiovascular dysfunction, and metabolic syndrome. They contributed the human evidence that transformed Hashab gum from promising traditional remedy into evidence-based therapeutic candidate. The university has also trained multiple generations of researchers who carry expertise into other Sudanese institutions and into international collaborations, creating multiplier effects where initial institutional investment continues generating returns through alumni networks.

University of Wales / North East Wales Institute / University of Edinburgh / University of Birmingham / University of Leeds (UK) represents perhaps the most sustained institutional commitment to Acacia research, with programs spanning chemical taxonomy, emulsification science, rheology, product development, and health applications running continuously from the 1960s through present day. This Welsh research cluster produced innovations like SUPER GUM™ (optimized fractions with enhanced functional properties), established analytical methods that became industry standards, and trained food scientists and materials engineers who spread Acacia gum expertise globally through their subsequent careers. University of Leeds research is heavily cited by food scientists and material engineers globally who need theoretical frameworks explaining Acacia's behavior and predicting how it will perform in novel applications. The longevity matters as institutional memory preserved across decades enables current researchers to build on deep foundations rather than starting fresh, and established international collaborations create pipelines for sharing samples, methods, and findings that accelerate progress for everyone involved.

415

King Saud University (Saudi Arabia) has emerged as a dominant institution for biomedical research on Acacia's therapeutic effects, with particularly strong programs investigating nephroprotection, hepatoprotection, cardioprotection, pharmaceutical toxin protection and protection against environmental toxins. The university's research follows rigorous protocols, uses sophisticated analytical techniques, and publishes in high-impact journals, establishing credibility that helps Acacia gain serious consideration from medical researchers globally who might otherwise dismiss natural products as unproven folk remedies. King Saud's work often involves dose-response studies, mechanistic investigations using molecular biology techniques, and systematic comparisons against pharmaceutical standards; generating the data that evidence-based medicine requires.

Sultan Qaboos University (Oman) has built remarkable focused expertise in chronic kidney disease, producing consistent output over 15+ years investigating how Acacia gum affects renal function markers, inflammatory pathways, oxidative stress, and progression of kidney damage in various disease models. The focused specialization creates depth and authority. When nephrologists worldwide want to understand whether Acacia might benefit their patients, Sultan Qaboos research provides the most comprehensive evidence base available.

INRA / University of Montpellier (France) excels at deep structural characterization and at connecting structure to biological function, particularly regarding prebiotic properties and gut microbiota interactions. Their research on arabinogalactan-protein fractions (how different molecular-weight distributions ferment differently) and on the immunological consequences of fermentation products has advanced mechanistic understanding beyond simple prebiotic-feeds-bacteria models. Their sophisticated elevated Acacia gum as an immunomodulator operating through multiple pathways.

416

The University of Minnesota, Al-Neelain University, University of Tübingen, Cairo University, and others each contribute essential research in their domains of expertise. Minnesota in encapsulation and food-science applications, Al-Neelain in clinical trials for sickle cell and inflammatory conditions, Tübingen in renal physiology and diabetes, Cairo in reproductive health and organ protection. The collective global research infrastructure represents billions of dollars of investment (when you count facilities, equipment, personnel salaries, and operating costs across decades) that no single institution could have justified for one ingredient.

The institutional story reveals how research capacity concentrates where natural advantages (proximity to source material in Sudan), historical advantages (established scientific infrastructure in UK and France), strategic priorities (health crisis response in Saudi Arabia and Oman), and sustained commitment (long-running programs that survived changes in leadership, funding, and scientific fashion) combine to create centers of excellence that enhances the field forward. The heroes aren't just the individuals but the institutions that hired them, supported their work, invested in infrastructure, and maintained the programs.

V. The Individual Researcher Heroes: Scientists Who Dedicated Careers to Understanding a Tree Exudate

While institutions and nations provide infrastructure and resources, individual researchers provided the creativity, dedication, and intellectual persistence that transformed materials into knowledge and knowledge into application. The researcher heroes profiled here represent scientific careers substantially devoted to Acacia gum investigations. These are the people who saw the promise in this ancient natural remedy and pursued it with enough commitment that their names are now inseparably linked to Acacia gum's scientific story. This list is based on the 540+ studies I was able to access, and I understand it's possible I missed many others. That said, these individuals undeniably stand among the most important contributors to current knowledge.

D.M.W. Anderson stands as one of the quiet architects of trust and standards in Acacia gum, he is someone whose name rarely appears in popular accounts, but whose work created the foundation enabling everything that followed. Working across major British research and industrial institutions, Anderson approached this ancient material with the determination that it deserved. He incorporated modern scientific precision to the traditional approximations. He built chemical taxonomy that defines how we classify different Acacia gums in addition to distinguishing Acacia from the dozens of other plant exudates that superficially resemble it but don't share its safety and chemical properties. He established analytical methods for quality control, purity assessment, and authentication that protect consumers and manufacturers from adulteration and substitution. He contributed important safety evidence, authoring controlled toxicology and ultrastructure studies in animals and collating the broader safety literature. His data underpinned international evaluations in which JECFA confirmed an ADI "not specified" for Acacia gum and the U.S. FDA affirmed it as GRAS in 21 CFR 184.1330.

Glyn O. Phillips was a driving force in modern hydrocolloid science and a major reason Gum arabic moved from "commodity emulsifier" to a rigorously characterized, high-performance natural ingredient. Trained at the University of Wales, he later shaped the field as Chief Executive Editor of Food Hydrocolloids and co-editor of the Handbook of Hydrocolloids. Within that broader leadership, he pursued Gum arabic with unusual focus. He showed how selective fractionation and control of the arabinogalactan-protein (AGP) component could boost emulsification efficiency and stability. He collaborated with industry (e.g., San-Ei Gen's Acacia(sen) SUPERGUM™) to demonstrate performance gains without synthetic modification. His team mapped Gum arabic's key fractions (AG, AGP, GP), linked composition to function, and provided practical routes to more consistent, clean-label behavior. Just as important, Phillips synthesized scattered knowledge across disciplines through authoritative editing and review, helping reposition Acacia gum as a versatile, evidence-based platform ingredient for food and related applications.

Badreldin H. Ali represents the pivotal transition from "Acacia gum is interesting chemistry" toward "Acacia gum is protective medicine". A researcher whose systematic toxicology and pharmacology research revealed the biological face of this desert tree exudate and validated its potential for therapeutic application. A Sudanese researcher working from Sultan Qaboos University in Oman; Ali and his teams used established renal-injury models (most prominently adenine-induced chronic kidney disease and gentamicin nephrotoxicity) to show that Acacia gum can blunt oxidative stress, dampen inflammatory signaling, and mitigate histologic damage in rat kidneys. Those experiments, together with follow-ups on genetic damage and other endpoints, helped define plausible mechanisms for organ protection. Ali's work complemented the safety foundation. His contributions aroused the curiosity of many researchers contributing immensely to the field.

Peter A. Williams brought hard-nosed polymer/colloid physics to Acacia gum. As Professor of Polymer and Colloid Chemistry at NEWI/Glyndŵr University and head of the Centre for Water-Soluble Polymers, he and collaborators (notably Glyn O. Phillips) treated Acacia gum like an engineered material. They measured its interfacial adsorption, mapped how the protein-rich arabinogalactan-protein (AGP) fraction stabilizes oil droplets, and showed how effective emulsion stability can arise from interfacial films and steric/electrostatic repulsion even when bulk viscosity is low. They coupled rheology, process-relevant characterization, and structure–function work that fractionated Acacia gum (AG/AGP/GP) and related compositional differences (including A. senegal vs A. seyal) to performance. William's group also examined modified variants (e.g., DDSA-derivatized GA) alongside native material, providing the predictive data sets industry uses for equipment design, process optimization, and QC. In short, he helped give Gum arabic a clear structural and interfacial identity, elevating it from "interesting natural gum" to a specifiable, scalable ingredient for real-world manufacturing.

Amal M. Saeed has been instrumental in moving Acacia gum from background chemistry into human clinical investigation. Based at the University of Khartoum, she helped run and publish trials in three high-burden conditions. In type 2 diabetes, a double-blind, placebo-controlled trial in Sudan showed favorable changes in adiposity indices and lipids. In sickle-cell disease, her team's studies showed that daily Gum arabic increased fetal hemoglobin and improved antioxidant status. In rheumatoid arthritis, a phase-II trial found significant reductions in TNF-α, ESR, and disease activity (DAS-28), supporting an anti-inflammatory effect. Collectively, this program reframed Gum arabic as a plausible adjunct for metabolic, inflammatory, and hematologic disorders, grounded in human data from the region where the material originates.

Christian Sanchez represents the deep, molecular investigation that turns Acacia gum from a black box into a predictable material. His program asks (and answers) structure-function questions with sophisticated analytical chemistry and soft-matter physics. Asking which arabinogalactan-protein (AGP) motifs control interfacial behavior; how molecular heterogeneity resolved by fractionation maps onto emulsifying efficiency; and why nominally similar gums perform differently in real products. This work established that Gum arabic's standout emulsification does not come from bulk viscosity but from AGP-rich species that adsorb at oil–water interfaces and form protective, steric/electrostatic barriers.

Beyond general mechanisms, Sanchez and colleagues linked source/composition to use-case performance. In beverages and wine technology, they showed that A. senegal and A. seyal gums can shift foamability and stability. Sanchez gave Acacia gum a rigorous molecular identity card (AGP architecture, fractionation, and interfacial behavior tied to measurable properties) so formulators can select, standardize, and scale the right gum for the job, and scientists can reason from composition to performance rather than tradition alone.

Lamis Kaddam represents the courage to study hard diseases in resource-limited settings, demonstrating that high-quality clinical inquiry can thrive wherever committed investigators pursue questions systematically. At Al-Neelain University in Sudan, Kaddam focused on sickle cell disease and rheumatoid arthritis. These are conditions that bring chronic pain, organ damage, fatigue, social cost, and shortened lifespan. Conditions that are often underfunded and undertreated, especially in regions carrying disproportionate global disease burden.

Her team engaged directly with patients living with these burdens, measuring validated laboratory and disease-activity markers that matter for care. The work is scientifically careful (prospective protocols, defined dosing, standardized assays, appropriate statistics, and publication in peer-reviewed journals) while remaining focused on practical questions for patient care and public health where access to biologics and advanced procedures is constrained. Kaddam's legacy includes not just the specific human biomarker and disease-activity findings with Acacia, but the broader demonstration that research sovereignty and capacity-building in source nations benefit global science. When clinical research occurs in communities most familiar with traditional uses (where investigators share cultural context with participants and understand local priorities) that research often asks more relevant questions and produces more practically applicable answers than studies conducted far from use settings by investigators unfamiliar with implementation realities.

Rasha Babiker connected Acacia gum to today's dominant metabolic burdens (type 2 diabetes, cardiovascular risk, and metabolic-syndrome profiles) by running human trials that treated Acacia as an intervention, not just a food additive. From the University of Khartoum, her studies asked practical questions and measured clinical markers. Her randomized trials evaluated glycemia, lipids, adiposity indices, and blood pressure. By reframing Acacia gum as a metabolic partner, Babiker's work positioned it within population-level challenges rather than niche symptom control. The emphasis on validated anthropometry, lipid ratios, and glycemic readouts aligned with emerging trials in adults at risk of metabolic syndrome. Babiker's legacy is methodological and translational.

Mohamed E. Osman represents the essential role of source-nation scientists who ensure that knowledge about natural resources is generated, defended, and transmitted by those closest to the trees, the trade, and the traditions. Working from Sudan University of Science and Technology (SUST); and collaborating closely with UK hydrocolloid groups. Osman helped move Gum arabic from folklore and commodity status into rigorously characterized material science. His name sits on foundational analytical papers that many later studies build on, including "Characterization of Commercial Samples of Gum Arabic" (1993) with Williams, Menzies, and Phillips, and earlier immunochemical work developing an ELISA for Acacia senegal gum; the kind of practical assay that lets regulators and buyers tell authentic material from substitutes.

From within Sudan's gum belt, Osman's program helped define how A. senegal and A. seyal differ in composition and function, and how those differences show up in processing and performance. The 1993 J. Agric. Food Chem. paper systematically compared commercial and authenticated samples using sugar profiles, nitrogen/amino-acid content, and molecular-mass distributions, creating a comparative baseline that QC labs still cite. Follow-on work with the same UK collaborators mapped the molecular characterization of Acacia senegal polysaccharide and fed into the broader "structure ↔ function" story that explains why some lots emulsify reliably while others do not.

Equally important is what this meant for Sudanese research capacity. Osman's CV and professional profiles trace decades of local training, supervision, and industry-facing projects (from characterization of Sudanese gums to mechanized tapping and collection initiatives) plus service on national bodies concerned with the gum sector. Osman and his colleagues played a critical role sustaining active labs, publishing steadily, and joining international networks.

VI. Why This Book Prioritizes Health Benefits Over Industrial Applications

Hashab gum has extensive and growing industrial applications that represent substantial research effort, commercial value, and technical sophistication. Emulsification studies demonstrate how Hashab stabilizes oil-in-water systems at lower concentrations than synthetic alternatives, with superior long-term stability and sensory neutrality.

Microencapsulation research shows how Acacia protects sensitive ingredients (probiotics, omega-3 fatty acids, polyphenols, pharmaceutical actives) through processing, storage, and delivery to target sites. Nanotechnology investigations explore how Hashab can be engineered into sophisticated drug delivery systems enabling targeted release, controlled kinetics, and enhanced bioavailability. Materials science research examines applications in tissue engineering scaffolds, wound dressings, biodegradable films, and advanced biomaterials. These applications are scientifically impressive and economically valuable. So why did this book ignore these applications and focused on health benefits only?

The answer is strategic priority based on three considerations: First, complexity and accessibility. Explaining health benefits is already enormously challenging given their mechanistic complexity and their manifestation across multiple simultaneous pathways rather than through single mechanisms. Adding equally complex explanations of interfacial chemistry, emulsion thermodynamics, encapsulation optimization, and controlled-release kinetics would overwhelm readers and obscure the health messages that motivated writing this book. Industrial applications, while fascinating to specialists, serve primarily technical functions that don't directly address the urgent health crises driving this work.

Second, the synthetic replacement imperative. Industrial applications do matter critically for health when viewed through specific lens. Hashab's potential to replace harmful synthetic food additives with ingredients that actively adds health rather than subtracting it is established and globally accepted. Most of the current demand for Hashab gum is specifically toward these applications and is not secret. This book, however, is concerned with resolving a health crises and the "Synergy" chapter was an effort to combine the functional properties from a health benefit perspective rather than a pure formulation perspective.

Third, urgent priority hierarchy. The developed world faces interlinked crises in metabolic health (obesity, diabetes, cardiovascular disease affecting billions), gut health (dysbiosis driven by antibiotics, ultra-processed foods, chronic stress), inflammatory disease (autoimmune conditions, inflammatory bowel disease, chronic systemic inflammation), and organ dysfunction (chronic kidney disease, fatty liver disease, neurodegeneration). These crises create more human suffering, more premature death, and more healthcare cost than most infectious diseases.

Critically, dietary interventions that are safe, affordable, accessible, and tolerable enough for sustained daily use remain remarkably scarce. Hashab gum represents a potential solution, and this book is an effort in that direction.

CHAPTER 25

The Future and a Call for Collaboration

Projecting forward from current trajectories and analyzing the frontier research appearing in 2023-2025 publications reveals three probable futures converging:

The Clinical Integration Future. Within five to ten years, Hashab gum recommendations will likely appear in clinical practice guidelines for chronic kidney disease, metabolic syndrome, inflammatory bowel conditions, and diabetes management; not as alternative medicine but as evidence-based adjunctive care supported by meta-analyses of randomized controlled trials demonstrating measurable benefit on patient-centered outcomes. Nephrologists will routinely discuss Hashab supplementation with CKD patients, not because traditional medicine says so but because Level 1 evidence shows it slows progression and improves quality of life. Gastroenterologists will recommend it for IBS and inflammatory bowel disease based on tolerability and efficacy data from large trials. Endocrinologists will incorporate it into diabetes management protocols because postprandial glucose control data meet evidence thresholds for guideline inclusion.

This integration requires completing the large-scale trials currently in planning or early execution. It requires multicenter studies with five hundred to one thousand participants, 12-24 month durations, hard clinical endpoints (disease progression, hospitalization rates, quality-of-life measures), and rigorous methodology meeting standards for Cochrane reviews and guideline development. Those trials are coming because regulatory recognition and commercial interest now justify the multi-million-dollar investments required.

The Food Infrastructure Future. Major food manufacturers will increasingly replace synthetic emulsifiers and stabilizers with Hashab gum in products consumed by billions daily. This will be a result of emerging evidence demonstrating the harm of synthetic emulsifiers. The ensuing liability exposure will make Hashab indispensable as it delivers equivalent technical performance plus health benefits. This shift will be gradual, limited by Hashab production capacity and cost differentials, but the trajectory is clear. When Hashab becomes standard ingredient in healthy bread, yogurt, plant-based beverages, protein supplements, and similar foundational foods, billions will receive prebiotic benefits passively through baseline diet rather than requiring active supplementation. This infrastructure approach is how dietary interventions achieve population impact.

Realizing this future requires production scaling beyond current 100,000 tons annually. Sudanese industry experts believe 200,000 tons are achievable if a concentrated effort takes place without additional planting. With additional planting production can increase to 300,000 tons over ten to fifteen years. This demands agricultural investment in Acacia-producing regions, sustainable intensification of harvesting practices, development of processing capacity closer to source regions rather than shipping raw gum for processing elsewhere, and quality standardization ensuring material consistency. These are solvable challenges given sufficient investment and coordination.

The Precision Medicine Future. As microbiome sequencing becomes cheaper and more routine, personalized Acacia gum recommendations will emerge based on individual microbiome composition, genetic variants, baseline metabolic profiles, and specific health goals. Some individuals will be identified as "super-responders" who gain exceptional benefit from Hashab gum due to favorable microbial communities and genetic backgrounds. Others may be "slow-responders" who would benefit over longer time scales or might benefit more from Talha gum or alternative fibers or combinations. Rather than generic "everyone should take Acacia gum" recommendations, clinical practice will evolve toward precision prebiotic prescription matching fiber type, dose, and timing to individual biology.

This future requires research infrastructure and clinical implementation systems allowing practical translation of complex multi-omic data into simple recommendations physicians and patients can act on. The technology exists; what's needed is coordinated data collection and analysis at sufficient scale to train predictive models reliably.

These three futures aren't mutually exclusive; they're complementary visions that together describe Acacia's trajectory from niche ingredient toward a foundational tool supporting human health across clinical care, food infrastructure, and personalized optimization. The speed of arrival depends on continued research investment, successful completion of pivotal clinical trials, commercial commitments to reformulation and scaling, and effective translation of scientific findings into clinical practice and consumer awareness. All are probable; the question is timeline rather than possibility.

The Future We're Building Together: Your Invitation to Participate

After documenting Acacia gum's journey, we arrive at the question that matters most. What happens next? And crucially, do you want to help shape that answer? Here's the reality that should be simultaneously exciting and sobering. Despite all the evidence and validation documented in this book, most households globally have never heard of Hashab gum. Even more concerning is the fact that most people have never considered incorporating prebiotic fiber into daily routines. Most of the population continue relying on dietary patterns and supplement choices that don't serve their long-term metabolic, inflammatory, and systemic health needs.

The developed world faces a dysbiosis epidemic (massive disruption of gut microbial ecosystems through antibiotic overuse, ultra-processed food dominance, chronic stress, environmental toxins, and pharmaceutical side effects) driving rising rates of inflammatory bowel diseases, autoimmune conditions, metabolic syndrome, obesity, type 2 diabetes, cardiovascular disease, and neurodegenerative decline. The majority are suffering from chronic low-grade inflammation that doesn't fit neat diagnostic categories but that erodes quality of life and accelerates aging for hundreds of millions. We have a tool that could help (not as magic bullet or complete solution but an accessible, safe, tolerable, broadly beneficial prebiotic) yet that tool remains largely unknown outside specialized research, food technology, and clinical communities.

The gap between what's known in scientific literature and what's practiced in daily life is vast and closing that gap requires more than just academic publications or even regulatory recognition. It requires education, awareness, product development, distribution infrastructure, clinical adoption, consumer trust-building, and sustained commitment from people willing to invest time, energy, and resources into making Hashab gum accessible to families, friends, patients, clients, and communities who could benefit but who've never encountered it. That's where you come in, if you choose to accept this invitation.

The opportunity presenting itself: We stand at inflection point where scientific validation, regulatory recognition, commercial infrastructure, public health need, and communication technologies converge to create a unique opportunity for the rapid scaling of Hashab awareness and adoption. The research foundation is solid; five hundred forty studies and growing exponentially. Major institutions worldwide are actively investigating, clinical trials continue demonstrating measurable human benefits, and safety established beyond reasonable doubt. The regulatory permission exists with FDA recognition in United States, long-standing acceptance in Europe and elsewhere, GRAS status enabling food use, and petition processes available for expanded claims as additional evidence accumulates.

The commercial infrastructure is growing with major ingredient suppliers positioning Hashab as a premium health ingredient. Food manufacturers are incorporating it into functional products, supplement companies are adding it to their formulations, and grassroots brands like GumArabicUSA are creating direct consumer access to pure material with transparent sourcing. The public health need is worsening, and the cascading consequences currently affect billions of people as Western dietary patterns spread globally. The communication technologies enabling education and awareness exist at scale unprecedented in human history with platforms that can spread information about beneficial interventions far faster and broader than traditional medical publishing or public health campaigns ever could.

What participation might look like. I'm not sure about what should be done but I'm inviting you to register interest in participating. You can join the discussion about Hashab's journey toward accessible household use by simply stating that you are interested and present any ideas you might have. This can be easily done by filling out a simple form providing your information and any idea you propose. I created a QR code at the end of this chapter for you to scan and access this form on a webpage. The form asks basic information about who you are, and a message from you to me. Tell us how you can contribute and what ideas you may have and maybe something will come out of it. This isn't a commitment to specific action or investment; it's an expression of interest for potentially being involved if opportunities emerge that match your capabilities and interests.

What happens with that information? It creates a list of interested people who can be informed when opportunities arise. It also creates potential for connection and collaboration; introducing researchers to clinicians, connecting entrepreneurs to investors, linking educators to content platforms, enabling spontaneous partnerships and initiatives that nobody planned but that emerge when interested people discover each other.

I can't promise specific outcomes or timeline. I don't know exactly what opportunities will develop or when. What I can promise is that if you indicate interest, you'll be included in communications as things develop. You will have a chance to participate in ways matching your situation, and you'll be part of a community that didn't exist before. A network of people worldwide who understand Hashab's value and seek to make it accessible to the hundreds of millions who could benefit. This is your invitation to move from passive reader to active participant, from learning about Hashab to helping build its future.

The vision worth pursuing: Imagine households globally where Hashab prebiotics are as common as whey protein supplements. Imagine supporting metabolic health, inflammatory control, organ protection, and gut-brain axis function as routine as multivitamins or morning coffee. Not as medical interventions but as ordinary nutritional foundations that everyone understands and that everyone can access affordably. Imagine clinical guidelines routinely incorporating Hashab recommendations for chronic kidney disease, diabetes, inflammatory bowel conditions, and metabolic syndrome; not as alternative medicine but as evidence-based adjunctive care improving outcomes and quality of life alongside pharmaceutical management. Imagine food supply broadly incorporating Hashab as replacement for synthetic emulsifiers and stabilizers, passively delivering prebiotic benefits to billions through everyday products.

Imagine research communities worldwide investigating Hashab's mechanisms, applications, and optimal use with resources and attention proportionate to its potential impact. Imagine turning this initiative into a major health-sciences priority commanding funding, talent, and institutional commitment matching infectious disease, cancer, or cardiovascular research. Imagine source nations like Sudan capturing fair share of value from research, innovation, and commercialization rather than remaining primarily raw-material suppliers.

That vision is achievable. The scientific foundation exists. The regulatory permission exists. The commercial infrastructure is growing. The public health needs are urgent, and communication gaps can be closed by the growing reach of technology. What's needed is human commitment; enough people willing to contribute energy, skills, and resources toward making vision reality.

You're invited to be among them.

Scan the QR code, fill out the form, and join the journey toward making Hashab gum accessible to all households worldwide

[   ]

Form URL: [www.AcaciaGumArabic.com]

By participating, you're not committing specific actions or investments. You're simply indicating interest in staying informed and potentially being involved as opportunities develop that match your situation and capabilities. Your participation might be the connection, the insight, the resource, or the energy that makes the difference. Or it might simply add one more voice to a growing chorus saying this matters, this deserves attention, and this is worth pursuing. Either way, you're invited to be part of what happens next.

Scan the code. Fill in the form. Join the journey.

The future is an invitation, not a prediction. Whether it becomes reality depends on who accepts the invitation and what they do with it. Welcome to the journey. We're glad you're here.

ACKNOWLEDGEMENTS

I would like to give special thanks to Dr. Isam Sidig and his proteges Taric Khalil, Fawaz Abbaro, and Mohamed Bakhit. They were instrumental in the knowledge and experience I accumulated over the years whilst working on this book.

I would also like to thank UNCTAD organization for coordinating, planning and executing strategies that maintain Acacia gum production throughout Sudan. Their relentless work will be of prime importance as the country transitions into peace and Acacia gum production scales back to pre-war heights. Additionally, they are the main force on the ground that can exact real progress regarding increasing Acacia gum production and fighting desertification. A coordinated international effort to accomplish these 2 goals will be of immense priority to solve the dysbiosis epidemic of the first world while fighting environmental catastrophe in the 3rd world.

ABOUT THE AUTHOR

Mohamad Alnoor is an Acacia gum expert. He is also a consultant in IT systems, Real estate, Import & Export, Marketing, Logistics and E-commerce.

www.MohamadAlnoor.com

Support me by Tipping 😊 Thanks in Advance

https://paypal.me/RealMohamadAlnoor

GLOSSARY

Acacia – Originally a genus of trees and shrubs, native to Africa and used for their medicinal resin. Botanical authorities changed this to an Australian species.

Acetate - A short-chain fatty acid produced when gut bacteria break down fiber, helping to nourish colon cells and reduce inflammation.

Adiponectin - A hormone released by fat tissue that helps regulate blood sugar and break down fatty acids, with higher levels generally indicating better metabolic health.

Adiposity - The state of having excess body fat; a measure of obesity.

AGE (Advanced Glycation End Products) - Harmful compounds formed when proteins or fats combine with sugar, contributing to aging and chronic disease.

Albumin - The main protein in blood that helps maintain fluid balance and transport nutrients; low levels can indicate kidney or liver problems.

Alkaline phosphatase - An enzyme found in the liver and bones; elevated levels may indicate liver disease or bone disorders.

ALT (Alanine Aminotransferase) - A liver enzyme; elevated levels in blood indicate liver damage or inflammation.

Amino acids - The building blocks of proteins, essential for cell growth and repair throughout the body.

Amylase - An enzyme that breaks down starches into sugars, produced by the salivary glands and pancreas.

Anemia - A condition where the body lacks enough healthy red blood cells to carry adequate oxygen to tissues.

Anthocyanins - Plant compounds with antioxidant properties found in colorful fruits and vegetables.

Antibacterial - Capable of inhibiting the growth of harmful bacteria.

Antioxidants - Substances that protect cells from damage caused by free radicals, helping prevent disease and aging.

Antitumor - Having the ability to prevent or slow the growth of tumors.

Apoptosis - Programmed cell death, a natural process that removes damaged or unwanted cells from the body.

Arabinogalactan - A type of soluble fiber found in acacia gum that acts as a prebiotic to feed beneficial gut bacteria.

Arginase - An enzyme involved in breaking down the amino acid arginine, playing a role in immune function and wound healing.

AST (Aspartate Aminotransferase) - A liver enzyme; elevated blood levels can indicate liver or heart damage.

Atherosclerosis - The buildup of fats and cholesterol in artery walls, leading to narrowed blood vessels and increased risk of heart disease.

Atopic dermatitis - A chronic inflammatory skin condition characterized by itchy, red, and dry skin patches; commonly called eczema.

Bacterial translocation - The movement of bacteria from the gut through the intestinal wall into the bloodstream, which can trigger inflammation.

Bacteroides - A genus of beneficial bacteria commonly found in the human gut that help break down complex carbohydrates.

Bifidobacteria - A type of beneficial bacteria in the gut that aids digestion, produces vitamins, and supports immune function.

Bioavailability - The degree to which nutrients or drugs are absorbed and become available to the body.

Biofilm - A protective layer formed by bacteria that helps them stick to surfaces and resist antibiotics.

Bioflavonoids - Plant compounds with antioxidant and anti-inflammatory properties that support overall health.

Blood urea nitrogen (BUN) - A waste product filtered by the kidneys; elevated levels indicate kidney problems.

BMI (Body Mass Index) - A measure of body fat based on height and weight, used to assess if someone is underweight, normal weight, overweight, or obese.

Butyrate - A short-chain fatty acid produced by gut bacteria from fiber that nourishes colon cells and reduces inflammation.

C-reactive protein (CRP) - A marker of inflammation in the body; elevated levels indicate increased risk of chronic disease.

Candida - A type of yeast that naturally lives in the body but can overgrow and cause infections, particularly in the gut and mouth.

Carcinogenic - Capable of causing cancer.

Cardiovascular - Relating to the heart and blood vessels.

Cariogenic - Capable of causing tooth decay.

Catalase - An enzyme that breaks down harmful hydrogen peroxide into water and oxygen, protecting cells from damage.

CCL2 (MCP-1) - A protein that attracts immune cells to sites of inflammation, playing a role in inflammatory diseases.

Celiac disease - An autoimmune disorder where consuming gluten damages the small intestine.

Cholesterol - A waxy substance in blood needed for cell function; high levels increase heart disease risk.

Chronic kidney disease (CKD) - Progressive loss of kidney function over time, affecting the body's ability to filter waste from blood.

Chyme - The semi-fluid mixture of partially digested food and digestive juices in the stomach and small intestine.

Cirrhosis - Severe scarring of the liver caused by chronic damage, leading to impaired liver function.

Colitis - Inflammation of the colon (large intestine), causing abdominal pain and diarrhea.

Colon - The large intestine, where water is absorbed and waste is prepared for elimination.

Commensal bacteria - Beneficial bacteria that live in the body without causing harm, often providing health benefits.

Creatinine - A waste product from muscle metabolism filtered by the kidneys; elevated levels indicate kidney problems.

Crohn's disease - A chronic inflammatory bowel disease that can affect any part of the digestive tract.

Cytokines - Proteins released by cells that regulate immune responses and inflammation.

Dental plaque - A sticky film of bacteria that forms on teeth and can lead to cavities and gum disease.

Diabetes mellitus - A chronic condition where the body cannot properly regulate blood sugar levels.

Diarrhea - Loose, watery stools that occur more frequently than normal.

Digestion - The process of breaking down food into nutrients that the body can absorb and use.

DNA damage - Harm to the genetic material in cells that can lead to mutations and disease.

Dysbiosis - An imbalance in gut bacteria where harmful bacteria outnumber beneficial ones, leading to digestive and health problems.

Dyslipidemia - Abnormal levels of fats (lipids) in the blood, including high cholesterol or triglycerides.

E. coli - A type of bacteria commonly found in the intestines; some strains are beneficial while others can cause illness.

Eczema - See Atopic dermatitis.

Emulsifier - A substance that helps mix ingredients that normally don't combine, like oil and water.

Endothelial dysfunction - Impaired function of the inner lining of blood vessels, contributing to heart disease.

Endotoxemia - The presence of bacterial toxins in the bloodstream, often due to a leaky gut, causing inflammation.

Enterocytes - The cells lining the small intestine that absorb nutrients from digested food.

Enzyme - A protein that speeds up chemical reactions in the body, such as breaking down food during digestion.

Epithelial barrier - The protective layer of cells lining organs like the gut that prevents harmful substances from entering the body.

Eradication - Complete removal or elimination, such as removing harmful bacteria.

Fasting blood glucose - Blood sugar level measured after not eating for at least 8 hours, used to diagnose diabetes.

Fatty liver - Buildup of excess fat in liver cells, which can lead to inflammation and liver damage.

Fecal microbiota - The community of bacteria and other microorganisms found in stool.

Fermentation - The process by which gut bacteria break down undigested fiber, producing beneficial compounds.

Fiber - Indigestible plant material that passes through the digestive system, feeding gut bacteria and promoting regular bowel movements.

Fibrosis - The formation of excess scar tissue in organs, which can impair their function.

Firmicutes - A large group of bacteria commonly found in the gut; imbalances may be linked to obesity.

Free radicals - Unstable molecules that can damage cells and contribute to aging and disease.

Fructooligosaccharides (FOS) - A type of prebiotic fiber that feeds beneficial gut bacteria.

GALT (Gut-Associated Lymphoid Tissue) - Immune tissue in the digestive tract that protects against pathogens.

Gastric emptying - The process of food leaving the stomach and entering the small intestine.

Gastritis - Inflammation of stomach lining, causing pain and discomfort.

Gastrointestinal (GI) tract - The digestive system, including the stomach, intestines, and associated organs.

GFR (Glomerular Filtration Rate) - A measure of how well the kidneys filter waste from blood; low rates indicate kidney disease.

GLP-1 (Glucagon-like peptide-1) - A hormone that helps regulate blood sugar and promotes feelings of fullness.

Glucose - The main type of sugar in blood, used by cells for energy.

Glucose tolerance - The body's ability to process and regulate blood sugar levels.

Glutathione peroxidase - An antioxidant enzyme that protects cells from damage by breaking down harmful peroxides.

Glycation - The process where sugar molecules attach to proteins or fats, potentially causing damage.

Glycemic control - The regulation of blood sugar levels within a healthy range.

Glycemic index - A measure of how quickly foods raise blood sugar levels after eating.

Goblet cells - Cells in the intestinal lining that produce mucus to protect the gut wall.

GRAS (Generally Recognized As Safe) - A designation by the FDA indicating a substance is safe for consumption.

Gut barrier - The protective lining of the intestines that prevents harmful substances from entering the bloodstream.

Gut flora - See Gut microbiota.

Gut microbiota - The community of trillions of bacteria and other microorganisms living in the digestive tract.

Gut permeability - The degree to which the intestinal lining allows substances to pass through; increased permeability is called "leaky gut."

H. pylori (Helicobacter pylori) - A bacteria that infects the stomach and can cause ulcers and gastritis.

HbA1c (Hemoglobin A1c) - A measure of average blood sugar levels over the past 2-3 months, used to diagnose and monitor diabetes.

HDL (High-Density Lipoprotein) - "Good" cholesterol that helps remove harmful cholesterol from blood vessels.

Hematuria - The presence of blood in urine, which may indicate kidney or urinary tract problems.

Hemoglobin - The protein in red blood cells that carries oxygen throughout the body.

Hepatic - Relating to the liver.

Hepatotoxicity - Liver damage caused by chemicals, drugs, or toxins.

HOMA-IR (Homeostatic Model Assessment of Insulin Resistance) - A calculation used to measure insulin resistance and diabetes risk.

Homeostasis - The body's ability to maintain stable internal conditions despite external changes.

Hyperglycemia - Abnormally high blood sugar levels, a characteristic of diabetes.

Hyperlipidemia - Elevated levels of fats (lipids) in the blood, including cholesterol and triglycerides.

Hypertension - High blood pressure, a major risk factor for heart disease and stroke.

IBS (Irritable Bowel Syndrome) - A common disorder causing abdominal pain, bloating, and changes in bowel habits.

IgA (Immunoglobulin A) - An antibody that plays a key role in immune function, particularly in the gut and respiratory tract.

IL-6 (Interleukin-6) - A cytokine involved in inflammation and immune responses; elevated levels indicate chronic inflammation.

Immune cells - White blood cells and other cells that protect the body from infection and disease.

Immune modulation - The adjustment or regulation of immune system activity to maintain balance.

Immune response - The body's reaction to foreign substances or infections, involving various cells and proteins.

Immunomodulatory - Having the ability to modify or regulate immune system function.

Immunosuppression - Reduction in the immune system's ability to fight infections and disease.

Inflammation - The body's response to injury or infection, involving redness, swelling, and heat; chronic inflammation contributes to many diseases.

Inflammatory bowel disease (IBD) - Chronic inflammation of the digestive tract, including Crohn's disease and ulcerative colitis.

Inflammatory markers - Substances in blood that indicate the presence of inflammation in the body.

Insoluble fiber - Fiber that doesn't dissolve in water, adding bulk to stool and promoting regular bowel movements.

Insulin - A hormone produced by the pancreas that helps cells absorb glucose from the blood.

Insulin resistance - A condition where cells don't respond properly to insulin, leading to elevated blood sugar.

Insulin sensitivity - How effectively cells respond to insulin; higher sensitivity is healthier.

Intestinal barrier - See Gut barrier.

Intestinal microbiota - See Gut microbiota.

Intestinal permeability - See Gut permeability.

Inulin - A type of prebiotic fiber found in plants that feeds beneficial gut bacteria.

LDL (Low-Density Lipoprotein) - "Bad" cholesterol that can build up in artery walls and increase heart disease risk.

Leaky gut - Increased intestinal permeability where the gut lining becomes damaged, allowing harmful substances to enter the bloodstream.

Leptin - A hormone that regulates appetite and energy balance; problems with leptin can lead to weight gain.

Lipid peroxidation - Damage to fats in cell membranes caused by free radicals, contributing to disease.

Lipids - Fats and fat-like substances in the body, including cholesterol and triglycerides.

Lipopolysaccharide (LPS) - A toxin found on the outer membrane of certain bacteria that can trigger inflammation if it enters the bloodstream.

Liver enzymes - Proteins produced by the liver; elevated levels in blood indicate liver damage.

Lymphocytes - A type of white blood cell that plays a key role in immune defense.

Macrophages - Immune cells that engulf and destroy pathogens and dead cells.

Malondialdehyde (MDA) - A compound formed during oxidative stress;

443

elevated levels indicate cellular damage.

Metabolic syndrome - A cluster of conditions including high blood pressure, high blood sugar, and abnormal cholesterol that increase disease risk.

Metabolism - The chemical processes in cells that convert food into energy and build or repair tissues.

Metabolites - Substances produced during metabolism, including beneficial compounds made by gut bacteria.

Metformin - A medication commonly used to treat type 2 diabetes by lowering blood sugar.

Microbe - A microscopic organism such as bacteria, fungi, or viruses.

Microbiome - The collection of all microorganisms living in a particular environment, such as the gut.

Microbiota - The community of microorganisms (bacteria, fungi, viruses) living in a specific location in the body.

Mitochondria - The "powerhouses" of cells that produce energy.

Mucin - A protein component of mucus that protects and lubricates body surfaces.

Mucus layer - A protective coating on the intestinal lining that prevents bacteria from directly contacting gut cells.

NAFLD (Non-Alcoholic Fatty Liver Disease) - Fat buildup in the liver not caused by alcohol consumption.

Nephropathy - Kidney disease or damage, often caused by diabetes or high blood pressure.

Neuropathy - Nerve damage causing pain, numbness, or weakness, commonly affecting the hands and feet.

Neutrophils - A type of white blood cell that is one of the body's first defenses against infection.

NF-κB (Nuclear Factor Kappa B) - A protein complex that controls inflammation and immune responses.

Obesity - Excessive accumulation of body fat that presents health risks.

Oxidative stress - An imbalance between free radicals and antioxidants in the body, leading to cell damage.

Pancreas - An organ that produces insulin and digestive enzymes.

Pathogen - A harmful microorganism that causes disease.

Pathogenic bacteria - Harmful bacteria that can cause infections and illness.

Pepsin - A digestive enzyme in the stomach that breaks down proteins.

Periodontal disease - Gum disease involving inflammation and infection of the tissues supporting teeth.

Permeability - The degree to which substances can pass through a barrier, such as the intestinal wall.

Phagocytosis - The process by which immune cells engulf and destroy pathogens and debris.

Phosphorus - A mineral important for bones and kidneys; elevated levels can indicate kidney problems.

Plaque - See Dental plaque or Atherosclerosis.

Plasma - The liquid component of blood that carries cells, nutrients, and waste products.

Polyphenols - Plant compounds with antioxidant and anti-inflammatory properties.

Polysaccharide - A complex carbohydrate made of many sugar molecules linked together, such as fiber.

Postprandial - Occurring after a meal, such as postprandial blood sugar levels.

Potassium - An essential mineral important for heart and muscle function; levels must be carefully managed in kidney disease.

Prebiotic - A type of fiber that feeds beneficial gut bacteria, promoting their growth and activity.

Probiotic - Live beneficial bacteria that support gut health when consumed.

Pro-inflammatory - Promoting or increasing inflammation in the body.

Propionate - A short-chain fatty acid produced by gut bacteria that helps regulate metabolism and reduce inflammation.

Protein - Essential nutrients made of amino acids, necessary for building and repairing tissues.

Proteinuria - The presence of excess protein in urine, indicating kidney damage.

Psyllium - A type of soluble fiber derived from plant seeds, commonly used as a laxative.

Reactive oxygen species (ROS) - Free radicals containing oxygen that can damage cells; overproduction leads to oxidative stress.

Renal - Relating to the kidneys.

Resistant starch - A type of starch that resists digestion and acts like fiber, feeding beneficial gut bacteria.

Saliva - Fluid in the mouth that contains enzymes to begin food digestion and protect teeth.

Satiety - The feeling of fullness and satisfaction after eating.

SCFA (Short-Chain Fatty Acids) - Beneficial compounds produced when gut bacteria ferment fiber, including acetate, propionate, and butyrate.

Serum - The clear liquid part of blood that remains after clotting.

SIBO (Small Intestinal Bacterial Overgrowth) - Excessive bacteria in the small intestine causing digestive symptoms.

Small intestine - The part of the digestive tract where most nutrient absorption occurs.

Soluble fiber - Fiber that dissolves in water to form a gel, helping lower cholesterol and regulate blood sugar.

SOD (Superoxide Dismutase) - An antioxidant enzyme that protects cells from damage by breaking down harmful free radicals.

Steatosis - See Fatty liver.

Stool - Solid waste eliminated from the body through bowel movements.

Streptococcus mutans - A bacteria that causes tooth decay by producing acid from sugar.

Synbiotic - A combination of prebiotics and probiotics that work together to support gut health.

Systemic inflammation - Body-wide inflammation that affects multiple organs and contributes to chronic disease.

T-cells - A type of white blood cell crucial for immune responses, including fighting infections and cancer.

Tight junctions - Connections between intestinal cells that regulate what passes through the gut barrier.

TNF-α (Tumor Necrosis Factor Alpha) - A cytokine involved in inflammation; elevated levels contribute to chronic inflammatory diseases.

Total cholesterol - The combined amount of all types of cholesterol in the blood.

Toxin - A poisonous substance produced by living organisms or present in the environment.

Transit time - The time it takes for food to move through the digestive system from eating to elimination.

Triglycerides - A type of fat in blood; high levels increase risk of heart disease.

Ulcer - A sore or erosion in the lining of the stomach or intestines.

Ulcerative colitis - A chronic inflammatory bowel disease causing ulcers in the colon and rectum.

Uremia - Buildup of waste products in the blood due to kidney failure.

Uric acid - A waste product filtered by kidneys; high levels can cause gout and may indicate kidney problems.

Urinary tract - The system that produces and eliminates urine, including kidneys, bladder, and related structures.

Viscosity - The thickness or stickiness of a fluid; high-viscosity fiber can slow digestion.

VLDL (Very Low-Density Lipoprotein) - A type of cholesterol carrier in blood that transports triglycerides.

Weight management - The process of maintaining a healthy body weight through diet and lifestyle.

White blood cells - Immune cells that protect the body from infection and disease.

Xenobiotics - Foreign chemical substances found in the body that are not naturally produced, such as drugs or pollutants.

Zonulin - A protein that regulates tight junctions in the intestinal wall; elevated levels are associated with leaky gut.

DISCLAIMER

The author and publisher of "The Exceptional Acacia Gum Arabic" has made every effort to ensure that the information presented herein is accurate, complete, and current as of the date of publication. Nevertheless:

Informational Purpose Only
The Work is provided solely for educational, historical, and journalistic purposes. Nothing contained herein should be construed as legal, financial, medical, or other professional advice. Readers should consult qualified professionals before acting on any information.

No Warranty of Accuracy or Completeness
All facts, figures, and citations are presented "as is" without warranties of any kind (express or implied) including but not limited to warranties of accuracy, reliability, completeness, merchantability, or fitness for a particular purpose.

Evolving Science & Policy
Scientific classifications, regulatory frameworks, and legal standards referenced in the text may change over time. The author and publisher accept no responsibility for updates after the publication date.

Good-Faith Scholarship & Fair Use
Quotations, images, tables, and other materials reproduced from third-party sources are used under fair-use, academic, or license-based principles. All trademarks, service marks, and trade names are the property of their respective owners; use herein does not imply endorsement.

Opinions & Interpretations
Analyses, viewpoints, and conclusions expressed are those of the author and do not necessarily reflect the views of any affiliated institution, sponsor, or reviewer. Any resemblance to real persons, organizations, or events beyond documented facts is coincidental.

Limitation of Liability
To the maximum extent permitted by law, the author, publisher, editors, and distributors disclaim all liability for any loss, damage, or disruption (direct or indirect) that may arise from using, relying on, or acting upon information contained in the Work.

Notice of Potential Errors
Despite rigorous sourcing, errors or omissions may remain. Readers who identify possible inaccuracies are invited to contact the publisher so corrections can be considered for future editions.

www.ingramcontent.com/pod-product-compliance
Lightning Source LLC
Chambersburg PA
CBHW071959260326
41914CB00004B/858